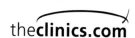

CARDIOLOGY CLINICS

CardioRenal Disease

GUEST EDITORS
Ragavendra R. Baliga, MD, MBA, FACC, FRCP(Edin)
Sanjay Rajagopalan, MD
Rajiv Saran, MD, MS, MRCP

CONSULTING EDITOR
Michael H. Crawford, MD

August 2005 • Volume 23 • Number 3

SAUNDERS

An Imprint of Elsevier, Inc.
PHILADELPHIA   LONDON   TORONTO   MONTREAL   SYDNEY   TOKYO

W.B. SAUNDERS COMPANY
A Division of Elsevier Inc.

Elsevier Inc. • 1600 John F. Kennedy Blvd., Suite 1800 • Philadelphia, Pennsylvania 19103-2899

http://www.theclinics.com

CARDIOLOGY CLINICS
August 2005
Editor: Karen Sorensen

Volume 23, Number 3
ISSN 0733-8651
ISBN 1-4160-2700-9

Reprints. For copies of 100 or more, of articles in this publication, please contact the Commercial Reprints Department, Elsevier Inc., 360 Park Avenue South, New York, New York 10010-1710. Tel. (212) 633-3813 Fax: (212) 462-1935 email: reprints@elsevier.com

The ideas and opinions expressed in *Cardiology Clinics* do not necessarily reflect those of the Publisher. The Publisher does not assume any responsibility for any injury and/or damage to persons or property arising out of or related to any use of the material contained in this periodical. The reader is advised to check the appropriate medical literature and the product information currently provided by the manufacturer of each drug to be administered to verify the dosage, the method and duration of administration, or contraindications. It is the responsibility of the treating physician or other health care professional, relying on independent experience and knowledge of the patient, to determine drug dosages and the best treatment for the patient. Mention of any product in this issue should not be construed as endorsement by the contributors, editors, or the Publisher of the product or manufacturers' claims.

Cardiology Clinics (ISSN 0733-8651) is published quarterly by W.B. Saunders Company; Corporate and editorial Offices: Elsevier Inc., 1600 John F. Kennedy Blvd., Suite 1800, Philadelphia, PA 19103-2899. Accounting and circulation offices: 6277 Sea Harbor Drive, Orlando, FL 32887-4800. Periodicals postage paid at Orlando, FL 32862, and additional mailing offices. Subscription prices are $170.00 per year for US individuals, $266.00 per year for US institutions, $85.00 per year for US students and residents, $210.00 per year for Canadian individuals, $323.00 per year for Canadian institutions, $230.00 per year for international individuals, $323.00 per year for international institutions and $115.00 per year for Canadian and foreign students/residents. To receive student/resident rate, orders must be accompanied by name of affiliated institution, data of term, and the *signature* of program/residency coordinator on institution letterhead. Orders will be billed at individual rate until proof of status is received. Foreign air speed delivery is included in all *Clinics* subscription prices. All prices are subject to change without notice. POSTMASTER: Send address changes to *Cardiology Clinics*, W.B. Saunders Company, Periodicals Fulfillment, Orlando, FL 32887-4800. **Customer Service: 1-800-654-2452 (US). From outside of the US, call 1-407-345-1000.**

Cardiology Clinics is also published in Spanish by McGraw-Hill Interamericana Editores S. A., P.O. Box 5-237, 06500, Mexico D. F., Mexico; in Portuguese by Reichmann and Alfonso Editores Rio de Janeiro, Brazil; and in Greek by Dimitrios P. Lagos, 8 Pondon Street, GR115-28 Ilissia, Greece.

Cardiology Clinics is covered in *Index Medicus, Excerpta Medica, The Cumulative Index to Nursing and Allied Health Literature* (INAHL).

Printed in the United States of America.

CONSULTING EDITOR

MICHAEL H. CRAWFORD, MD, Professor of Medicine, Lucie Stern Chair in Cardiology at University of California at San Francisco; Chief of Clinical Cardiology, University of California San Francisco Medical Center, San Francisco, California

GUEST EDITORS

RAGAVENDRA R. BALIGA, MD, MBA, FACC, FRCP(Edin), Director of Cardiovascular Medicine, Ohio State University Hospital East; Clinical Professor of Medicine, Ohio State University, Columbus, Ohio

SANJAY RAJAGOPALAN, MD, Associate Professor, Zena and Michael A. Wiener Cardiovascular Institute and Marie-Josée and Henry R. Kravis Center for Cardiovascular Health, Mount Sinai Medical Center; Associate Professor & Director of Cardiac MRI, Mount Sinai School of Medicine, New York, New York

RAJIV SARAN, MD, MS, MRCP, Assistant Professor of Medicine, Division of Nephrology, University of Michigan, Ann Arbor, Michigan

CONTRIBUTORS

RAJIV AGARWAL, MD, Associate Professor of Medicine, Division of Nephrology, Department of Medicine, Indiana University School of Medicine, Indianapolis; Roudebush VA Medical Center, Indianapolis, Indiana

AARON D. BERMAN, MD, FACC, Department of Medicine, Divisions of Cardiology, Nutrition and Preventive Medicine, William Beaumont Hospital, Royal Oak, Michigan

CHRISTOPHER T. CHAN, MD, FRCPC, Staff Nephrologist, Medical Director – Home Hemodialysis, Division of Nephrology, Department of Medicine, Toronto General Hospital–University Health Network, Toronto, Ontario, Canada

BRYAN M. CURTIS, MD, FRCPC, Assistant Professor of Medicine, Division of Nephrology and Clinical Epidemiology Unit, Patient Research Centre, Health Sciences Centre, Memorial University of Newfoundland, St. John's, Newfoundland, Canada

SANTO DELLEGROTTAGLIE, MD, Post-doctoral Research Fellow, Zena and Michael A. Wiener Cardiovascular Institute and Marie-Josée and Henry R. Kravis Center for Cardiovascular Health, Mount Sinai Medical Center, New York, New York

PANKAJ DESAI, PhD, Professor, Department of Surgery, University of Cincinnati Medical Center, Cincinnati, Ohio

RALF DIKOW, MD, Staff Physician, Department of Nephrology, University Hospital of Heidelberg, Heidelberg, Germany

SUE C. HEFFELFINGER, MD, PhD, Associate Professor, Department of Pathology, University of Cincinnati Medical Center, Cincinnati, Ohio

WILLIAM L. HENRICH, MD, Professor and Chairman, Department of Medicine, University of Maryland School of Medicine, Baltimore, Maryland

JONATHAN HIMMELFARB, MD, Director, Division of Nephrology and Transplantation, Maine Medical Center, Portland, Maine

WILLIAM F. KEANE, MD, US Human Health, Merck & Co., Inc., North Wales, Pennsylvania

BURNETT S. KELLY, MD, Instructor, Department of Surgery, University of Cincinnati Medical Center, Cincinnati, Ohio

KIRAN KUNDHAL, MD, Nephrology Fellow, Division of Nephrology, Department of Medicine, Toronto General Hospital-University Health Network, Toronto, Ontario, Canada

JINSONG LI, MD, PhD, Post-doctoral Fellow, Division of Nephrology and Hypertension, University of Cincinnati Medical Center, Cincinnati, Ohio

PAULETTE A. LYLE, BS, Merck Research Laboratories, Horsham, Pennsylvania

PETER A. MCCULLOUGH, MD, MPH, FACC, FACP, FCCP, FAHA, Department of Medicine, Divisions of Cardiology, Nutrition and Preventive Medicine, William Beaumont Hospital, Royal Oak, Michigan

MURAD MELHEM, MS, Graduate Student, College of Pharmacy, University of Cincinnati Medical Center, Cincinnati, Ohio

RINO MUNDA, MD, Professor, Department of Surgery, University of Cincinnati Medical Center, Cincinnati, Ohio

ANN M. O'HARE, MA, MD, Assistant Professor of Medicine, Nephrology Division, University of California, San Francisco, San Francisco; Staff Physician, VA Medical Center, San Francisco, California

PATRICK S. PARFREY, MD, FRCPC, University Research Professor, Division of Nephrology and Clinical Epidemiology Unit, Patient Research Centre, Health Sciences Centre, Memorial University of Newfoundland, St. John's, Newfoundland, Canada

ANDREAS PIERRATOS, MD, FRCPC, Staff Nephrologist, Director of Home Hemodialysis, Division of Nephrology, Department of Medicine, Humber River Regional Hospital, Toronto, Ontario, Canada

SANJAY RAJAGOPALAN, MD, Associate Professor, Zena and Michael A. Wiener Cardiovascular Institute and Marie-Josée and Henry R. Kravis Center for Cardiovascular Health, Mount Sinai Medical Center, New York; Associate Professor & Director of Cardiac MRI, Mount Sinai School of Medicine, New York, New York

CLAUDIO RIGATTO, MD, Assistant Professor of Medicine, University of Manitoba, Winnipeg; Nephrologist, Manitoba Renal Program, Winnipeg, Manitoba, Canada

EBERHARD RITZ, MD, Professor of Internal Medicine, Chief, Department of Nephrology, University Hospital of Heidelberg, Heidelberg, Germany

PRABIR ROY-CHAUDHURY, MD, PhD, Associate Professor, Division of Nephrology and Hypertension, University of Cincinnati Medical Center, Cincinnati, Ohio

RAJIV SARAN, MD, MS, MRCP, Assistant Professor of Medicine, Division of Nephrology, University of Michigan, Ann Arbor, Michigan

AUSTIN G. STACK, MD, MSc, MRCPI, FASN, Internal Medicine, University of Texas Health Science Center, Houston, Texas; Consultant Nephrologist, Regional Kidney Centre, Department of Medicine, Letterkenny General Hospital, North West Area, County Donegal; Health Services Executive, North West Area, County Donegal, Ireland

RAVINDER K. WALI, MD, Assistant Professor of Medicine, Division of Nephrology, Department of Medicine, University of Maryland School of Medicine, Baltimore, Maryland

MARTIN ZEIER, MD, Chief, Division of Nephrology, Department of Nephrology, University Hospital of Heidelberg, Heidelberg, Germany

JIANHUA ZHANG, BS, Research Assistant, Division of Nephrology and Hypertension, University of Cincinnati Medical Center, Cincinnati, Ohio

CONTRIBUTORS

CONTENTS

> This article underlines the high prevalence and incidence of lower extremity peripheral arterial disease (PAD) as well as the considerable morbidity and mortality associated with PAD in persons with chronic kidney disease (CKD). It also draws attention to the paucity of information available to guide management of PAD among patients with CKD and reviews relevant literature from the general population.

> Hypertension affects 24% of the adult US population. In the United States, 3% of the adult population has an elevated serum creatinine level, and 70% of these patients have hypertension. The prevalence of hypertension in chronic kidney disease (CKD) depends on the patient's age and the severity of renal failure, proteinuria, and underlying renal disease. As patients with CKD progress to end-stage renal disease (ESRD), 86% are diagnosed with hypertension. It has long been recognized that kidney function affects and is affected by hypertension. This article discusses the pathophysiology and management of hypertension in patients with CKD.

> This article (1) identifies the types of hemodialysis access, (2) summarizes the clinical standard of care for dialysis access grafts and fistulae, (3) describes the pathology and pathogenesis of venous stenosis in dialysis access grafts and fistulae, (4) tabulates available therapies for hemodialysis vascular access dysfunction and speculates on the reasons for the lack of effective therapies, and (5) discusses the development and application of novel therapeutic interventions for this difficult clinical problem. The possibility that dialysis access grafts and fistulae could be the ideal clinical model for testing novel local therapies to block neointimal hyperplasia is discussed.

FORTHCOMING ISSUES

RECENT ISSUES

CARDIOLOGY CLINICS

Cardiol Clin 23 (2005) xi

Foreword

CardioRenal Disease

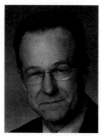

Michael H. Crawford, MD
Consulting Editor

Cardiologists are frequently confronted with patients who have kidney disease from chronic renal insufficiency to end-stage renal disease and patients pre– and post–kidney transplant. This issue of the *Cardiology Clinics* is devoted to the management of such patients. Doctors Babiga, Rajagopalan, and Saran represent the expertise of three different institutions and have recruited an excellent group of expert authors in this area. The topics range from the highly practical, such as revascularization in renal disease patients, to potential new approaches to renal disease management that may improve cardiovascular outcomes.

Clearly this is an important area, because renal dysfunction is now recognized as a risk factor for atherosclerotic vascular disease just as diabetes and rheumatologic diseases are. Also, all of these diseases interact with one compounding the risks of the others. The common thread here is blood vessels—all of these diseases are vasculitides. Hopefully, approaches that benefit one vascular disease will ultimately benefit the others. In this vein, prevention of reno-vascular disease is critical, and optimal management is essential to prevent further vascular disease of other organs. I am sure that this issue of the *Cardiology Clinics* will provide new insights and practical approaches to patients who have renal disease.

Michael H. Crawford, MD
Division of Cardiology
Department of Medicine
University of California
San Francisco Medical Center
505 Parnassus Avenue, Box 0124
San Francisco, CA 94143-0124, USA

E-mail address: michael.crawford@ucsfmedctr.org

Preface

CardioRenal Disease

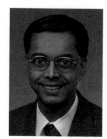 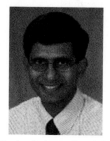 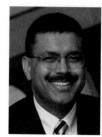

Ragavendra R. Baliga,
MD, MBA, FACC, FRCP(Edin)

Sanjay Rajagopalan, MD

Rajiv Saran, MD, MS, MRCP

Guest Editors

The increasing prevalence of obesity, hypertension, and diabetes has meant that practitioners are increasingly encountering patients who have both chronic renal disease and cardiovascular disease. Diabetes and hypertension remain the most common causes of end-stage renal disease (ESRD) in most countries. Most patients who have chronic kidney disease die before they reach ESRD. There is a considerable amount of data to suggest that chronic renal disease accelerates atherosclerosis, myocardial disease, and valvular and arterial calcification and promotes cardiac arrhythmias. Moreover, with the aging population it is important to have a better understanding of the impact of worsening renal function on cardiovascular disease. The idea fast emerging from a review of the current literature is that the kidney not only mirrors changes in the cardiovascular system but also negatively impacts the evolution of cardiovascular disease.

To promote the awareness and understanding of the most pertinent issues, we have assembled a panel of international experts, both cardiologists and nephrologists, to write on major areas of interface between cardiovascular and kidney disease. The articles focus on topics that are directly relevant to the patient and include articles that discuss the pathophysiology, management, and newer paradigms of treatment for patients who exhibit clinical manifestations of both cardiovascular and renal disease, including those who have end-stage renal failure on dialysis or after kidney transplantation.

The management of patients who have both cardiovascular and renal disease remains a challenge, despite significant advances and burgeoning interest. Research in this field is a work in progress, and it is our hope that this issue of the *Cardiology Clinics* will not only provide insight into the day-to-day management of such patients but will also provide an impetus for future research. Clearly, it is high time that nephrologists and cardiologists join forces in the fight against the vicious circle of cardiorenal disease.

Ragavendra R. Baliga, MD, MBA,
FACC, FRCP(Edin)
Director of Cardiovascular Medicine
Ohio State University Hospital East
Ohio State University
Columbus, OH, USA

E-mail address: rrbaliga@gmail.com

Sanjay Rajagopalan, MD
Division of Cardiology
Mount Sinai School of Medicine
New York, NY, USA

Rajiv Saran, MD, MS, MRCP
Division of Nephrology
University of Michigan
Ann Arbor, MI, USA

ELSEVIER
SAUNDERS

CARDIOLOGY
CLINICS

Cardiol Clin 23 (2005) 225–236

Management of Peripheral Arterial Disease in Chronic Kidney Disease

Ann M. O'Hare, MD, MA[a,b,*]

[a]VA Medical Center, San Francisco, 4150 Clement Street, San Francisco, CA 94121, USA
[b]Nephrology Division, University of California, San Francisco, 513 Parnassus Avenue,
Health Sciences East, Room 672, San Francisco, CA 94143-0532, USA

Lower extremity peripheral arterial disease (PAD) has not been examined in most prior studies of the epidemiology of cardiovascular disease among patients with chronic kidney disease (CKD) [1–5], and very few epidemiologic studies of PAD have considered CKD as a potential risk factor [6–11]. Thus, knowledge of the epidemiology, outcomes, and treatment options for PAD among patients with CKD lags behind that for other forms of cardiovascular disease. This article underlines the high prevalence and incidence of PAD as well as the considerable morbidity and mortality associated with PAD in persons with CKD. It also draws attention to the paucity of information available to guide management of PAD among patients with CKD and reviews relevant literature from the general population.

Epidemiology of peripheral arterial disease in patients with chronic kidney disease

Prevalence of peripheral arterial disease in chronic kidney disease

Prevalence estimates for PAD are highly dependent on the diagnostic method selected and population of interest [12]. In the adult population,

Dr. O'Hare is supported by a Research Career Development Award from the Department of Veterans Affairs Health Services Research and Development Service.

* VA Medical Center, San Francisco, Box 111j (Nephrology), 4150 Clement Street, San Francisco, CA 94121.

E-mail address: Ann.O'Hare@med.va.gov

0733-8651/05/$ - Published by Elsevier Inc.
doi:10.1016/j.ccl.2005.03.006

PAD diagnosed using an ankle brachial index (ABI) cutoff of less than 0.90 has an estimated prevalence of 12%, with approximately one third of these patients having classic symptoms of claudication [13,14]. As is true for the general population, prevalence estimates among patients with CKD are much lower when PAD is defined by the presence of intermittent claudication than when it is defined using the ABI.

Prevalence of intermittent claudication

Intermittent claudication is often considered a cardinal symptom of PAD. Prior epidemiologic studies have reported the prevalence of typical intermittent claudication in the adult population to be less than 5% and in many cases less than 2% [6,16–18]. Although several studies have examined risk factors for intermittent claudication, few have included renal insufficiency as a potential correlate or have examined the prevalence of intermittent claudication among patients with renal insufficiency [9,19,20]. Webb et al [21] reported a 19% prevalence of intermittent claudication among 325 chronic dialysis patients in the United Kingdom. Leskinen et al [22] found that among 59 predialysis patients, 36 dialysis patients, 41 renal transplant recipients, and 59 control subjects in Finland the prevalence of intermittent claudication was 6.8%, 2.8%, 10%, and 0%, respectively. Both of these studies, however, focused on a small sample of patients with advanced CKD.

In the Cardiovascular Health Study (CHS), a cohort study of 5888 community-dwelling adults aged 65 years or older, the baseline prevalence of classic intermittent claudication (by the Rose Claudication Questionnaire) was 1.68% among patients with normal renal function and 4.46% among patients with renal insufficiency defined as a serum creatinine measurement of 1.3 mg/dL or higher among women and 1.5 mg/dL or higher among men (O'Hare et al, unpublished work based on CHS public use data). Among patients aged 45 to 64 years enrolled in the Atherosclerosis Risk in Communities (ARIC) study, the prevalence of Rose intermittent claudication was 0.68% among those with normal renal function and 1.63% among those with an estimated creatinine clearance of less than 60 mL/min (O'Hare et al, unpublished work based on ARIC public use data). In summary, the prevalence of intermittent claudication seems to be substantially higher among patients with CKD than in the general population, although the exact prevalence varies according to the population studied and may reflect the older age and higher prevalence of diabetes and hypertension in patients with CKD as well as other risk factors for claudication in this population.

Prevalence of ankle brachial index less than 0.90

In the general population, an ABI of less than 0.90 correlates well with the presence of angiographic evidence of PAD [23]. PAD prevalence estimates that are based on ABI measurement are consistently higher than those based on the presence of intermittent claudication. In community-cohort studies, the prevalence of an ABI of less than 0.90 has ranged from less than 5% among ARIC participants to as high as 12.4% among CHS participants [8,10,18,24]. Prevalence estimates among patient cohorts recruited from medical clinics tend to be considerably higher [15,25]. For example 29% of high-risk patients enrolled from primary care clinics as part of the PAD Awareness, Risk and Treatment: New Resources for Survival program had an ABI of less than 0.90 [25]. Patients eligible for this study included those over 70 years old and those between the ages of 50 and 69 years who had diabetes or a smoking history.

A small number of studies have reported ABI measurements in relation to renal function. Newman et al [24] documented an inverse association between serum creatinine level and ABI of less than 0.90 that was independent of potential confounders. Among the subset of CHS patients who underwent baseline serum creatinine measurement, 12% with renal insufficiency (defined as a serum creatinine level $\geq$ 1.3 mg/dL in women and $\geq$ 1.5 mg/dL in men) and 7% with normal

renal function had an ABI of less than 0.90 [26]. Based on data from the most recent National Health and Nutrition Examination Survey (1999–2000), 24% of the noninstitutionalized civilian population aged 40 years and older with an estimated creatinine clearance of less than 60 mL/min/1.73 m^2 are estimated to have an ABI of less than 0.90, compared with 3.7% of those with a clearance of 60 mL/min/1.73 m^2 or higher [27]. As for the CHS sample, renal insufficiency was independently associated with a low ABI even after adjustment for differences in patient age, diabetes, and other potential confounders. In the small study by Leskinen [22] described previously, 15.3% of Predialysis patients, 8.3% of dialysis patients, and 2.6% of transplant patients had an ABI below 0.90, whereas none of the control patients in this study had an ABI below 0.90.

Among dialysis patients, several larger cross-sectional studies have examined the prevalence of a low ABI. With the exception of a study in Japanese dialysis patients in which 16.9% of patients had an ABI below 0.90 [28], all other studies have reported the prevalence of an ABI below 0.90 among hemodialysis patients to be in the range of 30% to 38% [29–31]. Hence, the prevalence of PAD seems to be much higher among dialysis-dependent patients than among the general population and those with milder forms of CKD.

Sensitivity and specificity of diagnostic testing for peripheral arterial disease

In the general population, claudication detected by the Rose Claudication Questionnaire has a high specificity and positive predictive value but extremely low sensitivity for detecting large-vessel PAD [12]. The Edinburgh Claudication questionnaire seems to be somewhat more sensitive [32]. A low ABI is highly sensitive and specific for the presence of more than 50% stenosis of lower extremity vessels on angiography [23].

The sensitivity and specificity for the Rose and Edinburgh claudication questionnaires are unknown among patients with CKD. There is a theoretical concern that a high prevalence of vascular calcification, particularly in patients with advanced CKD, may render an ABI below 0.90 a less sensitive measure of lower extremity PAD in this population. In support of this possiblity, Leskinen et al [22] reported an extremely high prevalence of ABIs above 1.30 among Finnish predialysis patients, hemodialysis patients, and post–renal transplant patients (23.7%, 41.7%, and 23.1%, respectively). These numbers are much higher than those reported for several larger dialysis-patient cohorts. For example, 7% among a sample of 132 United States hemodialysis patients [30] and 10.9% among a sample of 1010 Japanese hemodialysis patients had an ABI higher than 1.30. For comparison, in the latter study, 0.67% of patients in an age- and gender-matched control group of healthy volunteers had an ABI higher than 1.30 [28]. Collectively, these findings suggest that a broader range of ABI measurements may be encountered in dialysis patients than in the general population.

Incidence of peripheral arterial disease in chronic kidney disease

CKD has not traditionally been viewed as a possible risk factor for PAD, and most previous epidemiologic studies of PAD have not even included information on renal function [6–11]. Conversely, although many studies have now demonstrated that CKD is a risk factor for all-cause mortality, cardiovascular death, and cardiovascular events such as coronary heart disease and stroke [1–5], most of these studies did not examine the association of CKD with lower extremity PAD.

Among patients enrolled in the United Kingdom Prospective Diabetes Study, albuminuria was associated with the development of PAD during study follow-up in univariate but not in multivariate analysis [33]. This analysis examined only albuminuria, not renal function. Renal insufficiency, defined as a serum creatinine level $\geq$ 1.3 g/dL in women and $\geq$ 1.5 mg/dL in men, was independently associated with the development of intermittent claudication among participants in the CHS [1]. Secondary analysis of data from the Heart and Estrogen/Progestin Replacement Study showed that both moderate and severe CKD, defined respectively as an estimated creatinine clearance of 30 to 59 and less than 30 mL/min/1.73m^2, were associated with an increased risk of arriving at a predefined PAD end point (revascularization, amputation, or lower extremity sympathectomy) during follow-up [34]. This study did not adjust for the baseline prevalence of PAD among study participants. Thus, although patients with even moderate CKD are at risk for PAD events, it is unclear whether this risk simply reflects a higher baseline prevalence of subclinical PAD in this population (as described previously) or whether CKD is a true risk factor for PAD.

Risk factors for peripheral arterial disease among patients with chronic kidney disease

Established risk factors for PAD include male sex, older age, diabetes, smoking, hypertension, dyslipidemia (low HDL and high LDL and triglyceride levels), lipoprotein (a), hyperhomocysteinemia, and chronic inflammation, whereas alcohol intake and physical activity seem to be protective [6–11,35–43]. Among dialysis patients, many of the risk factors for PAD are the same as for the general population, but there also seem to be associations that are unique to dialysis patients. Webb et al [21] reported that among 325 hemodialysis patients, intermittent claudication was associated with older age, smoking, hypertension, and hypertriglyceridemia. Among a subgroup of patients enrolled in the HEMO study, Cheung et al [44] reported cross-sectional associations of baseline PAD with smoking, older age, diabetes, and non-black race. In this study, hypertension and cholesterol were not associated with PAD. Among patients enrolled in Waves 1, 3, and 4 of the United States Renal Data System's (USRDS) Dialysis Morbidity and Mortality Study (DMMS), coronary artery disease, cerebrovascular disease, smoking, lower diastolic blood pressure, left ventricular hypertrophy, lower serum albumin, malnourished status, lower parathyroid hormone level, and longer time since initiation of dialysis were associated with baseline PAD, in addition to age, gender, diabetes, and race as reported for the HEMO study [45]. The lack of association of PAD with either hypertension or dyslipidemia in these last two studies is striking. A limitation of these studies is that they were cross-sectional in nature and did not define PAD using objective measures of lower extremity perfusion such as the ABI. There is currently a paucity of studies examining risk factors for PAD among patients with CKD who are not receiving dialysis.

Few longitudinal analyses have examined risk factors for incident (rather than prevalent) PAD among patients with CKD. In a study of the association of smoking with cardiovascular end points among patients enrolled in DMMS2, active smokers had an increased risk of peripheral arterial events [46]. This outcome, however, was defined broadly to include arterial aneurisms, Raynaud's phenomenon, and arterial embolic events in addition to lower extremity atherosclerotic disease. On the other hand, smoking was not a risk factor for lower extremity amputation among hemodialysis patients enrolled in DMMS 3 and 4 [47] (although the study outcome was not restricted to amputations performed for PAD), nor was it a risk factor for amputation following revascularization among dialysis patients enrolled in DMMS 1, 3, and 4 [48]. No studies have examined risk factors for the development of PAD among CKD patients.

Impact of chronic kidney disease on peripheral arterial disease outcomes

In the general population, patients with intermittent claudication are at increased risk for death and for cardiovascular events, although the course of their lower extremity disease is often benign [49,50]. In fact, even patients with subclinical PAD are at increased risk for all-cause and cardiovascular mortality along with myocardial infarction, stroke, and peripheral arterial events [18,24,51–57]. Furthermore, although most of the aforementioned studies have focused on the prognostic value of a low ABI, it has recently been shown that the presence of a high ABI (>1.40)—generally indicative of arterial incompressibility—is also predictive of mortality [58]. Finally, in addition to its well-documented associations with mortality and cardiovascular events, lower extremity PAD is also associated with lower extremity functional impairment [29,59–62] and with depression [63,64].

Although the natural history of claudication in the general population is characterized by high cardiovascular mortality but relatively benign lower extremity outcomes, it is unclear whether this is also the case in CKD. Relatively more information is available on the prognostic importance of a low ABI in patients with CKD. Several studies have now reported an association between an ABI below 0.90 and increased risk of both cardiovascular and all-cause mortality among hemodialysis patients [28,29,31]. In fact, in one study, patients with a high ABI (>1.30) and those with a borderline low ABI (0.90–1.10) were also at increased risk for all-cause and cardiovascular mortality when compared with patients who had ABIs between 1.10 and 1.30 [28].

The ABI–mortality association has not been examined among patients with milder forms of CKD. Most information on mortality among patients with CKD and PAD comes from studies of operative outcomes among patients undergoing lower extremity revascularization (as discussed later). Furthermore, the impact of PAD on functional status and other health-related quality-of-life outcomes likewise has not been explored among patients with CKD. Compared with the general population, dialysis patients seem to have lower self-assessed physical function, demonstrate poorer physical performance [65–67], and have a high prevalence of depression [68]. The associations of PAD with physical function, physical performance, or depression among patients with CKD have not been measured, however.

Medical therapy for peripheral arterial disease

Statin therapy

Cholesterol lowering with statin therapy seems to reduce overall frequency of cardiovascular events among high-risk patients in the general population [69,70]. Thus, statin therapy is frequently recommended for patients with PAD based solely on their elevated risk of cardiovascular death, myocardial infarction, and stroke [71]. Recently, however, the Medical Research Council\British Heart Foundation (MRC\BHF) Heart Protection Study has demonstrated a specific benefit of statin therapy in reducing PAD events among those at high risk for cardiovascular events. In this trial, patients randomly assigned to receive treatment with simvastatin, 40 mg, versus placebo experienced fewer peripheral vascular events in follow-up [72,73]. This benefit was seen among participants with and without diabetes and, importantly, in patients with PAD who had no prior history of other cardiovascular disease. Furthermore, statin therapy may also be associated with improved health-related quality-of-life outcomes in patients with PAD. For example, statin therapy seems to improve pain-free walking distance in patients with claudication [74] and is associated with superior leg function in patients with PAD [75]. In an observational study of 293 patients undergoing infrainguinal bypass operations, statin therapy was associated with superior graft patency and lower amputation rates, although it was not associated with improved survival [76].

Among dialysis patients, low rather than high serum cholesterol levels seem to be predictive of mortality [77,78]. At least one observational study has shown that dialysis patients receiving statin therapy nevertheless have lower overall cardiovascular mortality [79]. Although there have been no published randomized, controlled trials of the impact of statin therapy on cardiovascular events focusing specifically on dialysis patients or patients with CKD, several larger trials have included participants with mild CKD. In the Cholesterol and Recurrent Events study, pravastatin was equally effective in reducing secondary cardiovascular events in patients with mild chronic renal insufficiency (defined as an estimated creatinine clearance < 75 mL/min) as among the overall study population [80]. Peripheral arterial events were not included as an outcome in this study, however. Likewise in the MRC/BHF Heart Protection Study, a reduction in major vascular and coronary events has been documented for the 1329 participants with mild CKD, but the peripheral arterial disease outcome (noncoronary revascularization) examined in the primary analysis was not included in this subgroup analysis [73]. Therefore, it remains unclear whether statin therapy also reduces PAD events among patients with CKD; the overall frequency of these events in this cohort was fairly low, and the study was not powered to examine this outcome. The impact of statin therapy on lower extremity function also has not been studied in patients with CKD. Although patients with CKD were not specifically excluded from the study by McDermott et al [75], no information is provided on the prevalence of CKD in this cohort or on the association of statin therapy with lower extremity function in this subgroup.

Blood pressure–lowering agents

In the general population, hypertension is a risk factor for PAD. The Appropriate Blood-Pressure Control in Diabetes study was a prospective, randomized, controlled trial among persons with diabetes of the effects of intensive blood pressure control with either enalapril or nisoldipine versus moderate blood pressure control in the placebo group. In this trial, intensive blood pressure control resulted in fewer cardiovascular events among those with and without PAD [81]. Furthermore, although there was an inverse relationship between ABI and the odds of a cardiovascular event among those randomly assigned to placebo, no such relationship existed among patients randomly assigned to intensive blood pressure control [81]. Although this study demonstrates that intensive blood pressure lowering reduces cardiovascular events in patients with PAD, it does not address the question of whether tight blood pressure control can reduce

the incidence of these events, because PAD events were not evaluated. Although some participants had CKD (a creatinine level above 3.0 mg/dL was an exclusion criteria), the impact of intensive blood pressure control on cardiovascular events among persons with CKD and PAD has not been reported.

In the Heart Outcomes Prevention Evaluation study, persons aged 55 years or older with prevalent cardiovascular disease were randomly assigned to receive ramipril versus placebo. All-cause and cardiovascular mortality, stroke, and myocardial infarction were decreased among participants who received ramipril. This effect was seen among participants with and without PAD at baseline [82]. Ramipril was also associated with a decreased need for lower extremity revascularization or amputation in the overall study population. In subgroup analysis, however, a statistically significant protective effect was present only for patients without clinical evidence of PAD and with an ABI higher than 0.90 [82]. Although further subgroup analysis has not been conducted among those with PAD and CKD, ramipril was equally protective against the primary outcome of stroke, myocardial infarction, or cardiovascular death among participants with and without CKD (defined as a serum creatinine level between 1.4 and 2.3 mg/dL) [83]. Finally, in an observational study of patients undergoing infrainguinal bypass, overall mortality was lower among patients who were receiving angiotensin-converting enzyme (ACE) inhibitors, but graft patency and amputation rates were similar in the two arms [76].

Smoking cessation

Current and former smoking is associated with PAD in cross-sectional analysis [10,84], and smoking increases the risk of amputation in patients with claudication [85] and decreases patency rates after lower extremity bypass [86]. Smoking cessation seems to result in an increase in exercise tolerance and in ankle pressure among patients with intermittent claudication [87]. Although these studies did not focus specifically on patients with CKD, Foley et al [46] have shown that, among dialysis patients, current smoking is predictive of future cardiovascular events, including PAD. Although smoking remains a modifiable risk factor, it is noteworthy that among several large cohorts undergoing lower extremity revascularization smoking was less common among those with CKD than among those with normal renal function [88,89].

Nevertheless, smoking cessation should be strongly encouraged in patients with CKD and PAD given their high incidence of PAD and other cardiovascular events.

Antiplatelet agents

In a meta-analysis of clinical trials using antiplatelet agents (aspirin, clopidogrel, ticlopidine, picotamide, and dipyridamole), use of any antiplatelet agent resulted in a 23% risk reduction of the chosen outcome of nonfatal myocardial infarction, nonfatal stroke, or vascular death among the subgroup of 9214 patients with PAD [90]. The benefit was similar among patients with intermittent claudication, those having peripheral grafting, and those having peripheral angioplasty. In the Clopidogrel versus Aspirin in Patients at Risk for Ischemic Events (CAPRIE) trial—a randomized, blinded, clinical trial designed to assess the relative efficacy of clopidogrel (75 mg once daily) and aspirin (325 mg once daily) in reducing the risk of a composite outcome cluster of ischemic stroke, myocardial infarction, or vascular death—there was a 23.8% risk reduction in these outcomes in the clopidogrel-treated group among the subgroup of patients with PAD at baseline [91]. The risk of amputation (a secondary study outcome) was not significantly different between treatment groups, although the study was underpowered to test that outcome. Severe renal insufficiency was an exclusion criterion for the CAPRIE trial, and subgroup analysis among patients with milder forms of renal insufficiency enrolled in the trial has not been conducted.

Cilostazol

Cilostazol is a phosphodiesterase inhibitor that has both antiplatelet and vasodilating properties. Cilostazol has been shown to increase pain-free and maximal walking distance among persons with claudication caused by PAD but does not seem to affect mortality or cardiovascular morbidity in this group [92–94]. Persons with CKD were not explicitly excluded from these trials, but no subgroup analyses are presented. Furthermore, it is unclear whether cilostazol is a safe drug for dialysis patients. It has not been tested in this population, and its metabolism may be affected by altered protein binding in dialysis patients.

Exercise

Exercise therapy is considered first-line therapy for intermittent claudication, although its value in asymptomatic PAD and critical ischemia is unknown [95]. A number of prospective studies have shown that exercise improves walking ability and quality of life in patients with claudication. A meta-analysis of studies of exercise to reduce claudication demonstrated that programs that use intermittent walking to near-maximal pain over at least 6 months are most likely to be effective [96]. The safety and efficacy of exercise therapy for claudication among patients with CKD have not been reported. A high prevalence of claudication among dialysis patients [21], documented low activity levels in this population [97], and the rarity of exercise counseling in the dialysis unit setting [98] suggest that exercise therapy could be an important area for intervention. Less is known about the activity levels and exercise counseling practices among patients with milder forms of CKD.

Surgical therapy for peripheral arterial disease

Revascularization

Lower extremity surgical or percutaneous revascularization may be performed for disabling claudication or for critical limb ischemia (rest pain, ischemic ulceration, or gangrene). Many small retrospective surgical case series have demonstrated higher mortality rates and lower limb salvage rates among patients with advanced CKD [99–105]. In larger series of patients undergoing lower extremity revascularization, postoperative and 1-year mortality seem to increase with declining renal function [88,89].

A recent retrospective study of 800 hemodialysis patients enrolled in the USRDS DMMS 1, 3, and 4 who underwent lower extremity revascularization demonstrated high mortality and amputation rates after this procedure [48]. Mortality and limb salvage rates were more favorable among study patients who underwent percutaneous rather than surgical revascularization. Although this finding may reflect selection bias, it suggests a need for randomized, controlled clinical trials to explore the possibility that lower extremity angioplasty may result in better outcomes than surgical revascularization among dialysis patients. In this study, amputation rates after revascularization were higher among black patients, those without insurance or receiving Medicaid, and those with diabetes. Although dialysis patients seem to be at singularly increased risk for limb loss after lower extremity revascularization, this does not seem to be true for patients with milder forms of CKD based on a retrospective study of lower extremity revascularization procedures performed nationally within the Department of Veterans Affairs [89].

Amputation

Amputation rates among end-stage renal disease (ESRD) patients seem to be disproportionately high, and, along with diabetes, the presence of diagnosed PAD is one of the strongest risk factors for amputation [47,106]. Based on national Medicare data, lower extremity amputation is associated with extraordinarily high mortality rates among ESRD patients. Those at greatest risk include older patients, Native American and African-American (compared with white) patients, those whose primary renal disease was diabetes or hypertension, and those undergoing dialysis (versus transplant recipients) [106]. Dialysis patients seem to be at particularly high risk for bilateral amputations [107]. In general, there has been little interest in efforts to prevent amputation among ESRD patients, although provision of preventive foot care in the dialysis unit setting does seem to be effective in lowering amputation rates among patients with diabetes [108,109].

Unfortunately, observational studies do not provide clear guidance for surgical decision making in patients with CKD and limb-threatening ischemia. The increased risk of death after amputation and revascularization attributable to CKD are quite similar [88,110]. Crude postoperative mortality rates are considerably higher after amputation than after revascularization [110], and mortality rates are lower after percutaneous than after surgical revascularization among dialysis patients [48]. These findings, however, may simply reflect the impact of selection bias. Further studies are needed to evaluate the risks and benefits of amputation over revascularization (and type of revascularization) among patients with CKD and to investigate reasons for the high mortality associated with these procedures in this population.

Impact of chronic kidney disease on surgical management of limb ischemia

Several studies have suggested that the clinical indications for lower extremity revascularization may differ for patients with normal renal function and those with CKD. In a case-control study of patients undergoing lower extremity revascularization at two surgical centers, rest pain and claudication were the most common reasons for revascularization among non-ESRD controls, whereas ulceration and gangrene were the most common reason among dialysis patients [111]. In addition, dialysis patients were more likely to undergo more distal revascularization procedures. Similar patterns existed in a national sample of veterans undergoing initial lower extremity revascularization [89]. Even after adjustment for other patient characteristics, when compared with all other veterans undergoing bypass procedures, dialysis patients were more likely to present with wound infection, gangrene, infection or ischemic ulceration, elevated white blood cell count, and preoperative sepsis at the time of initial revascularization. They were also more likely to have a preoperative hospital stay longer than 1 week, to undergo concurrent minor amputation, and to undergo a more distal procedure. These findings may indicate more rapid disease progression among dialysis patients or may reflect different referral and care patterns for this population.

Few studies have evaluated the impact of CKD on procedure choice for limb-threatening ischemia. Collins et al [112] found a higher prevalence of dialysis patients among a national sample of veterans undergoing amputation than among those undergoing lower extremity revascularization for PAD, and this finding seemed to be independent of other patient characteristics such as age or prevalence of diabetes [112]. In a smaller study of all amputations and revascularizations performed at a single medical center over a 3-ear period, Abou-Zamzam [113] also found that dialysis patients seemed to be overrepresented in the group undergoing amputation. In multivariate analysis, dialysis status was the only independent predictor of amputation versus revascularization, although this study did include patients undergoing secondary procedures.

Summary

PAD has been overlooked in many epidemiologic studies evaluating cardiovascular risk associated with renal disease. Conversely, CKD has not been evaluated as a potential risk factor in epidemiologic studies of PAD. PAD, however, seems to be more prevalent among patients with even moderate CKD than in the general population and is most common among chronic dialysis patients, one third or more of whom have a low ABI. Patients with CKD also seem to be at increased risk for developing claudication and for requiring surgical intervention for lower extremity PAD. Furthermore, even moderate CKD seems to be a risk factor for postoperative death and complications after both lower extremity amputation and revascularization procedures. Conversely, even asymptomatic PAD seems to be a risk factor for death among dialysis patients.

In the general population, statins, antiplatelet agents (particularly clopidogrel), antihypertensive agents, and ACE inhibitors all have a proven benefit in reducing cardiovascular events in patients with PAD and in some instances may also reduce PAD events. Available evidence suggests that patients with CKD also experience cardiovascular risk reduction with statin and ACE-inhibitor therapy, but these therapies have not been shown to reduce PAD events specifically in patients with CKD. Further studies are needed to identify interventions that can specifically reduce the incidence of PAD complications in patients with CKD.

Although it is clear that mortality and complication rates after both lower extremity amputation and revascularization are increased in patients with even moderate CKD, currently available observational studies do not provide clear guidance for surgical decision making in CKD patients with limb-threatening ischemia. Further studies are needed to evaluate the risks and benefits of amputation over revascularization among patients with CKD and to investigate reasons for the high mortality associated with these procedures in this patient group. Further studies are also needed to measure the impact of CKD on care processes for PAD with the goal of identifying target areas for improvement.

Acknowledgments

The author thanks Dr. William R. Hiatt for valuable comments on an earlier draft of this article.

References

[1] Fried LF, Shlipak MG, Crump C, et al. Renal insufficiency as a predictor of cardiovascular outcomes and mortality in elderly individuals. J Am Coll Cardiol 2003;41:1364–72.

[2] Garg AX, Clark WF, Haynes RB, et al. Moderate renal insufficiency and the risk of cardiovascular mortality: results from the NHANES I. Kidney Int 2002;61:1486–94.

[3] Manjunath G, Tighiouart H, Coresh J, et al. Level of kidney function as a risk factor for cardiovascular outcomes in the elderly. Kidney Int 2003;63: 1121–9.

[4] Muntner P, He J, Hamm L, et al. Renal insufficiency and subsequent death resulting from cardiovascular disease in the United States. J Am Soc Nephrol 2002;13:745–53.

[5] Shlipak MG, Simon JA, Grady D, et al. Renal insufficiency and cardiovascular events in postmenopausal women with coronary heart disease. J Am Coll Cardiol 2001;38:705–11.

[6] Belch JJ, Topol EJ, Agnelli G, et al. Critical issues in peripheral arterial disease detection and management: a call to action. Arch Intern Med 2003;163: 884–92.

[7] Criqui MH, Langer RD, Fronek A, et al. Mortality over a period of 10 years in patients with peripheral arterial disease. N Engl J Med 1992;326:381–6.

[8] Fowkes FG, Housley E, Cawood EH, et al. Edinburgh Artery Study: prevalence of asymptomatic and symptomatic peripheral arterial disease in the general population. Int J Epidemiol 1991;20:384–92.

[9] Murabito JM, D'Agostino RB, Silbershatz H, et al. Intermittent claudication. A risk profile from The Framingham Heart Study. Circulation 1997;96: 44–9.

[10] Murabito JM, Evans JC, Nieto K, et al. Prevalence and clinical correlates of peripheral arterial disease in the Framingham Offspring Study. Am Heart J 2002;143:961–5.

[11] Ridker PM, Stampfer MJ, Rifai N. Novel risk factors for systemic atherosclerosis: a comparison of C-reactive protein, fibrinogen, homocysteine, lipoprotein(a), and standard cholesterol screening as predictors of peripheral arterial disease. JAMA 2001;285:2481–5.

[12] Criqui MH, Fronek A, Klauber MR, et al. The sensitivity, specificity, and predictive value of traditional clinical evaluation of peripheral arterial disease: results from noninvasive testing in a defined population. Circulation 1985;71:516–22.

[13] Hiatt WR, Hoag S, Hamman RF. Effect of diagnostic criteria on the prevalence of peripheral arterial disease. The San Luis Valley diabetes study. Circulation 1995;91:1472–9.

[14] Criqui MH, Fronek A, Barrett-Connor E, et al. The prevalence of peripheral arterial disease in a defined population. Circulation 1985;71:510–5.

[15] Collins TC, Petersen NJ, Suarez-Almazor M, et al. The prevalence of peripheral arterial disease in a racially diverse population. Arch Intern Med 2003;163:1469–74.

[16] Diehm C, Schuster A, Allenberg JR, et al. High prevalence of peripheral arterial disease and comorbidity in 6880 primary care patients: cross-sectional study. Atherosclerosis 2004;172:95–105.

[17] Newman AB, Naydeck BL, Sutton-Tyrrell K, et al. The role of comorbidity in the assessment of intermittent claudication in older adults. J Clin Epidemiol 2001;54:294–300.

[18] Zheng ZJ, Sharrett AR, Chambless LE, et al. Associations of ankle-brachial index with clinical coronary heart disease, stroke and preclinical carotid and popliteal atherosclerosis: the Atherosclerosis Risk in Communities (ARIC) Study. Atherosclerosis 1997;131:115–25.

[19] Kannel WB, Skinner JJ Jr, Schwartz MJ, et al. Intermittent claudication. Incidence in the Framingham Study. Circulation 1970;41:875–83.

[20] Kannel WB, McGee DL. Update on some epidemiologic features of intermittent claudication: the Framingham Study. J Am Geriatr Soc 1985;33: 13–8.

[21] Webb AT, Franks PJ, Reaveley DA, et al. Prevalence of intermittent claudication and risk factors for its development in patients on renal replacement therapy. Eur J Vasc Surg 1993;7:523–7.

[22] Leskinen Y, Salenius JP, Lehtimaki T, et al. The prevalence of peripheral arterial disease and medial arterial calcification in patients with chronic renal failure: requirements for diagnostics. Am J Kidney Dis 2002;40:472–9.

[23] Carter SA. Indirect systolic pressures and pulse waves in arterial occlusive diseases of the lower extremities. Circulation 1968;37:624–37.

[24] Newman AB, Shemanski L, Manolio TA, et al. Ankle-arm index as a predictor of cardiovascular disease and mortality in the Cardiovascular Health Study. The Cardiovascular Health Study Group. Arterioscler Thromb Vasc Biol 1999;19:538–45.

[25] Hirsch AT, Criqui MH, Treat-Jacobson D, et al. Peripheral arterial disease detection, awareness, and treatment in primary care. JAMA 2001;286: 1317–24.

[26] Shlipak MG, Fried LF, Crump C, et al. Cardiovascular disease risk status in elderly persons with renal insufficiency. Kidney Int 2002;62:997–1004.

[27] O'Hare AM, Glidden DV, Fox CS, et al. High prevalence of peripheral arterial disease in persons with renal insufficiency: results from the National Health and Nutrition Examination Survey 1999–2000. Circulation 2004 Jan 27;109(3): 320–3.

[28] Ono K, Tsuchida A, Kawai H, et al. Ankle-brachial blood pressure index predicts all-cause and cardiovascular mortality in hemodialysis patients. J Am Soc Nephrol 2003;14:1591–8.

[29] Al Zahrani HA, Al Bar HM, Bahnassi A, et al. The distribution of peripheral arterial disease in a defined population of elderly high-risk Saudi patients. Int Angiol 1997;16:123–8.

[30] Fishbane S, Youn S, Flaster E, et al. Ankle-arm blood pressure index as a predictor of mortality in hemodialysis patients. Am J Kidney Dis 1996; 27:668–72.

[31] Testa A, Ottavioli JN. [Ankle-arm blood pressure index (AABPI) in hemodialysis patients]. Arch Mal Coeur Vaiss 1998;91:963–5 [in French].

[32] Leng GC, Fowkes FG. The Edinburgh Claudication Questionnaire: an improved version of the WHO/Rose Questionnaire for use in epidemiological surveys. J Clin Epidemiol 1992;45:1101–9.

[33] Adler AI, Stevens RJ, Neil A, et al. UKPDS 59: hyperglycemia and other potentially modifiable risk factors for peripheral vascular disease in type 2 diabetes. Diabetes Care 2002;25:894–9.

[34] O'Hare AM, Vittinghoff E, Hsia J, et al. Renal insufficiency and the risk of lower extremity peripheral arterial disease: results from the heart and estrogen/progestin replacement study (HERS). J Am Soc Nephrol 2004;15:1046–51.

[35] Fowkes FG, Housley E, Riemersma RA, et al. Smoking, lipids, glucose intolerance, and blood pressure as risk factors for peripheral atherosclerosis compared with ischemic heart disease in the Edinburgh Artery Study. Am J Epidemiol 1992; 135:331–40.

[36] Lowe GD, Fowkes FG, Dawes J, et al. Blood viscosity, fibrinogen, and activation of coagulation and leukocytes in peripheral arterial disease and the normal population in the Edinburgh Artery Study. Circulation 1993;87:1915–20.

[37] MacGregor AS, Price JF, Hau CM, et al. Role of systolic blood pressure and plasma triglycerides in diabetic peripheral arterial disease. The Edinburgh Artery Study. Diabetes Care 1999;22: 453–8.

[38] Price JF, Mowbray PI, Lee AJ, et al. Relationship between smoking and cardiovascular risk factors in the development of peripheral arterial disease and coronary artery disease. Edinburgh Artery Study. Eur Heart J 1999;20:344–53.

[39] Price JF, Lee AJ, Rumley A, et al. Lipoprotein (a) and development of intermittent claudication and major cardiovascular events in men and women: the Edinburgh Artery Study. Atherosclerosis 2001;157:241–9.

[40] Smith FB, Lee AJ, Hau CM, et al. Plasma fibrinogen, haemostatic factors and prediction of peripheral arterial disease in the Edinburgh Artery Study. Blood Coagul Fibrinolysis 2000;11:43–50.

[41] Housley E, Leng GC, Donnan PT, et al. Physical activity and risk of peripheral arterial disease in the general population. Edinburgh Artery Study. J Epidemiol Community Health 1993;47:475–80.

[42] Jepson RG, Fowkes FG, Donnan PT, et al. Alcohol intake as a risk factor for peripheral arterial disease in the general population in the Edinburgh Artery Study. Eur J Epidemiol 1995;11:9–14.

[43] Hsia J, Simon JA, Lin F, et al. Peripheral arterial disease in randomized trial of estrogen with progestin in women with coronary heart disease: the Heart and Estrogen/Progestin Replacement Study. Circulation 2000;102:2228–32.

[44] Cheung AK, Sarnak MJ, Yan G, et al. Atherosclerotic cardiovascular disease risks in chronic hemodialysis patients. Kidney Int 2000;58:353–62.

[45] O'Hare AM, Hsu CY, Bacchetti P, et al. Peripheral vascular disease risk factors among patients undergoing hemodialysis. J Am Soc Nephrol 2002;13:497–503.

[46] Foley RN, Herzog CA, Collins AJ. Smoking and cardiovascular outcomes in dialysis patients: the United States Renal Data System Wave 2 study. Kidney Int 2003;63:1462–7.

[47] O'Hare AM, Bacchetti P, Segal M, et al. Factors associated with future amputation among patients undergoing hemodialysis: results from the Dialysis Morbidity and Mortality Study Waves 3 and 4. Am J Kidney Dis 2003;41:162–70.

[48] Jaar BG, Astor BC, Berns JS, et al. Predictors of amputation and survival following lower extremity revascularization in hemodialysis patients. Kidney Int 2004;65:613–20.

[49] McDermott MM, McCarthy W. Intermittent claudication. The natural history. Surg Clin North Am 1995;75:581–91.

[50] Aquino R, Johnnides C, Makaroun M, et al. Natural history of claudication: long-term serial follow-up study of 1244 claudicants. J Vasc Surg 2001;34:962–70.

[51] Leng GC, Lee AJ, Fowkes FG, et al. Incidence, natural history and cardiovascular events in symptomatic and asymptomatic peripheral arterial disease in the general population. Int J Epidemiol 1996;25:1172–81.

[52] Tsai AW, Folsom AR, Rosamond WD, et al. Ankle-brachial index and 7-year ischemic stroke incidence: the ARIC study. Stroke 2001;32:1721–4.

[53] Sikkink CJ, van Asten WN, van 't Hof MA, et al. Decreased ankle/brachial indices in relation to morbidity and mortality in patients with peripheral arterial disease. Vasc Med 1997;2:169–73.

[54] Newman AB, Sutton-Tyrrell K, Vogt MT, et al. Morbidity and mortality in hypertensive adults with a low ankle/arm blood pressure index. JAMA 1993;270:487–9.

[55] Murabito JM, Evans JC, Larson MG, et al. The ankle-brachial index in the elderly and risk of stroke, coronary disease, and death: the Framingham Study. Arch Intern Med 2003;163:1939–42.

[56] Abbott RD, Petrovitch H, Rodriguez BL, et al. Ankle/brachial blood pressure in men > 70 years of age and the risk of coronary heart disease. Am J Cardiol 2000;86:280–4.

[57] Abbott RD, Rodriguez BL, Petrovitch H, et al. Ankle-brachial blood pressure in elderly men and the risk of stroke: the Honolulu Heart Program. J Clin Epidemiol 2001;54:973–8.

[58] Resnick HE, Lindsay RS, McDermott MM, et al. Relationship of high and low ankle brachial index to all-cause and cardiovascular disease mortality:

the Strong Heart Study. Circulation 2004;109:733–9.

[59] McDermott MM, Greenland P, Liu K, et al. The ankle brachial index is associated with leg function and physical activity: the Walking and Leg Circulation Study. Ann Intern Med 2002;136:873–83.

[60] McDermott MM, Mehta S, Liu K, et al. Leg symptoms, the ankle-brachial index, and walking ability in patients with peripheral arterial disease. J Gen Intern Med 1999;14:173–81.

[61] McDermott MM, Liu K, Guralnik JM, et al. The ankle brachial index independently predicts walking velocity and walking endurance in peripheral arterial disease. J Am Geriatr Soc 1998;46:1355–62.

[62] McDermott MM, Fried L, Simonsick E, et al. Asymptomatic peripheral arterial disease is independently associated with impaired lower extremity functioning: the Women's Health and Aging Study. Circulation 2000;101:1007–12.

[63] Arseven A, Guralnik JM, O'Brien E, et al. Peripheral arterial disease and depressed mood in older men and women. Vasc Med 2001;6:229–34.

[64] McDermott MM, Greenland P, Guralnik JM, et al. Depressive symptoms and lower extremity functioning in men and women with peripheral arterial disease. J Gen Intern Med 2003;18:461–7.

[65] Blake C, Codd MB, Cassidy A, et al. Physical function, employment and quality of life in end-stage renal disease. J Nephrol 2000;13:142–9.

[66] Johansen KL, Chertow GM, da Silva M, et al. Determinants of physical performance in ambulatory patients on hemodialysis. Kidney Int 2001;60:1586–91.

[67] Mittal SK, Ahern L, Flaster E, et al. Self-assessed physical and mental function of haemodialysis patients. Nephrol Dial Transplant 2001;16:1387–94.

[68] Watnick S, Kirwin P, Mahnensmith R, et al. The prevalence and treatment of depression among patients starting dialysis. Am J Kidney Dis 2003;41:105–10.

[69] Sacks FM, Pfeffer MA, Moye LA, et al. The effect of pravastatin on coronary events after myocardial infarction in patients with average cholesterol levels. Cholesterol and Recurrent Events Trial investigators. N Engl J Med 1996;335:1001–9.

[70] Pedersen TR, Kjekshus J, Pyorala K, et al. Effect of simvastatin on ischemic signs and symptoms in the Scandinavian Simvastatin Survival Study (4S). Am J Cardiol 1998;81:333–5.

[71] Hirsch AT, Gotto AM Jr. Undertreatment of dyslipidemia in peripheral arterial disease and other high-risk populations: an opportunity for cardiovascular disease reduction. Vasc Med 2002;7:323–31.

[72] Collins R, Armitage J, Parish S, et al. MRC/BHF Heart Protection Study of cholesterol-lowering with simvastatin in 5963 people with diabetes:

a randomised placebo-controlled trial. Lancet 2003;361:2005–16.

[73] MRC/BHF Heart Protection Study of cholesterol lowering with simvastatin in 20,536 high-risk individuals: a randomised placebo-controlled trial. Lancet 2002;360:7–22.

[74] Mohler ER III, Hiatt WR, Creager MA. Cholesterol reduction with atorvastatin improves walking distance in patients with peripheral arterial disease. Circulation 2003;108:1481–6.

[75] McDermott MM, Guralnik JM, Greenland P, et al. Statin use and leg functioning in patients with and without lower-extremity peripheral arterial disease. Circulation 2003;107:757–61.

[76] Henke PK, Blackburn S, Proctor MC, et al. Patients undergoing infrainguinal bypass to treat atherosclerotic vascular disease are underprescribed cardioprotective medications: effect on graft patency, limb salvage, and mortality. J Vasc Surg 2004;39:357–65.

[77] Liu Y, Coresh J, Eustace JA, et al. Association between cholesterol level and mortality in dialysis patients: role of inflammation and malnutrition. JAMA 2004;291:451–9.

[78] Kalantar-Zadeh K, Block G, Humphreys MH, et al. Reverse epidemiology of cardiovascular risk factors in maintenance dialysis patients. Kidney Int 2003;63:793–808.

[79] Seliger SL, Weiss NS, Gillen DL, et al. HMG-CoA reductase inhibitors are associated with reduced mortality in ESRD patients. Kidney Int 2002;61:297–304.

[80] Tonelli M, Moye L, Sacks FM, et al. Pravastatin for secondary prevention of cardiovascular events in persons with mild chronic renal insufficiency. Ann Intern Med 2003;138:98–104.

[81] Mehler PS, Coll JR, Estacio R, et al. Intensive blood pressure control reduces the risk of cardiovascular events in patients with peripheral arterial disease and type 2 diabetes. Circulation 2003;107:753–6.

[82] Ostergren J, Sleight P, Dagenais G, et al. Impact of ramipril in patients with evidence of clinical or subclinical peripheral arterial disease. Eur Heart J 2004;25:17–24.

[83] Mann JF, Gerstein HC, Pogue J, et al. Renal insufficiency as a predictor of cardiovascular outcomes and the impact of ramipril: the HOPE randomized trial. Ann Intern Med 2001;134:629–36.

[84] Newman AB, Siscovick DS, Manolio TA, et al. Ankle-arm index as a marker of atherosclerosis in the Cardiovascular Health Study. Cardiovascular Heart Study (CHS) Collaborative Research Group. Circulation 1993;88:837–45.

[85] Juergens JL, Barker NW, Hines EA Jr. Arteriosclerosis obliterans: review of 520 cases with special reference to pathogenic and prognostic factors. Circulation 1960;21:188–95.

[86] Myers KA, King RB, Scott DF, et al. The effect of smoking on the late patency of arterial reconstructions in the legs. Br J Surg 1978;65:267–71.

[87] Quick CR, Cotton LT. The measured effect of stopping smoking on intermittent claudication. Br J Surg 1982;69(Suppl):S24–6.

[88] O'Hare AM, Feinglass J, Sidawy AN, et al. Impact of renal insufficiency on short-term morbidity and mortality after lower extremity revascularization: data from the Department of Veterans Affairs' National Surgical Quality Improvement Program. J Am Soc Nephrol 2003;14:1287–95.

[89] O'Hare AM, Sidawy AN, Feinglass J, et al. Influence of renal insufficiency on limb loss and mortality after initial lower extremity surgical revascularization. J Vasc Surg 2004;39:709–16.

[90] Collaborative meta-analysis of randomised trials of antiplatelet therapy for prevention of death, myocardial infarction, and stroke in high risk patients. BMJ 2002;324:71–86.

[91] A randomised, blinded, trial of clopidogrel versus aspirin in patients at risk of ischaemic events (CAPRIE). CAPRIE Steering Committee. Lancet 1996;348:1329–39.

[92] Beebe HG, Dawson DL, Cutler BS, et al. A new pharmacological treatment for intermittent claudication: results of a randomized, multicenter trial. Arch Intern Med 1999;159:2041–50.

[93] Money SR, Herd JA, Isaacsohn JL, et al. Effect of cilostazol on walking distances in patients with intermittent claudication caused by peripheral vascular disease. J Vasc Surg 1998;27:267–74.

[94] Dawson DL, Cutler BS, Meissner MH, et al. Cilostazol has beneficial effects in treatment of intermittent claudication: results from a multicenter, randomized, prospective, double-blind trial. Circulation 1998;98:678–86.

[95] Stewart KJ, Hiatt WR, Regensteiner JG, et al. Exercise training for claudication. N Engl J Med 2002;347:1941–51.

[96] Gardner AW, Poehlman ET. Exercise rehabilitation programs for the treatment of claudication pain. A meta-analysis. JAMA 1995;274:975–80.

[97] Johansen KL, Chertow GM, Ng AV, et al. Physical activity levels in patients on hemodialysis and healthy sedentary controls. Kidney Int 2000;57:2564–70.

[98] Johansen KL, Sakkas GK, Doyle J, et al. Exercise counseling practices among nephrologists caring for patients on dialysis. Am J Kidney Dis 2003;41:171–8.

[99] Harrington EB, Harrington ME, Schanzer H, et al. End-stage renal disease—is infrainguinal limb revascularization justified? J Vasc Surg 1990;12:691–5.

[100] Johnson BL, Glickman MH, Bandyk DF, et al. Failure of foot salvage in patients with end-stage renal disease after surgical revascularization. J Vasc Surg 1995;22:280–5.

[101] Korn P, Hoenig SJ, Skillman JJ, et al. Is lower extremity revascularization worthwhile in patients with end-stage renal disease? Surgery 2000;128: 472–9.

[102] Lantis JC, Conte MS, Belkin M, et al. Infrainguinal bypass grafting in patients with end-stage renal disease: improving outcomes? J Vasc Surg 2001;33: 1171–8.

[103] Lumsden AB, Besman A, Jaffe M, et al. Infrainguinal revascularization in end-stage renal disease. Ann Vasc Surg 1994;8:107–12.

[104] Wassermann RJ, Saroyan RM, Rice JC, et al. Infrainguinal revascularization for limb salvage in patients with end-stage renal disease. South Med J 1991;84:190–2.

[105] Whittemore AD, Donaldson MC, Mannick JA. Infrainguinal reconstruction for patients with chronic renal insufficiency. J Vasc Surg 1993;17: 32–9.

[106] Eggers PW, Gohdes D, Pugh J. Nontraumaticlower extremity amputations in the Medicare end-stage renal disease population. Kidney Int 1999;56:1524–33.

[107] Dossa CD, Shepard AD, Amos AM, et al. Results of lower extremity amputations in patients with end-stage renal disease. J Vasc Surg 1994;20:14–9.

[108] McMurray SD, Johnson G, Davis S, et al. Diabetes education and care management significantly improve patient outcomes in the dialysis unit. Am J Kidney Dis 2002;40:566–75.

[109] McMurray SD, McDougall K. Improving diabetes foot care in the dialysis facility. Nephrol News Issues 2003;17:566–75.

[110] O'Hare AM, Feinglass J, Reiber GE, et al. Postoperative mortality after nontraumatic lower extremity amputation in patients with renal insufficiency. J Am Soc Nephrol 2004;15:427–34.

[111] Reddan DN, Marcus RJ, Owen WF Jr. Long-term outcomes of revascularization for peripheral vascular disease in end-stage renal disease patients. Am J Kidney Dis 2001;38:57–63.

[112] Collins TC, Johnson M, Henderson W, et al. Lower extremity nontraumatic amputation among veterans with peripheral arterial disease: is race an independent factor? Med Care 2002;40:I106–16.

[113] Abou-Zamzam AMJ, Teruya TH, Killeen JD, et al. Major lower extremity amputation in an academic vascular center. Ann Vasc Surg 2003; 17:86–90.

CARDIOLOGY CLINICS

Cardiol Clin 23 (2005) 237–248

Hypertension in Chronic Kidney Disease and Dialysis: Pathophysiology and Management

Rajiv Agarwal, MD[a,b,]*

[a]*Division of Nephrology, Department of Medicine, Emerson Hall Room 520, Indiana University School of Medicine, 1481 West 10th Street, Indianapolis, IN 46202, USA*
[b]*Roudebush VA Medical Center, 1481 West 10th Street 111 N, Indianapolis, IN 46202, USA*

Hypertension affects 24% of the adult United States population [1]. In the United States, 3% of the adult population has an elevated serum creatinine level, and 70% of these patients have hypertension [2]. The prevalence of hypertension in chronic kidney disease (CKD) depends on the patient's age and the severity of renal failure, proteinuria, and underlying renal disease [3]. As patients with CKD progress to end-stage renal disease (ESRD), 86% are diagnosed with hypertension [4]. It has long been recognized that kidney function affects and is affected by hypertension. This article discusses the pathophysiology and management of hypertension in patients with CKD.

Pathophysiology of hypertension

Sodium and water

It has been recognized for at least 50 years that increasing sodium intake leads to a variable but consistent increase in blood pressure in animals. Dahl et al [5] thought this heterogeneity in response resulted from the interaction between genetic and environmental factors and that by ingenious inbreeding experiments in Sprague-Dawley rats fed a high-sodium diet, within three generations they could create colonies that were hypertensive. The

predisposed animals did not develop increased blood pressure when fed a sodium-poor diet, but a sodium-rich diet caused an elevation in blood pressure in the sodium-sensitive animals. This finding confirmed the importance of the interaction between sodium intake and genetic predisposition in causing hypertension.

The most definitive experiments investigating the significance of sodium in hypertension in primates were performed over a span of 2.5 years in chimpanzees fed a high-sodium diet [6]. Chimpanzees, who typically consume a vegetarian, potassium-rich, sodium-poor diet, were fed a diet that was gradually supplemented with dietary sodium to a level of 15 g/d that was sustained over 16 months. At the end of supplementation period, blood pressure had increased by 10/33 mm Hg together with suppression of plasma renin activity. Within 20 weeks after sodium supplementation was stopped, blood pressure returned to baseline.

Human data support the findings in animals. In primitive societies, such as the New Guinea Highlanders, Yanomamo Indians in Amazon rain forest [7], Bushmen in the Kalahari, or Kenyan tribal farmers, sodium content in the diet is extremely low (1–10 mEq/d). Hypertension and age-related increase in blood pressure is not seen in these populations. In contrast, the mean dietary intake of sodium in Akita, Japan, is 450 mEq/d (26 g/d) and a high incidence of hypertension and strokes is seen. Furthermore, the increase in dietary sodium intake that occurs when members of primitive societies move to an urban area is associated with rapid increase in blood pressure.

Guyton et al [8] studied the hemodynamic basis of the development of hypertension in

Dr. Agarwal's work is supported by a research award from the National Institutes of Health (NIDDK 5 RO1- 062030-02).

* Division of Nephrology, Department of Medicine, Emerson Hall Room 520, Indiana University School of Medicine, 545 Barnhill Drive, Indianapolis, IN 46202.

E-mail address: ragarwal@iupui.edu

response to volume overload. Guyton's group studied the time course of change in cardiac output and vascular resistance in dogs after removing 40% of one kidney and infusing isotonic saline for 13 days. During the first 3 days of saline administration, blood pressures increased together with a rise in cardiac output, but peripheral vascular resistance fell. Subsequently, cardiac output dropped, but peripheral vascular resistance increased and resulted in hypertension. These results were explained by an increase in blood volume, an increase in mean circulatory filling pressure, and a higher cardiac output at the initial stages of volume expansion. These effects were followed by autoregulatory vasoconstriction that resulted in increased peripheral vascular resistance. Perfusion of kidneys at higher pressures caused pressure natriuresis and restoration of cardiac output. Because of persistently elevated peripheral vascular resistance, hypertension was sustained even after the reduction in cardiac output [8,9].

It is increasingly being recognized that sodium has an important influence on vascular endothelial and adventitial function. For example, cultured vascular smooth muscle cells undergo hypertrophy when exposed to high concentrations of sodium chloride [10]. In Dahl salt-resistant rats, a high-sodium diet induced hypertrophy of the arterial wall and increased mortality compared with a normal-sodium diet, independent of hypertension [11]. Increased sodium intake impairs nitric oxide (NO) bioavailability and induces oxidative stress. Furthermore, increased sodium intake accelerates vascular production of angiotensin II despite reduction in plasma renin activity, suggesting that angiotensin II production in blood vessels is independent of plasma renin activity [12]. Finally, increased dietary sodium can increase the release of sodium-pump ligands that inhibit the sodium pump on cell membranes (eg, digoxin) and increase smooth muscle tone. Reducing dietary sodium to less than 60 mmol/d increases arterial compliance and reduces arterial stiffness within 1 to 2 weeks, with a concomitant reduction of 6 mm Hg in systolic ambulatory blood pressure [13]. It is clear that sodium has an effect on blood pressure and cardiac responses above and beyond its effect on plasma volume and hemodynamic responses.

The renin–angiotensin system

In addition to the hemodynamic actions of angiotensin II that include vasoconstriction,

sympathetic activation, and sodium retention, other nonhemodynamic effects are well recognized. These effects include endothelial, mesangial, and renal tubular activation and oxidative stress. Inflammation and fibrosis can occur with elevated levels of this angiotensin II in a variety of kidney diseases. For example, the activity of angiotensin-converting enzyme (ACE) can be higher in areas of renal injury than in noninjured areas [14]. The resultant overexpression of angiotensin II can lead to progressive renal damage and hypertension [15].

Oxidative stress

Reactive oxygen species, such as superoxide and hydrogen peroxide, are important signaling molecules. They participate in vascular smooth muscle cell growth and migration; modulation of endothelial function, including endothelium-dependent relaxation and expression of adhesion molecules, chemoattractant compounds, and cytokines rendering a proinflammatory phenotype; and modification of the extracellular matrix.

Haugen et al [16] examined three models to assess the direct effect of angiotensin II on the structure and function of the kidney by oxidative stress. In the first model, angiotensin II was administered using mini-osmotic pumps to rats maintained on standard diets. Oxidative stress and hypertension were observed. In the second model, rats were made hypertensive with deoxycorticosterone acetate and salt, but they were not given angiotensin II. In this model, suppression of the renin–angiotensin system would be expected, and hypertension without oxidative stress was noted. In the third model, rats maintained on antioxidant-deficient diets were studied while infused with angiotensin II. Proteinuria and decreased creatinine clearance were noted in addition to oxidative stress and hypertension. Others have demonstrated that rats with renin-mediated hypertension have AT1 receptor–mediated endothelial dysfunction associated with increased oxidative stress and increased vascular xanthine oxidase activity [17]. In contrast, knockout mice that are genetically deficient in gp91(phox), a nicotinamide adenine dinucleotide phosphate (NADPH) oxidase subunit protein, show lower baseline blood pressures and demonstrate less oxidative stress–mediated vascular injury in response to angiotensin II [18]. Nishiyama et al [19] have demonstrated that the effect of angiotensin II in elevating blood pressure is partly caused by inactivation of NO through the generation of oxygen-derived free radicals. In humans with CKD, the author and colleagues have found that blockade of the renin–angiotensin system can reduce oxidative stress [20] and profibrotic cytokines [21] independent of the reduction in proteinuria or blood pressure [22].

Taken together, these experiments offer direct evidence that angiotensin II induces oxidative stress in vivo, which contributes to renal injury. This injury seems to be predominantly localized to the renal proximal tubules. The NADPH oxidase–derived superoxide anion seems to be important for the regulation of basal blood pressure as well as in the pathogenesis of hypertension. Furthermore, these studies reveal a pressure-independent vascular hypertrophic response to angiotensin II and suggest that oxidative stress is causally important in the genesis of renal parenchymal hypertension.

Nitric oxide and circulating inhibitors of nitric oxide

Endothelial derived NO plays a critical role in the maintenance and regulation of vascular tone and modulates key processes mediating vascular disease including leukocyte adhesion, platelet aggregation, and vascular smooth muscle proliferation [23]. Endothelial NO synthase enzymatically produces NO from the substrate L-arginine. NO vasodilates the vasculature through activation of guanylate cyclase, which subsequently produces cyclic guanosine monophosphate (c-GMP) [24]. c-GMP activates a protein kinase enzyme that phosphorylates and activates a calcium-dependent potassium channel, leading to potassium efflux and vasodilation [25]. In hypertensive patients, this mechanism has been found to be defective [26–28]. Also, L-arginine supplementation can partially reverse renal failure–associated endothelial dysfunction [29]. Reactive oxygen species can impair the activity of NO. Superoxide quenches NO to produce peroxynitnitrite, which is devoid of vasodilating activity [30].

A circulating inhibitor of NO synthase, asymmetrical dimethyl arginine (ADMA), competes with L-arginine for NO synthase. In humans with salt-sensitive hypertension, a high-salt diet increases plasma ADMA and blood pressure [31]. Circulating ADMA is increased in persons with CKD [32] and ESRD [33] and may contribute to endothelial dysfunction and increased blood pressure. In patients with ESRD, ADMA is correlated with increased left ventricular thickness and reduced ejection fraction, consistent with its ability to increase systemic vascular resistance [34].

Of the 300 μmol/d ADMA normally generated, the kidneys in healthy volunteers excrete only 50 μmol/d. The remaining amount is degraded enzymatically by dimethylarginine dimethylaminohydrolase (DDAH) [35]. Pharmacologic inhibition of DDAH causes accumulation of ADMA and generalized vasoconstriction. In contrast, overexpression of DDAH reduces ADMA, improves NO bioavailability, and reduces systolic blood pressure. Oxidative stress that impairs DDAH activity by oxidizing a sulfhydryl moiety critical for its enzymatic activity leads to accumulation of ADMA and promotes endothelial dysfunction. The inflammation, increased homocysteine levels, reduced antioxidant defenses, and increased free radicals in ESRD therefore may explain the relationship between oxidative stress, endothelial dysfunction, and the generation of hypertension [33].

The sympathetic nervous system

Strong evidence has emerged that implicates enhanced sympathetic activity as a cause of hypertension in patients with CKD and ESRD [36]. Microvascular and tubulointerstitial damage induced by repeated injections of phenylephrine in animals leads to the development of sodium-sensitive hypertension [37]. On the other hand, there is also ample evidence that the sympathetic nervous system is activated in CKD. Diminished vascular response to norepinephrine in animal models of chronic renal failure provided initial indirect evidence of increased sympathetic nerve activity that decreased the expression of adrenergic receptors [38]. Later studies provided more direct evidence of elevated sympathetic tone in patients with ESRD [36] by direct measurement of efferent sympathetic nerve activity [39]. Using microneurography, investigators have demonstrated that the sympathetic activity is increased in patients receiving chronic hemodialysis who still have their native kidneys. In contrast, patients with bilateral nephrectomy have reduced sympathetic activity, lower vascular resistance in the calf, and lower mean arterial pressure [36]. Thus, the kidney, even when devoid of excretory function, serves as an afferent organ to signal the midbrain region to increase sympathetic activity. The central mechanisms of increased sympathetic activity may involve dopaminergic neuronal transmission. Experiments in hypertensive hemodialysis patients show that administration of the dopamine-releasing drug bromocriptine decreased plasma norepinephrine and lowered mean arterial pressure [40]. In animals with chronic renal failure, norepinephrine turnover rate is increased in the posterior hypothalamic nuclei, and endogenous NO may be an important regulator of sympathetic activity [41]. NO inactivation in the central nervous system by an arginine analogue resulted in higher blood pressures and increased renal sympathetic nerve activity in rabbits [42]. Baroreceptor desensitization has also long been recognized in hypertensive patients with ESRD and may contribute to elevated blood pressure [43].

Drugs and toxins

Erythropoietin

Erythropoietin (EPO) can cause hypertension in approximately 20% of patients. Originally, EPO-induced hypertension was attributed to the rise in hematocrit and blood viscosity that occurred with treatment [44,45]. In both animal and human studies, however, results have consistently shown that the rise in blood pressure with EPO administration is independent of hematocrit [46–49]. For example, Vaziri et al [50] have shown that if EPO is administered to anemic animals with chronic renal failure, but hemoglobin is kept stable by feeding these animals an iron-deficient diet, hypertension still occurs. In blood vessels harvested from these animals, vasodilatory responses to NO donors were impaired, but response to several vasoconstrictors was normal.

Vascular smooth muscle cells use intracellular calcium to initiate vasoconstriction [51]. Platelet cytosolic calcium concentrations have been shown to correlate with vascular smooth muscle cytosolic calcium concentrations and blood pressure [52]. Thus, platelet cytosolic calcium serves as a surrogate for smooth muscle calcium concentration. In this context, EPO increases platelet cytosolic calcium in animals [50] as well as in hypertensive patients [53]. EPO can activate calcium channels through tyrosine kinase [54]. Felodipine, a calcium-channel blocker, lowered platelet cytosolic calcium concentrations and blood pressures in rats treated with EPO [55].

Lead

Low-level lead exposure is associated with impaired renal function [56] and hypertension [57–60]. Oxidative stress and impaired endothelial vasodilation seem to be important in the mechanism of lead-induced hypertension. Lead-exposed rats had hypertension and biomarkers of oxidative stress that improved with the administration of an antioxidant [61]. Similarly, tempol, an antioxidant that reduces superoxide levels, lowered blood pressures in lead-exposed rats while having no effect in the control rats [62]. Finally, lead-exposed rats, in addition to having hypertension, have reduced endothelial guanylate cyclase expression, suggesting endothelial dysfunction [63].

Cocaine

Cocaine, blocks the uptake of catecholamines in presynaptic sympathetic nerves [64], leading to peripheral vasoconstriction and elevated blood pressure. Cocaine infusions in laboratory rats raised blood pressure in a biphasic manner: after a rapid initial increase in blood pressure, a more sustained response ensued. The blood pressure–raising effect of cocaine is caused, at least in part, by its ability to impair endothelial function [65].

Cyclosporine

Cyclosporine, a calcineurin immunosuppressive agent, causes afferent arteriolar vasoconstriction and tubulointerstitial fibrosis [66] that can lead to hypertension and a reduced glomerular filtration rate. Reduced NO bioavailability may play a primary role in the pathogenesis of cyclosporine's toxicity. In vitro, cyclosporine increases the production of reactive oxygen species, primarily superoxide and hydrogen peroxide, that can be reduced by free radical scavengers [67]. Administration of cyclosporine to laboratory rats increased angiotensin II superoxide levels and blood pressure [68]. Nephrotoxicity of cyclosporine can be abrogated in laboratory rats by antioxidant therapy [69].

Nonsteroidal anti-inflammatory drugs

Prostaglandins promote vasodilation and enhance natriuresis [70]. Nonsteroidal anti-inflammatory drugs (NSAIDs) block the synthesis of prostaglandins and lead to an elevation in blood pressure of about 5 mm Hg [70,71]. Elderly persons, hypertensive persons, and those with CKD carry an increased risk of developing hypertension when taking NSAIDs. Aspirin and sulindac seem to have the least effect on increasing blood pressure [71]. Increased vascular resistance and expanded extracellular volume have both been associated with the genesis of NSAID-induced hypertension. Like NSAIDS, the coxcibs can also increase blood pressure and cause renal injury [72,73].

The pathophysiology of hypertension and CKD can be summarized as follows. Renal injury occurs from a variety of reasons that include hypertension, diabetes mellitus, immunologic diseases, and drugs and toxins. The underlying abnormalities in a variety of kidney diseases include activation of the renin-angiotensin-aldosterone axis and the sympathetic nervous system. Some of these factors (eg, the renin–angiotensin system, sympathetic system, and cocaine use) can by themselves aggravate hypertension. Many of these processes are accompanied by tubulointerstitial disease. Tubulointerstitial inflammation results in the release of oxidants by the invading inflammatory cells, the inactivation of local NO, and the heterogeneous activation of the intrarenal renin–angiotensin system. Tubular and vascular barotrauma, characterized by afferent arteriolopathy, leads to a right-shifted pressure–natriuresis curve. This response relieves the renal ischemia but does so at the expense of higher blood pressure, leading to the development of hypertension that causes further renal injury. Dietary sodium excess, by inactivating DDAH, can reduce NO activity, cause vascular smooth muscle hypertrophy, and further accelerate tubular and microcirculatory damage. Extracellular volume expansion by sodium overload can, by itself, aggravate hypertension. Renal inflammation and hypertension eventually lead to renal fibrosis, progressive CKD, and target-organ damage, including ESRD.

Management of hypertension in chronic kidney disease

Ascertaining the blood pressure level is the essential first step in treating hypertension but can be particularly problematic in patients receiving hemodialysis, who have large swings in blood pressure related to the dialysis treatment [74]. In such patients, home [75] and ambulatory blood pressure monitoring [76,77] can be of particular value.

Life-style modifications can improve blood pressure levels per se and can enhance the efficacy of antihypertensive therapies. Reducing sodium intake, increasing physical activity, losing weight, limiting alcohol intake, and smoking cessation are recommended strategies [78].

A meta-analysis of trials of sodium restriction in normotensive and hypertensive individuals concluded that a 50 mEq/d reduction in dietary sodium (which can be achieved simply by taking away table salt), would lead to a decrease in systolic blood pressure of 5 mm Hg on average and 7 mm Hg in those who are more hypertensive [79]. At least 5 weeks of sodium restriction would be required to see such an effect.

Systolic hypertension, not diastolic blood pressure, is the key treatment target [80]. Systolic hypertension is more prevalent than diastolic hypertension [81], and reduction of systolic blood pressure is associated with improved cardiovascular outcomes [82,83]. The recommended target blood pressure is less than 130/80 mm Hg in patients with CKD and less than 125/75 mm Hg in those with proteinuria in excess of 1 g/d [78]. To achieve these goals, multiple agents are required—on average, three to four per day [84]. It is obvious that more medications are required if blood pressure goals are more aggressive [85]. The guidelines set forth in the seventh report of the Joint National Committee on Prevention, Detection, Evaluation, and Treatment of High Blood Pressure recommend combination therapy if blood pressure is more than 20/10 mm Hg above goal [78]. Drug interactions should be monitored, especially with polypharmacy. NSAIDs, cyclooxygenase inhibitors, nasal decongestants, and amphetaminelike drugs can markedly worsen blood pressure control and should be avoided in patients with kidney disease [71]. Over time, the number of agents required to achieve the goal is likely to increase, so continual monitoring and titration are needed.

Hypertension in dialysis patients

Once a patient reaches end-stage renal disease and requires hemodialysis, a procedure that is typically performed three times per week, the sodium and water removed during the treatment must at least match the interdialysis gain of sodium and water. Furthermore, the absolute content of total body water and sodium must be at a level that does not cause signs and symptoms of volume overload, including hypertension, or signs and symptoms of sodium and water depletion, such as dizziness and hypotension. The assessment of total body water and sodium that is associated neither with volume overload nor with volume depletion is imperfect. The optimal level is called the dry weight.

Observational studies in dialysis patients show an association between large interdialysis weight gain and total mortality in patients with diabetes mellitus and poor nutritional status [86]. Foley et al [87] reported results from a historically prospective study of 11,142 patients receiving dialysis on December 31, 1993 randomly selected from the US Renal Data System Dialysis Morbidity and Mortality Study Waves 3 and 4. After accounting for multiple comorbid factors, they reported an interdialysis weight gain greater than 4.8% was associated with increased mortality. Dietary salt restriction, a strategy to limit interdialysis weight gain that is as old as dialysis itself, would, if practiced diligently, facilitate the achievement of dry weight. Like many other lifestyle modifications, however, it is not practiced widely [88]. Nevertheless, centers that have encouraged dietary salt restriction have been rewarded with less use of antihypertensives and better blood pressure control [89,90].

Another strategy to limit interdialysis weight gain and thirst is to lower the dialysate sodium concentration. Whereas increased dialysate sodium concentration increases interdialysis weight gain [91,92], the data supporting the reverse phenomenon are not as strong. Nevertheless, in one preliminary study, dialysate sodium was reduced at a rate of 1 mEq/L over 3 or 4 weeks, from 140 mEq/L to 135 mEq/L, in combination with a prescription sodium diet of less than 6 g/d [93]. Predialysis blood pressure improved from 147/88 mm Hg to 136/80 mm Hg (mean decrease in arterial pressure from 108 to 98 mm Hg; $P = 0.02$) without change in dry weight. Furthermore, four of the eight patients were able to stop using blood pressure medications completely. Others, in a study involving six hemodialysis patients, have not observed such an improvement [94]. In another study, sodium intakes of 15 dialysis patients were restricted so that their estimated dietary sodium intakes were reduced from 10 g/d to 7 g/d [95]. Dialysis parameters and dry body weight were kept constant. Predialysis blood pressure decreased with dietary salt restriction, from 139/79 to 132/75 mm Hg ($P < 0.01$ systolic; $P < 0.05$ diastolic), and mean arterial pressure was reduced from 99 to 94 mm Hg ($P < 0.01$). Interdialysis weight gain decreased with salt restriction from 2.3 ± 0.73 kg to 1.8 ± 0.52 kg ($P < 0.001$), whereas postdialysis weight did not change, (66.1 ± 11.9 kg to 66.1 ± 11.8 kg; not statistically significant). Clearly, these data need to be confirmed in adequately powered larger trials, but it seems that dietary sodium restriction may provide blood pressure lowering.

In another study, lowering the sodium concentration of the dialysate by individualizing dialysate prescriptions reduced thirst and interdialysis weight gain, improved hemodynamic stability, and reduced intradialysis symptoms [96]. In persons who were initially hypertensive, this strategy improved blood pressure control. In individuals with limited cardiovascular reserve relative to the ultrafiltration rates, a high sodium dialysate confers hemodynamic stability [91]. Lowering dialysate sodium may, at least theoretically, cause intradialysis hypotension; if the hypotension results in a limited ability to ultrafilter, lowering dialysate sodium may, paradoxically, increase blood pressure. Drug therapies for hypertension in hemodialysis patients are discussed elsewhere [97].

Choice of agent

In a meta-analysis of 15 studies to assess the impact of race on antihypertensive response, Sehgal et al [98] reported that for drug-associated changes in diastolic blood pressure, the mean difference between whites and blacks ranged from 0.6 to 3.0 mm Hg, whereas the SD within each race ranged from 5.0 to 10.1 mm Hg. On average, beta blockers and ACE inhibitors produced a greater reduction in blood pressure in white patients than in black patients (mean reduction in systolic blood pressure, 6 versus 4.6 mm Hg). In contrast, diuretics and calcium-channel blockers achieved greater mean reductions in black patients than in white patients (3.5 versus 2.4 mm Hg). In all the studies analyzed, however, the difference the size of the blood pressure reduction between white patients and black patients was smaller than the SD in each group. For example, the difference in systolic blood pressure between black and white patients after treatment with ACE inhibitors was 4.6 mm Hg, whereas the SD within each group was approximately 12 to 14 mm Hg. Thus, the small difference between whites and blacks in response to certain antihypertensives is dwarfed by the variation within each race. Furthermore, combination therapies such as diuretics plus ACE inhibitors or calcium-channel blockers plus ACE inhibitors nullify the effect of race. Thus, the choice of antihypertensive therapy should be an ACE inhibitor or angiotensin-receptor blocker in patients with kidney disease, regardless of race [85]. Water-soluble ACE inhibitors such as lisinopril and enalapril can be dosed less frequently because of their reduced renal clearance. In hemodialysis patients, postdialysis administration of lisinopril controls hypertension effectively [99].

In patients with a glomerular filtration rate below 30 mL/min, loop diuretics are effective in reducing blood pressure and have a synergistic response when used in combination with an ACE inhibitor, angiotensin-receptor blocker, or beta blocker. Torsemide and furosemide are equally effective in effecting natriuresis and reducing blood pressure, but torsemide has the advantage of once-daily administration [100]. Three to 4 weeks are required before maximal blood pressure reduction is achieved [101].

Water-soluble beta blockers such as atenolol should be reduced in dose and titrated to heart rate. They can accumulate with progressive renal failure, but atenolol given after hemodialysis three times per week effectively controls hypertension [102]. Some studies suggest that nondihydropyridine calcium-channel blockers can have incremental reduction in proteinuria compared with dihydropyridine calcium-channel blockers [103,104]. Direct vasodilators [105] and centrally acting agents [106] are commonly used and are effective in reducing blood pressure. Short-acting vasodilators should be avoided to prevent large swings in blood pressure and sympathetic activation.

In proteinuric patients, combination therapy with ACE inhibitors and angiotensin-receptor blockers can have incremental reduction in proteinuria [107], oxidative stress [20], and urinary excretion of fibrogenic cytokines [21], but definitive studies to support their use in preventing progression of renal disease have not yet been performed. Hyperkalemia and renal failure are potential complications of such combination therapies [108]. Antihypertensive medications are frequently titrated to achieve reduction in proteinuria. Although post hoc analyses of randomized, controlled trials find an association between reduction in proteinuria and reduction in cardiorenal end points [109], a cause-and-effect relationship remains to be firmly established. Other cardioprotective therapies such as aspirin and statins should be considered for cardiorenal protection in this high-risk population [110].

Reverse epidemiology of hypertension in hemodialysis?

High blood pressure has a continuous, graded, and etiologically significant relationship with cardiovascular outcomes in the general population [78], but studies in hemodialysis patients have found an inverse relationship between high blood

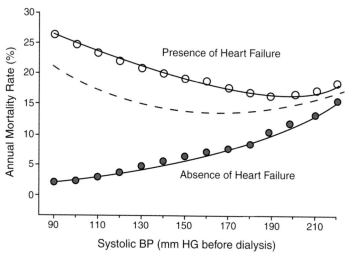

Fig 1. Impact of confounding variables influencing the relationship between hypertension and mortality: consideration of confounding variables, such as heart failure, can help explain the U-shaped relationship between blood pressure and total mortality (*dotted line*) seen in some studies. Well-controlled blood pressure in the presence of poor cardiac function is likely to be associated with high cardiovascular mortality (*open circles, upper line*). In contrast, poorly controlled blood pressure with intact cardiac function is expected to be associated with increased mortality (*solid circles, lower line*). If patients with impaired cardiac function constitute a large part of an observational cohort, a U-shaped relationship between blood pressure and total mortality is seen (*dotted line*). (*From* Agarwal R. Exploring the paradoxical relationship of hypertension with mortality in chronic hemodialysis. Hemodialysis Int 2004;8:208.)

pressure and outcomes [111,112]. Thus, patients with high blood pressures have a lower mortality than those with low blood pressures. It is intellectually troublesome to find such an association, because high blood pressure, which was such an important risk factor for cardiovascular disease before onset of dialysis, suddenly becomes a protective factor. Clinicians strive to lower blood pressure more aggressively in patients with chronic kidney disease who are not yet receiving hemodialysis than in patients with uncomplicated essential hypertension. If the observation of reverse epidemiology is etiologically significant, is treating high blood pressure in hemodialysis patients a wise practice?

Analyzing a prognostic value of blood pressure in observational cohort studies requires consideration of various other factors. One factor that is often ignored in considering hypertension as a prognostic variable in dialysis patients is reverse causation. Reverse causation means that the dependent process has a direct or indirect effect on the independent predictor. Fig. 1 shows the hypothesized relationship between hypertension and mortality when a confounding variable is considered [113]. Long-standing, poorly controlled hypertension may lead to heart failure, which may lower blood pressure, an example of reverse causation. If the confounding variable of heart failure is not considered, the conclusion that lower blood pressure is damaging would be inappropriate.

Thus, the author believes that, in hemodialysis patients, hypertension should be considered in the context of cardiovascular function and other parameters that modify blood pressure. In those who are otherwise healthy, complacence about high blood pressure would be inappropriate.

References

[1] Burt VL, Whelton P, Roccella EJ, et al. Prevalence of hypertension in the US adult population. Results from the Third National Health and Nutrition Examination Survey, 1988–1991. Hypertension 1995; 25:305–13.

[2] Coresh J, Wei GL, McQuillan G, et al. Prevalence of high blood pressure and elevated serum creatinine level in the United States: findings from the third National Health and Nutrition Examination Survey (1988–1994). Arch Intern Med 2001;161: 1207–16.

[3] Ridao N, Luno J, Garcia D, et al. Prevalence of hypertension in renal disease. Nephrol Dial Transplant 2001;16(Suppl 1):70–3.

[4] Agarwal R, Nissenson AR, Batlle D, et al. Prevalence, treatment, and control of hypertension in chronic hemodialysis patients in the United States. Am J Med 2003;115:291–7.

[5] Dahl LK, Heine M, Tassinari L. Effects of chronic excess salt ingestion. Evidence that genetic factors play an important role in susceptibility to experimental hypertension. J Exp Med 1962;115:1173–90.

[6] Denton D, Weisinger R, Mundy NI, et al. The effect of increased salt intake on blood pressure of chimpanzees. Nat Med 1995;1:1009–16.

[7] Oliver WJ, Cohen EL, Neel JV. Blood pressure, sodium intake, and sodium related hormones in the Yanomamo Indians, a "no-salt" culture. Circulation 1975;52:146–51.

[8] Guyton AC, Coleman TG, Cowley AV Jr, et al. Arterial pressure regulation. Overriding dominance of the kidneys in long-term regulation and in hypertension. Am J Med 1972;52(5):584–94.

[9] Coleman TG, Guyton AC. Hypertension caused by salt loading in the dog. 3. Onset transients of cardiac output and other circulatory variables. Circ Res 1969;25(2):153–60.

[10] Gu JW, Anand V, Shek EW, et al. Sodium induces hypertrophy of cultured myocardial myoblasts and vascular smooth muscle cells. Hypertension 1998; 31:1083–7.

[11] Tobian L, Hanlon S. High sodium chloride diets injure arteries and raise mortality without changing blood pressure. Hypertension 1990;15:900–3.

[12] Boddi M, Poggesi L, Coppo M, et al. Human vascular renin-angiotensin system and its functional changes in relation to different sodium intakes. Hypertension 1998;31:836–42.

[13] Gates PE, Tanaka H, Hiatt WR, et al. Dietary sodium restriction rapidly improves large elastic artery compliance in older adults with systolic hypertension. Hypertension 2004;44:35–41.

[14] Rosenberg ME, Smith LJ, Correa-Rotter R, et al. The paradox of the renin-angiotensin system in chronic renal disease. Kidney Int 1994;45: 403–10.

[15] Johnson RJ, Alpers CE, Yoshimura A, et al. Renal injury from angiotensin II-mediated hypertension. Hypertension 1992;19:464–74.

[16] Haugen EN, Croatt AJ, Nath KA. Angiotensin II induces renal oxidant stress in vivo and heme oxygenase-1 in vivo and in vitro. Kidney Int 2000;58: 144–52.

[17] Mervaala EM, Cheng ZJ, Tikkanen I, et al. Endothelial dysfunction and xanthine oxidoreductase activity in rats with human renin and angiotensinogen genes. Hypertension 2001;37: 414–8.

[18] Wang HD, Xu S, Johns DG, et al. Role of NADPH oxidase in the vascular hypertrophic and oxidative stress response to angiotensin II in mice. Circ Res 2001;88:947–53.

[19] Nishiyama A, Fukui T, Fujisawa Y, et al. Systemic and regional hemodynamic responses to tempol in angiotensin II–infused hypertensive rats. Hypertension 2001;37:77–83.

[20] Agarwal R. Proinflammatory effects of oxidative stress in chronic kidney disease: role of additional angiotensin II blockade. Am J Physiol Renal Physiol 2003;284:F863–9.

[21] Agarwal R, Siva S, Dunn SR, et al. Add-on angiotensin II receptor blockade lowers urinary transforming growth factor-beta levels. Am J Kidney Dis 2002;39:486–92.

[22] Agarwal R. Role of add-on angiotensin receptor blockade with maximized ACE inhibition. Kidney Int 2001;59:2282–9.

[23] Fuchgott RF. The discovery of endothelium-derived relaxing factor and its importance in the identification of nitric oxide. JAMA 1996;276:1186–8.

[24] Moro MA, Russel RJ, Cellek S, et al. cGMP mediates the vascular and platelet actions of nitric oxide: confirmation using an inhibitor of the soluble guanylyl cyclase. Proc Natl Acad Sci U S A 1996;93:1480–5.

[25] Archer SL, Huang JM, Hampl V, et al. Nitric oxide and cGMP cause vasorelaxation by activation of a charybdotoxin-sensitive K channel by cGMP-dependent protein kinase. Proc Natl Acad Sci U S A 1994;91:7583–7.

[26] Higashi Y, Sasaki S, Nakagawa K, et al. Endothelial function and oxidative stress in renovascular hypertension. N Engl J Med 2002;346:1954–62.

[27] Panza JA, Casino PR, Kilcoyne CM, et al. Role of endothelium-derived nitric oxide in the abnormal endothelium-dependent vascular relaxation of patients with essential hypertension. Circulation 1993;87:1468–74.

[28] Panza JA, Quyyumi AA, Brush JE Jr, et al. Abnormal endothelium-dependent vascular relaxation in patients with essential hypertension. N Engl J Med 1990;323:22–7.

[29] Hand MF, Haynes WG, Webb DJ. Hemodialysis and L-arginine, but not D-arginine, correct renal failure-associated endothelial dysfunction. Kidney Int 1998;53:1068–77.

[30] Welch WJ, Tojo A, Wilcox CS. Roles of NO and oxygen radicals in tubuloglomerular feedback in SHR. Am J Physiol Renal Physiol 2000;278:F769–76.

[31] Fujiwara N, Osanai T, Kamada T, et al. Study on the relationship between plasma nitrite and nitrate level and salt sensitivity in human hypertension: modulation of nitric oxide synthesis by salt intake. Circulation 2000;101:856–61.

[32] Vallance P, Leone A, Calver A, et al. Accumulation of an endogenous inhibitor of nitric oxide synthesis in chronic renal failure. Lancet 1992;339:572–5.

[33] Mallamaci F, Tripepi G, Maas R, et al. Analysis of the relationship between norepinephrine and asymmetric dimethyl arginine levels among patients with end-stage renal disease. J Am Soc Nephrol 2004;15:435–41.

[34] Zoccali C, Mallamaci F, Maas R, et al. Left ventricular hypertrophy, cardiac remodeling and asymmetric dimethylarginine (ADMA) in hemodialysis patients. Kidney Int 2002;62:339–45.

[35] Cooke JP. Asymmetrical dimethylarginine: the uber marker? Circulation 2004;109:1813–8.

[36] Converse RL Jr, Jacobsen TN, Toto RD, et al. Sympathetic overactivity in patients with chronic renal failure. N Engl J Med 1992;327:1912–8.

[37] Johnson RJ, Gordon KL, Suga S, et al. Renal injury and salt-sensitive hypertension after exposure to catecholamines. Hypertension 1999;34:151–9.

[38] Rascher W, Schomig A, Kreye VA, et al. Diminished vascular response to noradrenaline in experimental chronic uremia. Kidney Int 1982;21:20–7.

[39] Wallin BG, Elam M. Insights from intraneural recordings of sympathetic nerve traffic in humans. News Physiol Sci 1994;9:203–7.

[40] Degli Esposti E, Sturani A, et al. Effect of bromocriptine treatment on prolactin, noradrenaline and blood pressure in hypertensive haemodialysis patients. Clin Sci (Colch) 1985;69:51–6.

[41] Ye S, Nosrati S, Campese VM. Nitric oxide (NO) modulates the neurogenic control of blood pressure in rats with chronic renal failure (CRF). J Clin Invest 1997;99:540–8.

[42] Hilton PJ, Lavender S, Roth Z, et al. Creatinine clearance in patients with proteinuria. Lancet 1969;2:1215–6.

[43] Lazaurs JM, Hampers CL, Lowrie EG, et al. Baroreceptor activity in normotensive and hypertensive uremic patients. Circulation 1973;47:1015–21.

[44] Raine AE. Hypertension, blood viscosity, and cardiovascular morbidity in renal failure: implications of erythropoietin therapy. Lancet 1988;1:97–100.

[45] Linde T, Sandhagen B, Danielson BG, et al. Impaired erythrocyte fluidity during treatment of renal anemia with erythropoietin. J Intern Med 1992;231:601–6.

[46] Muntzel M, Hannedouche T, Lacour B, et al. Erythropoietin increases blood pressure in normotensive and hypertensive rats. Nephron 1993;65:601–4.

[47] Schmieder RE, Langenfeld MR, Hilgers KF. Endogenous erythropoietin correlates with blood pressure in essential hypertension. Am J Kidney Dis 1997;29:376–82.

[48] Jones MA, Kingswood JC, Dallyn PE, et al. Changes in diurnal blood pressure variation and red cell and plasma volumes in patients with renal

failure who develop erythropoietin-induced hypertension. Clin Nephrol 1995;44:193–200.

[49] Kaupke CJ, Kim S, Vaziri ND. Effect of erythrocyte mass on arterial blood pressure in dialysis patients receiving maintenance erythropoietin therapy. J Am Soc Nephrol 1994;4:1874–8.

[50] Vaziri ND, Zhou XJ, Naqvi F, et al. Role of nitric oxide resistance in erythropoietin-induced hypertension in rats with chronic renal failure. Am J Physiol 1996;271:E113–22.

[51] Inscho EW, Cook AK, Mui V, et al. Calcium mobilization contributes to pressure-mediated afferent arteriolar vasoconstriction. Hypertension 1998;31:421–8.

[52] Erne P, Bolli P, Burgisser E, et al. Correlation of platelet calcium with blood pressure. Effect of antihypertensive therapy. N Engl J Med 1984;310:1084–8.

[53] Tepel M, Wischniowski H, Zidek W. Erythropoietin induced transmembrane calcium influx in essential hypertension. Life Sci 1992;51:161–7.

[54] Marrero MB, Venema RC, Ma H, et al. Erythropoietin receptor-operated Ca2 + channels: activation by phospholipase C-gamma 1. Kidney Int 1998;53:1259–68.

[55] Ni Z, Wang XQ, Vaziri ND. Nitric oxide metabolism in erythropoietin-induced hypertension: effect of calcium channel blockade. Hypertension 1998;32:724–9.

[56] Kim R, Rotnitsky A, Sparrow D, et al. A longitudinal study of low-level lead exposure and impairment of renal function. The Normative Aging Study. JAMA 1996;275:1177–81.

[57] Cheng Y, Schwartz J, Sparrow D, et al. Bone lead and blood lead levels in relation to baseline blood pressure and the prospective development of hypertension: the Normative Aging Study. Am J Epidemiol 2001;153:164–71.

[58] Glenn BS, Stewart WF, Links JM, et al. The longitudinal association of lead with blood pressure. Epidemiology 2003;14:30–6.

[59] Vupputuri S, He J, Muntner P, et al. Blood lead level is associated with elevated blood pressure in blacks. Hypertension 2003;41:463–8.

[60] Nash D, Magder L, Lustberg M, et al. Blood lead, blood pressure, and hypertension in perimenopausal and postmenopausal women. JAMA 2003;289:1523–32.

[61] Vaziri ND, Ding Y, Ni Z, et al. Altered nitric oxide metabolism and increased oxygen free radical activity in lead-induced hypertension: effect of lazaroid therapy. Kidney Int 1997;52:1042–6.

[62] Vaziri ND, Ding Y, Ni Z. Compensatory up-regulation of nitric-oxide synthase isoforms in lead-induced hypertension; reversal by a superoxide dismutase-mimetic drug. J Pharmacol Exp Ther 2001;298:679–85.

[63] Marques M, Millas I, Jimenez A, et al. Alteration of the soluble guanylate cyclase system in the vascular wall of lead-induced hypertension in rats. J Am Soc Nephrol 2001;12:2594–600.

[64] Williams RG, Kavanagh KM, Teo KK. Pathophysiology and treatment of cocaine toxicity: implications for the heart and cardiovascular system. Can J Cardiol 1996;12:1295–301.

[65] Mo W, Singh AK, Arruda JA, et al. Role of nitric oxide in cocaine-induced acute hypertension. Am J Hypertens 1998;11:708–14.

[66] Andoh TF, Bennett WM. Chronic cyclosporine nephrotoxicity. Curr Opin Nephrol Hypertens 1998;7:265–70.

[67] Lopez-Ongil S, Hernandez-Perera O, Navarro-Antolin J, et al. Role of reactive oxygen species in the signalling cascade of cyclosporine A-mediated up-regulation of eNOS in vascular endothelial cells. Br J Pharmacol 1998;124:447–54.

[68] Nishiyama A, Kobori H, Fukui T, et al. Role of angiotensin II and reactive oxygen species in cyclosporine A-dependent hypertension. Hypertension 2003;42:754–60.

[69] Andoh TF, Gardner MP, Bennett WM. Protective effects of dietary L-arginine supplementation on chronic cyclosporine nephrotoxicity. Transplantation 1997;64:1236–40.

[70] de Leeuw PW. Nonsteroidal anti-inflammatory drugs and hypertension. The risks in perspective. Drugs 1996;51:179–87.

[71] Johnson AG, Nguyen TV, Day RO. Do nonsteroidal anti-inflammatory drugs affect blood pressure? A meta-analysis. Ann Intern Med 1994;121:289–300.

[72] Harris RC Jr. Cyclooxygenase-2 inhibition and renal physiology. Am J Cardiol 2002;89:10D–7D.

[73] Eras J, Perazella MA. NSAIDs and the kidney revisited: are selective cyclooxygenase-2 inhibitors safe? Am J Med Sci 2001;321:181–90.

[74] Agarwal R. Assessment of blood pressure in hemodialysis patients. Semin Dial 2002;15:299–304.

[75] Agarwal R. Role of home blood pressure monitoring in hemodialysis patients. Am J Kidney Dis 1999;33:682–7.

[76] Peixoto AJ, Santos SF, Mendes RB, et al. Reproducibility of ambulatory blood pressure monitoring in hemodialysis patients. Am J Kidney Dis 2000;36:983–90.

[77] Agarwal R, Lewis RR. Prediction of hypertension in chronic hemodialysis patients. Kidney Int 2001;60:1982–9.

[78] Chobanian AV, Bakris GL, Black HR, et al. The seventh report of the Joint National Committee on Prevention, Detection, Evaluation, and Treatment of High Blood Pressure: the JNC 7 report. JAMA 2003;289:2560–72.

[79] Law MR, Frost CD, Wald NJ. By how much does dietary salt reduction lower blood pressure? III—

analysis of data from trials of salt reduction. BMJ 1991;302:819–24.

[80] Gabay C, Kushner I. Acute-phase proteins and other systemic responses to inflammation [published erratum appears in N Engl J Med 1999;340(17):1376]. N Engl J Med 1999;340:448–54.

[81] Franklin SS, Jacobs MJ, Wong ND, et al. Predominance of isolated systolic hypertension among middle-aged and elderly US hypertensives: analysis based on National Health and Nutrition Examination Survey (NHANES) III. Hypertension 2001;37:869–74.

[82] Benetos A, Thomas F, Bean K, et al. Prognostic value of systolic and diastolic blood pressure in treated hypertensive men. Arch Intern Med 2002;162:577–81.

[83] Kjeldsen SE, Dahlof B, Devereux RB, et al. Effects of losartan on cardiovascular morbidity and mortality in patients with isolated systolic hypertension and left ventricular hypertrophy: a Losartan Intervention for Endpoint Reduction (LIFE) substudy. JAMA 2002;288:1491–8.

[84] Brenner BM, Cooper ME, de Zeeuw D, et al. Effects of losartan on renal and cardiovascular outcomes in patients with type 2 diabetes and nephropathy. N Engl J Med 2001;345:861–9.

[85] Wright JT Jr, Bakris G, Greene T, et al. Effect of blood pressure lowering and antihypertensive drug class on progression of hypertensive kidney disease: results from the AASK trial. JAMA 2002;288:2421–31.

[86] Szczech LA, Reddan DN, Klassen PS, et al. Interactions between dialysis-related volume exposures, nutritional surrogates and mortality among ESRD patients. Nephrol Dial Transplant 2003;18:1585–91.

[87] Foley RN, Herzog CA, Collins AJ. Blood pressure and long-term mortality in United States hemodialysis patients: USRDS Waves 3 and 4 Study. Kidney Int 2002;62:1784–90.

[88] Shaldon S. Dietary salt restriction and drug-free treatment of hypertension in ESRD patients: a largely abandoned therapy. Nephrol Dial Transplant 2002;17:1163–5.

[89] Ozkahya M, Ok E, Cirit M, et al. Regression of left ventricular hypertrophy in haemodialysis patients by ultrafiltration and reduced salt intake without antihypertensive drugs. Nephrol Dial Transplant 1998;13:1489–93.

[90] Charra B. "Dry weight" in dialysis: the history of a concept. Nephrol Dial Transplant 1998;13:1882–5.

[91] Henrich WL, Woodard TD, McPhaul JJ Jr. The chronic efficacy and safety of high sodium dialysate: double-blind, crossover study. Am J Kidney Dis 1982;2:349–53.

[92] Oliver MJ, Edwards LJ, Churchill DN. Impact of sodium and ultrafiltration profiling on hemodialysis-related symptoms. J Am Soc Nephrol 2001;12:151–6.

[93] Krautzig S, Janssen U, Koch KM, et al. Dietary salt restriction and reduction of dialysate sodium to control hypertension in maintenance haemodialysis patients. Nephrol Dial Transplant 1998;13:552–3.

[94] Kooman JP, Hendriks EJ, van Den Sande FM, et al. Dialysate sodium concentration and blood pressure control in haemodialysis patients. Nephrol Dial Transplant 2000;15:554.

[95] Maduell F, Navarro V. Dietary salt intake and blood pressure control in haemodialysis patients. Nephrol Dial Transplant 2000;15:2063.

[96] de Paula FM, Peixoto AJ, Pinto LV, et al. Clinical consequences of an individualized dialysate sodium prescription in hemodialysis patients. Kidney Int 2004;66:1232–8.

[97] Horl MP, Horl WH. Drug therapy for hypertension in hemodialysis patients. Semin Dial 2004;17:288–94.

[98] Sehgal AR. Overlap between whites and blacks in response to antihypertensive drugs. Hypertension 2004;43:566–72.

[99] Agarwal R, Lewis RR, Davis JL, et al. Lisinopril therapy for hemodialysis hypertension—hemodynamic and endocrine responses. Am J Kidney Dis 2001;38:1245–50.

[100] Vasavada N, Saha C, Agarwal R. A double-blind randomized crossover trial of two loop diuretics in chronic kidney disease. Kidney Int 2003;64:632–40.

[101] Vasavada N, Agarwal R. Role of excess volume in the pathophysiology of hypertension in chronic kidney disease. Kidney Int 2003;64:1772–9.

[102] Agarwal R. Supervised atenolol therapy in the management of hemodialysis hypertension. Kidney Int 1999;55:1528–35.

[103] Bakris GL, Barnhill BW, Sadler R. Treatment of arterial hypertension in diabetic humans: importance of therapeutic selection. Kidney Int 1992;41:912–9.

[104] Abbott K, Smith A, Bakris GL. Effects of dihydropyridine calcium antagonists on albuminuria in patients with diabetes. J Clin Pharmacol 1996;36:274–9.

[105] Camel GH, Carmody SE, Perry HM Jr. Use of minoxidil in the azotemic patient. J Cardiovasc Pharmacol 1980;2(Suppl 2):S173–80.

[106] Lowenthal DT, Saris SD, Paran E, et al. The use of transdermal clonidine in the hypertensive patient with chronic renal failure. Clin Nephrol 1993;39:37–42.

[107] Laverman GD, Navis G, Henning RH, et al. Dual renin-angiotensin system blockade at optimal doses for proteinuria. Kidney Int 2002;62:1020–5.

[108] Nakao N, Yoshimura A, Morita H, et al. Combination treatment of angiotensin-II receptor blocker and angiotensin-converting-enzyme inhibitor in non-diabetic renal disease (COOPERATE): a randomised controlled trial. Lancet 2003;361:117–24.

[109] de Zeeuw D, Remuzzi G, Parving HH, et al. Proteinuria, a target for renoprotection in patients with type 2 diabetic nephropathy: lessons from RENAAL. Kidney Int 2004;65:2309–20.

[110] Tonelli M, Moye L, Sacks FM, et al. Pravastatin for secondary prevention of cardiovascular events in persons with mild chronic renal insufficiency. Ann Intern Med 2003;138:98–104.

[111] Port FK, Hulbert-Shearon TE, Wolfe RA, et al. Predialysis blood pressure and mortality risk in a national sample of maintenance hemodialysis patients. Am J Kidney Dis 1999;33:507–17.

[112] Zager PG, Nikolic J, Brown RH, et al. "U" curve association of blood pressure and mortality in hemodialysis patients. Medical Directors of Dialysis Clinic, Inc [published erratum appears in Kidney Int 1998;54(4):1417]. Kidney Int 1998;54:561–9.

[113] Agarwal R. Exploring the paradoxical relationship of hypertension with mortality in chronic hemodialysis. Hemodialysis Int 2004;8:207–13.

ELSEVIER
SAUNDERS

Cardiol Clin 23 (2005) 249–273

CARDIOLOGY
CLINICS

Vascular Access in Hemodialysis: Issues, Management, and Emerging Concepts

Prabir Roy-Chaudhury, MD, PhD[a],*, Burnett S. Kelly, MD[b],
Murad Melhem, MS[c], Jianhua Zhang, BS[a], Jinsong Li, MD, PhD[a],
Pankaj Desai, PhD[b], Rino Munda, MD[b],
Sue C. Heffelfinger, MD, PhD[d]

[a]Division of Nephrology and Hypertension, University of Cincinnati Medical Center,
231 Albert Sabin Way, Cincinnati, OH 45267, USA
[b]Department of Surgery, University of Cincinnati Medical Center,
231 Albert Sabin Way, Cincinnati, OH 45267, USA
[c]Department of Pathology, University of Cincinnati Medical Center,
231 Albert Sabin Way, Cincinnati, OH 45267, USA
[d]College of Pharmacy, University of Cincinnati, 136 E Health Professions Building,
Cincinnati, OH 45267-0004, USA

The inclusion of an article on hemodialysis vascular access dysfunction in a series on cardiorenal disease is an interesting paradox. Neointimal hyperplasia, which lies at the heart of hemodialysis vascular access dysfunction, traditionally is thought to be a problem for cardiologists and vascular surgeons. This clinicopathologic entity has emerged in a new role for the practicing nephrologist, namely as the Achilles' heel of hemodialysis.

Hemodialysis vascular access dysfunction is the single most important cause of morbidity in the hemodialysis population (currently more than 260,000 persons and growing at a rate of 5.5% per annum) [1]. Medicare data indicate that vascular access dysfunction is responsible for approximately 20% of all hospitalizations of patients who have end-stage renal disease [2]. Indeed the annual cost of vascular access–related morbidity in the United States currently exceeds 1 billion dollars per year [2].

Types of hemodialysis access

The two most common forms of permanent vascular access in chronic hemodialysis patients are the native arteriovenous (AV) fistula and the AV polytetrafluoroethylene (PTFE) graft. Cuffed double-lumen silicone catheters are the third mode of permanent hemodialysis vascular access.

Arteriovenous fistulae

Creation of an AV fistula at the wrist was first described by Brescia and Cimino [3] in 1966 (Fig. 1) [3]. At present, AV fistulae at the wrist (radiocephalic) or at the elbow (brachiocephalic) are the preferred mode of dialysis vascular access. More recently, it has been shown that brachiobasilic transposition fistulae have a reasonable survival with a lower infection rate than seen with PTFE dialysis access grafts [4–6]. Thus, native AV fistulae (wrist, elbow, or transposition) should always be the dialysis access of choice (in preference to PTFE

This work was supported by funding from the Paul Teschan Research Foundation and from Dialysis Clinics, Inc, by a Scientist Development Grant from the American Heart Association, by a grant from the Kidney Foundation of Greater Cincinnati, and by National Institutes of Health grant NIH RO1DK61689-01.

* Corresponding author.
  E-mail address: roychap@ucmail.uc.edu
  (P. Roy-Chaudhury).

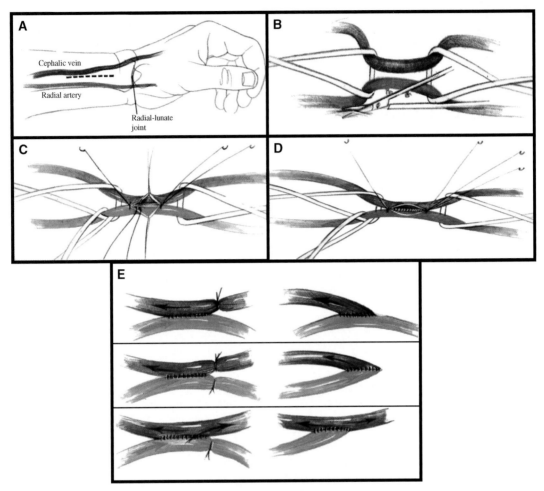

Fig. 1. Creation of a radiocephalic arteriovenous (Brescia-Cimino) fistula. (*A,B*) Dissection and isolation of the radial artery and cephalic vein at the wrist. (*C,D*) Creation of a side-to-side anastomosis. (*E*) Various techniques for tying off the distal vein to create a functional end-to-side anastomosis, thus preventing the occurrence of venous hypertension in the hand. (Courtesy of Dr. Michael J. Hanaway, University of Cincinnati, Cincinnati, OH.)

grafts and tunneled catheters). Native AV fistulae have a primary nonfunction rate [7,8] of about 20% (range, 10%–50%) that varies among centers depending on the aggressiveness of fistula placement and a maturation time between 1 and 4 months. Once a fistula matures, it has an excellent long-term primary patency (85% at 1 year and 75% at 2 years [9,10]) with a minimal infection rate (Fig. 2). Late fistula failure is caused primarily by neointimal hyperplasia that results in venous stenosis. Fig. 3 shows the most common sites of stenoses in patients who have wrist or elbow fistulae [11]. Note that the most common site of stenosis in the wrist fistula is at or around the anastomotic region; for upper arm (elbow fistula), most stenoses occur in a proximal (downstream) vein.

Polytetrafluoroethylene grafts

PTFE grafts are the second main form of permanent dialysis vascular access. They are often easier to create surgically, require a maturation time of only 2 to 3 weeks, and have a large cannulation area and are easy to cannulate [12]. Unfortunately, PTFE dialysis grafts have a poor primary patency rate (50% at 1 year and 25% at 2 years) (see Fig. 2) [9]. Every attempt should be made to create a primary AV fistula as the initial access and to reassess patients every time that they have access problems to see whether it is possible to place an AV fistula even though the initial access was a PTFE graft. Aggressive preemptive monitoring and intervention (discussed later and

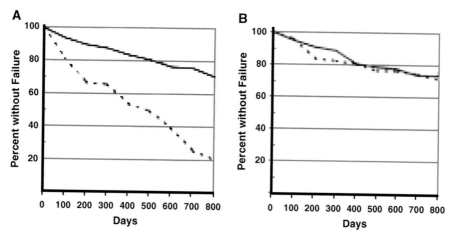

Fig. 2. Comparison of patency of arteriovenous fistulae (*solid lines*) versus PTFE dialysis grafts (*dashed lines*). (*A*) Unassisted primary patency of native arteriovenous fistulae versus PTFE grafts. (*B*) Cumulative patency in the setting of an active monitoring and intervention program. With prospective monitoring, the cumulative patency of PTFE grafts is similar to that for native arteriovenous fistulae but at the cost of a sixfold increase in the intervention rate. Graphs derived from the summed data analysis for the DOQI panel. (*From* Schwab SJ, Harrington JT, Singh A, et al. Vascular access for hemodialysis [clinical conference]. Kidney Int 1999;55(5):2083; with permission.)

shown in Fig. 2) can result in a cumulative patency for PTFE grafts that matches the results for AV fistulae. This increase in cumulative patency, however, requires a sixfold increase in interventions (thrombectomies and angioplasties) (see Fig. 2) [9]. Graft thrombosis is the cause of 80% of all vascular access dysfunction in PTFE dialysis grafts, and in more than 90% of thrombosed grafts the underlying pathology is a stenosis caused by venous neointimal hyperplasia (VNH)

at the venous anastomotic site or in the proximal vein (Fig. 4) [13]. Despite the enormity of this problem, there currently are no effective pharmacologic measures for the prevention or treatment of VNH in PTFE dialysis grafts [14,15].

Cuffed double-lumen silicone catheters

The main advantage of using double-lumen silicone catheters as a form of medium- to

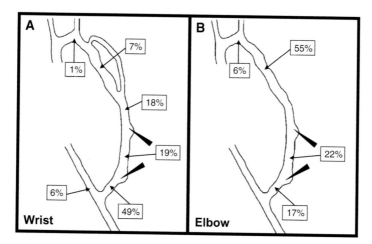

Fig. 3. Sites of venous stenoses for native arteriovenous fistulae (*A*) at the wrist and (*B*) at the elbow. (*From* Turmel-Rodrigues L, Pengloan J, Baudin S, et al. Treatment of stenosis and thrombosis in haemodialysis fistulas and grafts by interventional radiology. Nephrol Dial Transplant 2000;15(12):2032; with permission.)

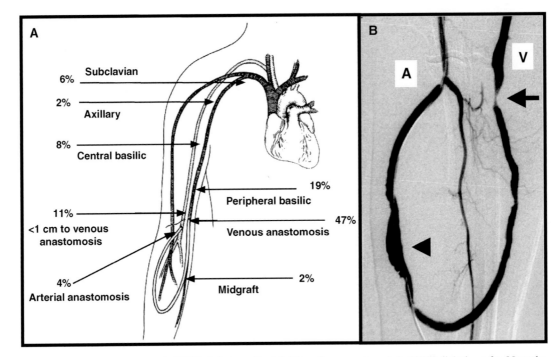

Fig. 4. Sites of venous stenoses in PTFE dialysis grafts. (*A*) Sites of venous stenosis in PTFE dialysis grafts. Note the preponderance of lesions at the graft–vein anastomosis or within 6 to 10 cm of the anastomosis. (*B*) Angiogram of a PTFE dialysis graft with a developing pseudoaneurysm (*arrowhead*) and stenosis (*arrow*) at the graft–vein anastomosis. (Courtesy of Dr. Tom Vesely, Malinckrodt Institute of Radiology, St. Louis. MO.)

long-term dialysis access (>3 weeks) is that they can be used immediately after placement. These catheters have many disadvantages, however, which include (1) a significant morbidity caused by thrombosis and infection, (2) a substantial risk of permanent central venous stenosis or occlusion, (3) a far shorter life span than with AV fistulae or PTFE grafts [16], and (4) low blood-flow rates resulting in inadequate dialysis. Ideally, these catheters should be used only as bridge catheters while an AV fistula matures. Early referral of patients who have chronic kidney disease to nephrologists for placement of permanent access should decrease the use of cuffed double-lumen silicon catheters significantly. A subcutaneous port (Life Site Hemodialysis System; VascA, Inc., Tewksbury, Massachusetts) has been licensed by the Food and Drug Administration in the United States. Initial studies suggest that the Life Site device results in higher blood flows, a lower infection rate, and a better survival than seen with Tessio catheters (Fig. 5) [17]. Many different cuffed double-lumen silicone catheters are available currently in the United States (Tessio, Vas-Cath, Split Ash). None have any major advantages

over their competitors, so cost should be considered in the selection process. Every attempt needs to be made to limit the use of cuffed double-lumen silicon catheters whenever possible.

Complications of dialysis access

Although some form of dialysis access is essential for the survival of the patient with end-stage renal disease, significant risks and complications are associated with all forms of dialysis access. Thus, early recognition and aggressive treatment of these complications is a critical aspect of the overall management of the hemodialysis patient.

Infection

After cardiovascular disease, infection is the second most important cause of mortality in the dialysis population, and it has been reported that the vascular access site is responsible for 23% to 73% of bacteremias in hemodialysis patients [18]. AV fistulae have the lowest rates of infection as compared with AV PTFE grafts (odds ratio [OR], 2.2), cuffed double-lumen silicone catheters (OR, 13.6), or temporary catheters (OR, 32.6) [19].

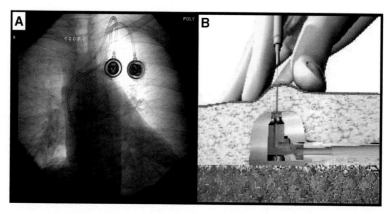

Fig. 5. Vascular access ports. (*A*) Two Vasca ports on a chest radiograph. (*B*) Schematic diagram of the Vasca port with a dialysis needle being inserted. (Courtesy Dr. Mark Sands, Cleveland Clinic Foundation, Cleveland, OH.)

Because vascular access infections usually begin at the cutaneous access site, the most common causative organisms are gram-positive cocci (*Staphylococcus aureus* and *Staphylococcus epidermidis*), with smaller contributions from gram-negative bacilli, enterococci, and fungi. The direct access into the blood stream (with the resulting high incidence of bacteremia), together with the frequency of *S aureus* infection, results in a disturbingly high incidence of metastatic complications such as endocarditis, osteomyelitis, septic arthritis, septic pulmonary emboli, and spinal epidural abscess. Clinicians caring for hemodialysis patients invariably have a very low threshold for searching for metastatic complications following access-related bacteremia. Detailed recommendations for the management of access infections in the setting of AV fistulae, PTFE grafts, and central vein dialysis catheters have been described in the Dialysis Outcomes Quality Initiative (DOQI) guidelines [20].

Cardiac failure

Hyperdynamic cardiac failure is a rare complication of fistulae created for hemodialysis access. For an AV fistula to cause cardiac compromise, it must have a blood flow that is at least 20% of the total cardiac output. Such a flow rate is almost never achieved in the setting of a Brescia-Cimino fistula at the wrist (300–500 mL/min) or in PTFE dialysis access grafts (800–1500 mL/min) [21]. These high flows can be achieved, however, in the context of upper arm autologous AV fistulae. At a physiologic level, creation of an AV fistula decreases peripheral vascular resistance and consequently leads to an increase in cardiac output, stroke volume, and contractility [21,22]. Over

a number of years, these increases result in left ventricular hypertrophy and dilatation followed by overt cardiac failure. At a molecular level, creation of a new AV fistula results in elevated levels of atrial natriuretic peptide, which decreases peripheral vascular resistance [23], and brain natriuretic peptide, which is thought to be a marker of diastolic dysfunction [22,24].

Most hemodialysis patients have significant pre-existing cardiac disease. It is, therefore, often difficult to tease out the exact contribution of an AV fistula to cardiac failure in a dialysis patient who has long-standing hypertension, diabetes, and coronary artery disease. Patients should be assessed for this complication on an individual basis. Temporary manual occlusion of the fistula followed by clinical assessment may help identify the patients most likely to benefit from permanent occlusion (patients who have a decreased pulse rate [Branham's sign] or an increase in peripheral arterial resistance and mean arterial blood pressure in response to temporary manual occlusion of the fistula). Patients who have increased peripheral arterial resistance and mean arterial blood pressure, in particular, have a more significant reduction in left ventricular end-diastolic diameter and left ventricular mass indexes when the fistula is permanently closed [22]. Occasionally, temporary manual occlusion can also result in a paradoxical worsening of cardiac performance in patients who have poor intrinsic left ventricular function [25].

Once it as been determined that the AV fistula is contributing to cardiac failure, two therapeutic options are available. The first is to try to constrict the fistula at its outflow, in the hope that this constriction will improve cardiac status but preserve vascular access. If constriction fails, the fistula is ligated completely, and an alternate access is placed. Unfortunately, at present there are no formal guidelines to screen hemodialysis patients for increased fistula flow and cardiac failure. MacRae and colleagues [22] have suggested that patients who have a high ratio of access flow (Qa) to cardiac output (CO) (>30%) should undergo regular biannual echocardiographic assessment for left ventricular end-diastolic and systolic dimensions, left ventricular mass index, and ejection fraction. Patients who have elevated Qa/CO ratios might be assessed for reduction of fistula flow, remembering, however, that vascular access is the lifeline of the hemodialysis patient. Finally, a recent study in the setting of renal transplantation [26] has demonstrated that surgical closure of an AV fistula after transplantation results in some beneficial effects on cardiac hemodynamics and left ventricular hypertrophy as compared with a control group of patients who had patent AV fistulae.

Vascular access modality, inflammation/infection, and mortality

A number of studies including data from the Dialysis Outcomes and Practice Patterns Study (DOPPS) have demonstrated an increase in all-cause mortality in hemodialysis patients that is related to the type of hemodialysis access (lowest mortality for fistulae, intermediate mortality for PTFE dialysis access grafts, and highest mortality for central venous dialysis catheters) [27–30]. Other authors, however, have suggested that this increase in mortality may be related to associated comorbidities in hemodialysis patients who have central catheters or PTFE grafts [31]. One of the mechanisms for this increased mortality in the setting of central venous catheters and PTFE dialysis access grafts as compared with native AV fistulae is thought to be linked to a possible proinflammatory state that results from the presence of prosthetic material combined with an increased infection rate [32–34]. Taking this train of thought one step further leads to speculation about whether the increased 1-year mortality for hemodialysis patients in the United States, as compared with those in other countries, is a function (at least in part) of the type of vascular access used. For example, AV fistulae are widely used in Japan, which has a low 1-year mortality. In the United States, PTFE grafts and catheters are widely used, and the 1-year mortality is high.

Superior vena cava thrombosis and atrial thrombus

The increasing prevalence of central venous catheters for hemodialysis (especially in the United States and the United Kingdom) has resulted in a marked increase in the number of patients who have superior vena cava (SVC) thrombosis and atrial thrombus. Both problems are potentially life-threatening complications. SVC thrombosis, which can result in SVC syndrome, is invariably secondary to an SVC stenosis. Such patients can be treated successfully with an SVC thrombectomy followed by placement of an appropriately sized SVC stent [35,36]. Right atrial clot formation is another serious complication linked to increased catheter usage. Removal of the catheter followed by thrombectomy yielded the best results in one series, as compared with removal and anticoagulation, removal alone, or no treatment [37,38]. Catheter infections and bacteremia seemed to be linked to the occurrence of right atrial clot [37,38].

Clinical standard of care for dialysis access grafts and fistulae

Increasing the prevalence of arteriovenous fistulae

Four decades of clinical experience with native AV fistulae and almost 3 decades of experience with PTFE dialysis grafts and cuffed double-lumen silicone catheters have repeatedly demonstrated the tremendous clinical and economic benefits of native AV fistulae over all other forms of dialysis access. At the clinical level, native AV fistulae have a significantly better primary patency rate after maturation (85% versus 50% at 1 year and 75% versus 25% at 2 years) and a much lower infection rate [9,39] than PTFE dialysis access grafts. In addition to clinical benefits, the placement of native AV fistulae has significant economic benefits. A multivariate analysis of Medicare costs per year after the initial placement of vascular access demonstrated that placing a PTFE graft resulted in an additional $10,000 per year in medical costs, whereas placing a cuffed double-lumen dialysis catheter resulted in an additional $23,000 in medical costs, as compared with patients who have an AV fistula (P. Eggers, personal communication, 2004).

Unfortunately, because of a lack of adequate veins, it may not be possible to create a primary AV fistula in all patients. This problem is seen particularly in women, African Americans, obese individuals, elderly patients, and patients who have peripheral vascular disease [40]. These factors have been used in the past to justify the marked differences in the incidence and prevalence rates of AV fistulae in the United States and in Europe/Japan. The DOPPS is a multicenter study that compares and contrasts dialysis practices in the United States/Canada (120 centers), Europe (140 centers), Japan (60 centers), and Australasia (20 centers). The most recent data (September 2003) from this study document a native fistula prevalence of 91% in Japan and between 70% and 90% in most European countries, compared with a dismal 30% in the United States (Fig. 6). Differences in the patient population in the United States and other countries cannot explain the appallingly low incidence of native AV fistulae in the United States. Specifically, after correction for clinical variables such as age, ethnicity, and peripheral vascular disease, the DOPPS data suggest that the United States should have a fistula prevalence rate of 75%. At a more practical level, individual centers in the United States have been able to achieve native AV fistula prevalence rates of greater than 80% through an aggressive approach that includes vein mapping before surgery, increased placement of upper arm and brachiobasilic transposition fistulae, and the creation of secondary native AV fistulae after failure of an initial PTFE dialysis graft (Fig. 7) [41].

At a clinical level, therefore, the single most important intervention that would improve hemodialysis vascular access care in the United States is a concerted attempt to increase the incidence (placement) and prevalence of native AV fistulae. The Centers for Medicare and Medicaid Services have recently set up a Vascular Access Improvement Initiative with goal of achieving 50% incidence and 40% prevalence for native AV fistulae in the United States. To achieve this goal the Vascular Access Improvement Initiative has developed and initiated a Fistula First project in association with the 18 end-stage renal disease networks that span the United States. Box 1 describes the 11 major conceptual changes targeted by the Fistula First project. These 11 proposals can be categorized as organizational, surgical, and dialysis unit issues.

Organizational issues include the development of a multidisciplinary vascular access team, early referral of patients who have chronic kidney disease to a nephrologist for initiation of access placement, continuous quality improvement meetings, and, most importantly, the availability of good-quality feedback data on fistula placement.

Surgical issues include the identification of surgeons who are interested in vascular access and the early referral of patients to these surgeons for placement of an AV fistula only. Other surgery-related issues are the use of a full range of surgical techniques, such as upper arm fistulae and brachial transpositions, rather than a rigid adherence to initial placement of a Brescia-Cimino wrist fistula, and, most importantly, the placement of secondary AV fistulae in patients who have PTFE grafts or cuffed double-lumen silicone catheters.

Issues related to dialysis units include the training of nurses and technicians in the cannulation of fistulae and continuing educational activities related to dialysis access.

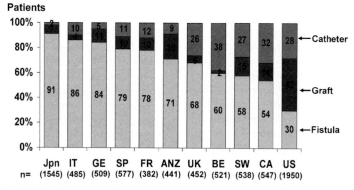

Fig. 6. Data from the Dialysis Outcomes and Practice Patterns Study. Note the dismal prevalence rate for native AV fistulae and the high prevalence rate for PTFE grafts in the United States as compared with other industrialized countries. ANZ, Australia and New Zealand; BE, Belgium; CA, Canada; FR, France; GE, Germany; IT, Italy; Jpn, Japan; SP, Spain; SW, Sweden; US, United States. (Data as of September, 2003; courtesy Dr. Rajiv Saran, University of Michigan, Ann Arbor, MI.)

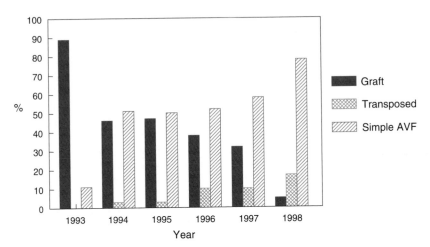

Fig. 7. High native arteriovenous (AV) fistula rates can be achieved in the United States. During a 5-year period, the prevalence of simple and transposed AV fistulae increased from 10% to 90% and the prevalence of PTFE grafts decreased from 90% to 10%. These and other data clearly demonstrate that native AV fistula rates similar to those of Europe and Japan can be achieved in the United States. (*Data from* Gibson KD, Caps MT, Kohler TR, et al. Assessment of a policy to reduce placement of prosthetic hemodialysis access. Kidney Int 2001;59(6):2335–45; with permission.)

Surveillance of dialysis grafts and fistulae

Rationale

Access thrombosis is the cause of 80% of all vascular access dysfunction. In more than 90% of thrombosed grafts and fistulae, the underlying pathology is a stenosis caused by VNH either at the venous anastomotic site (see Fig. 4B) or in the

---

Box 1. The 11 conceptual changes of the Fistula First program of the National Vascular Access Initiative

1. Routine (continuous quality improvement) review of vascular access
2. Early referral to nephrologist
3. Early referral to surgeon only for AV fistula
4. Selection of experienced surgeons
5. Use of the full range of appropriate surgical approaches
6. Creation of secondary AV fistulae in patients who have AV grafts
7. Placement of AV fistulae in patients who have catheters
8. Training in cannulation
9. Monitoring and surveillance
10. Continuing education of staff and patient
11. Feedback on outcomes

---

proximal vein [13]. These stenoses result in increased intra-access pressure and decreased access blood flow, which eventually result in thrombosis of the dialysis access. Numerous studies have demonstrated that PTFE grafts with decreased flow or increased intra-access pressures have a higher thrombosis rate than accesses with low pressures and high intra-access flows [42–44]. Other studies have reported similar results for AV fistulae [12,45,46]. Still other studies have shown a marked reduction in the thrombosis rate [47,48] and significant cost savings [49] when surveillance techniques have been instituted. (Most of these studies used historical or concurrent controls and were not randomized.) A randomized study by Ram and colleagues [50] did not demonstrate a difference in thrombosis rates between patients who had PTFE grafts who underwent prospective surveillance and those in whom intervention was based on clinical parameters alone (such as a change in the thrill over a graft). A meta-analysis conducted by the same investigators indicated that the association between surveillance of access blood flow and a reduction in thrombosis rates may not be as strong as suggested by other groups [51–53].

Current recommendations

At a clinical level, the current standard of care recommended by the DOQI is to monitor the function of dialysis grafts and fistulae prospectively using pressure- or flow-based techniques on a monthly basis [12,54]. If there is a significant decrease in intra-access flow or an increase in intra-access pressure, patients are referred for an angiogram. If the angiogram demonstrates a stenosis of greater than 50%, an angioplasty is performed. Routine angiograms to detect stenoses in the absence of a change in a functional parameter such as flow or pressure are not recommended currently.

Techniques for the prospective surveillance of dialysis access grafts and fistulae
Preferred techniques. The DOQI recommends the measurement of intra-access flow or static venous pressures as the optimal surveillance method for dialysis access. Measurement of intra-access flow using an ultrasound dilution technique (Transonics, Ithica, New York) [55], although not perfect, is perhaps the nearest to a reference standard. Current recommendations are to refer patients for an angiogram if the absolute access flow is less than 600 mL/min or the access flow is less than 1000 mL/min and has fallen by greater than 25% during the previous 4 months. Detailed recommendations for the measurement of static venous pressures and the threshold for intervention using this technique have been published in the DOQI guidelines [20].

Other techniques. Other methods that can be useful in prospectively detecting venous stenoses include

1. Measurement of dynamic venous pressures or access recirculation
2. Unexplained decreases in dialysis adequacy (Urea reduction ratio)
3. Physical findings (persistent swelling of the arm, prolonged bleeding after needle withdrawal, or altered characteristics of a pulse or thrill in a graft)
4. Doppler ultrasound studies

The DOQI guidelines have also provided detailed recommendations for the measurement of these parameters and recommended thresholds for intervention [56].

Surveillance of arteriovenous fistulae. Although the general rationale for surveillance remains valid for AV fistulae, direct measurement of flow is far more predictive of developing stenoses than is the measurement of venous pressures. The stenoses that develop in the setting of AV fistulae are often some distance away from the anastomotic site, allowing the development of collateral draining veins that prevent marked increases in pressure. This process does not occur in the setting of PTFE grafts. Measurement of recirculation, however, becomes a more useful screening tool for AV fistulae than for grafts, because flow in AV fistulae can drop to levels below the prescribed pump blood flow while maintaining access patency [56].

Pathology of arteriovenous fistula and polytetrafluoroethylene graft failure

Pathology of arteriovenous fistula failure

There are two main causes of AV fistula failure: early maturation failure and late venous stenosis caused by neointimal hyperplasia.

Early maturation failure
Early maturation failure usually is caused by the development of a juxta-anastomotic stenosis within a few centimeters of the artery–vein anastomosis. The pathophysiology of this early juxta-anastomotic stenosis, which results in maturation failure, is multifactorial. Contributing factors include the caliber and distensibility of the artery and the vein, the degree of venous and arterial manipulation, the exact surgical technique (and the skill of the surgeon), the magnitude of venous constriction, the integrity of the venous endothelium, and the propensity of individual veins to develop early neointimal hyperplasia. Unfortunately, no single therapy is available at present for the prevention or treatment of early maturation failure, perhaps because of its multifactorial pathogenesis. A multipronged effort that includes the use of duplex Doppler studies or venography to identify appropriate arteries and veins before surgery linked to a protocol that mandates angiography if a fistula is not maturing appropriately (followed by angioplasty or surgery for a juxta-anastomotic stenosis) can reduce maturation failure rates.

Late venous stenoses and thromboses
Studies of dysfunctional AV fistulae after initial maturation also demonstrate the presence of venous stenosis caused by venous neointimal hyperplasia composed primarily of smooth muscle cells [57]. Immunohistochemical studies have identified the expression of insulin-like growth factor 1 and transforming growth factor (TGF)-beta within the media and neointima of stenotic AV fistulae [57]. Other studies have demonstrated histologic colocalization between markers of oxidative stress

and molecules known to contribute to neointimal hyperplasia (endothelin, platelet-derived growth factor [PDGF] and TGF-beta) [58].

Pathology of venous stenosis in polytetrafluoroethylene dialysis grafts

Only a few studies have attempted to analyze the pathology of venous stenosis in PTFE dialysis grafts [59–61]. All these studies clearly demonstrated that the predominant lesion is a marked degree of VNH characterized by smooth muscle cell proliferation, extracellular matrix production, and angiogenesis (microvessel formation). Recently, the authors have performed a detailed histologic and immunohistochemical analysis of the different cell types, cytokines, and matrix proteins involved in the pathogenesis of

neointimal hyperplasia in human PTFE dialysis grafts [62]. The key features of VNH in the human specimens (Fig. 8) were:

1. Smooth muscle cell/myofibroblast proliferation within the neointima at the graft–vein anastomosis and in the downstream (proximal) vein.
2. Prominent angiogenesis in the adventitia and neointima at the graft–vein anastomosis and in the downstream (proximal) vein.
3. An active layer of macrophages (including macrophage giant cells) lining the adventitial and luminal sides of the PTFE graft and infiltrating into the interstices of the graft material.
4. Strong expression of cytokines such as basic fibroblast growth factor (bFGF), vascular

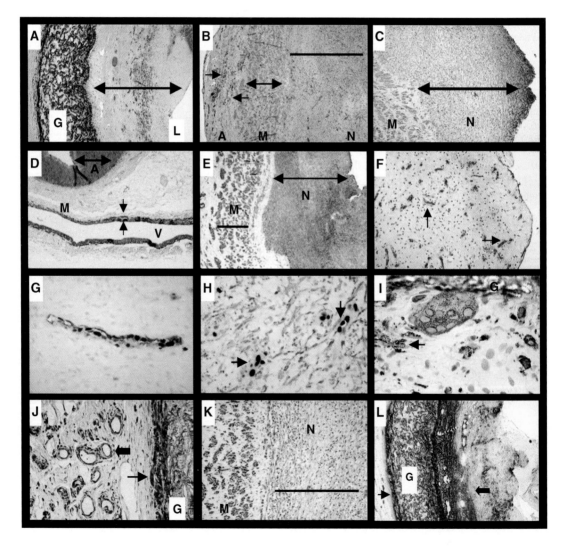

endothelial growth factor, and PDGF by smooth muscle cells and myofibroblasts, by microvessels within the neointima and adventitia, and by macrophages lining both sides of the graft.

5. The presence of extracellular matrix components such as collagen, fibronectin, and tenascin.

In addition, Weiss and colleagues [58] have demonstrated histologic colocalization between markers of oxidative stress and molecules known to contribute to neointimal hyperplasia (endothelin, PDGF, and TGF beta) in PTFE dialysis grafts and AV fistulae.

Differences between venous and arterial neointimal hyperplasia

Any discussion of the pathology and pathogenesis of venous stenosis and venous neointimal hyperplasia in dialysis access grafts and fistulae must address the potential differences between venous neointimal hyperplasia in this specific setting and the far more common arterial neointimal hyperplasia that occurs most commonly after balloon angioplasty of the coronary and peripheral arteries.

From a clinical standpoint, VNH in the setting of dialysis access grafts and fistulae is a far more aggressive lesion than arterial neointimal hyperplasia in the setting of peripheral vascular disease. This increased aggressiveness can be appreciated by comparing the 50% 1-year primary patency of PTFE dialysis access grafts with the 88% 5-year patency of aortoiliac grafts [63] and the 70% to 80% 1-year patency of femoro-popliteal grafts [64]. Venous stenoses in the setting of dialysis access grafts also have a poorer response to angioplasty (40% 3-month survival if thrombosed [65] and 50% 6-month survival if not thrombosed [66–68]) than do arterial stenoses. The greater clinical aggressiveness and poorer response to intervention for VNH, as compared with arterial neointimal hyperplasia, might be explained by the following differences:

1. Anatomy: At an anatomic level, the vein has a poorly defined internal elastic lamina that could facilitate the migration of smooth muscle cells and myofibroblasts from the media into the intima in response to endothelial shear stress.

2. Physiology: As compared with arteries, veins have relatively low nitric oxide and prostacyclin production, increased vasoconstrictor sensitivity, and relatively high numbers of bFGF receptors [69]. Molecular studies using gene-array techniques have demonstrated

Fig. 8. Venous neointimal hyperplasia in PTFE dialysis grafts (human samples). (*A*) PTFE graft (hematoxylin and eosin [H&E] stained × 200). Note the significant venous neointimal hyperplasia (*extent of arrow*) between the graft (G) and the lumen (L). (*B*) Downstream vein (H&E stained × 200). Note the presence of microvessels (*thin arrows*) within the adventitia (A). Also note the thickened (arterialized) media (M, *double-headed arrow*) and the significant amount of neointimal hyperplasia (N, *bar*). (*C*) Downstream (proximal) vein (alpha smooth muscle actin [SMA] × 400). The majority of cells in the downstream vein are smooth muscle cells. M, media; N, neointima. (*D*) Thickness of normal venous (V, *between thin arrows*) and arterial (A, *double-headed arrow*) intima-media (SMA × 117). (*E*) The thickness of the venous neointima (N, *double-headed arrow*) and media (M, *bar*) in a dialysis patient with venous stenosis (SMA × 117). At the same magnification as 3D, the venous neointima (N, *double-headed arrow*) is 20 times thicker than the intima-media of normal vein. This is an aggressive lesion. (*F*) Downstream vein (neointima) (von Willebrand factor (vWf) × 400). Note the prominent angiogenesis within the neointima (*arrows*) as assessed by this endothelial cell marker. (*G*) Downstream vein (neointima) (vWF + Ki67 × 800). High-power view of a microvessel within the neointima of downstream vein. Note the distinct colocalization of blue (endothelial) and brown (proliferating) cells indicating active endothelial cell proliferation (angiogenesis). (*H*) Downstream vein (neointima) (SMA + Ki67 × 1000). High-power view of a portion of the neointima stained for smooth muscle cells (brown) and proliferating cells (blue). Note that almost all the active cellular proliferation in this specimen (*arrows*) is occurring within the neointimal microvessels (angiogenesis). The large number of smooth muscle cells surrounding these microvessels is indicative of earlier smooth muscle cell proliferation and migration. (*I*) Upstream graft (neointima) (PG-M1 × 2000). High-power view of a macrophage giant cell adjacent to the neointimal surface of the PTFE graft (G). Also note the large number of macrophages in this area (*thin arrows*) in this area. (*J*) PTFE graft (adventitia) (bFGF × 500). Note the strong expression of bFGF in adventitial vessels (*thick arrow*) and by the macrophage giant cell layer (*thin arrow*) lining the graft. (*K*) Downstream vein (media and neointima) (PDGF × 400). There is strong expression of this cytokine in the venous media (M) and by smooth muscle cells/myofibroblasts within the neointima (N, *bar*). (*L*) PTFE graft (tenascin × 200). There is strong expression of tenascin in the region of the macrophage giant cell layer (*thin arrow*) surrounding PTFE graft (G) and on the abluminal side of the neointima (*thick arrow*). (*From* Roy-Chaudhury P, Kelly BS, Miller MA, et al. Venous neointimal hyperplasia in polytetrafluoroethylene dialysis grafts. Kidney Int 2001;59(6):2330; with permission.)

significant differences between arteries and veins in the expression of more than 50 genes [70].

3. Hemodynamics: The anastomosis between the relatively noncompliant PTFE graft and the compliant proximal vein (or between artery and vein in an AV fistula) is likely to result in a significant degree of turbulence and low shear stress at the graft–vein or artery–vein anastomosis, resulting in a more aggressive hyperplastic response (discussed later).

4. Dialysis factors: Factors that are specific to the dialysis patient include uremia as a modifying factor and the insertion of needles into PTFE dialysis grafts, which may result in platelet thrombi and the consequent downstream release of mediators of smooth muscle proliferation such as PDGF [10].

The authors believe that it is critical to identify the reasons for the clinical differences between venous and arterial neointimal hyperplasia at a cellular and molecular level. It is possible, for example, that the activation profile of venous endothelium in response to alterations in shear stress is different from that of arterial endothelium. From a practical standpoint, this difference could mean that interventions based on studies done in the context of arterial neointimal hyperplasia may not be effective in the setting of VNH occurring in an AV conduit.

Pathogenesis of venous stenosis in polytetrafluoroethylene dialysis grafts and arteriovenous fistulae

Although most of the information about the pathogenesis of neointimal hyperplasia comes from studies of arterial neointimal hyperplasia, there is an increasing amount of data on venous neointimal hyperplasia, especially in the setting of saphenous vein grafts. The following sections focus initially on the traditional view of the pathogenesis of venous neointimal hyperplasia, followed by a discussion on the influence of vascular remodeling and bone marrow–derived circulating cells on the final amount of luminal stenosis.

The traditional view

Initiating (upstream) events
Hemodynamic stress. The most important initiating event in the pathogenesis of venous stenosis in AV dialysis access grafts and fistulae is hemodynamic stress, especially regions of low shear stress

and turbulence at the graft–vein anastomoses. Shear stress [71,72] is probably the most critical hemodynamic parameter involved in the pathogenesis of neointimal hyperplasia and is defined as "the frictional force exerted by the circulating blood column on the intimal surface of the vessel." Atherosclerosis occurs mainly in regions of low flow and low shear stress [71,72] (which are usually regions of increased turbulence), and a similar paradigm holds true for venous [73] and arterial neointimal hyperplasia. In particular, an excellent experimental study by Mattsson and colleagues [74] has shown that increased flow and shear stress generated by creating an AV fistula downstream of an arterial interposition graft results in a decrease in neointimal hyperplasia. Ligation of the downstream AV fistula, however, results in a decrease in shear stress and an increase in neointimal hyperplasia at the upstream arterial interposition graft. It is likely that the transition from a noncompliant graft to a compliant vein at the graft–vein anastomosis (or from noncompliant artery to compliant vein, in the case of the AV fistula) results in marked turbulence and low shear stress in this region, predisposing the dialysis access to aggressive venous stenosis.

Polytetrafluoroethylene graft. The PTFE graft functions as a foreign body and stimulates a perigraft macrophage reaction (Fig. 8). These macrophages then produce a variety of cytokines (see Fig. 8) [62], which are likely to result in smooth muscle cell and endothelial cell activation.

Dialysis needles. The repeated placement of large-bore dialysis needles is also thought to contribute to VNH. It has been speculated that the platelet thrombi that form after the removal of dialysis needles produce PDGF and other cytokines, which then bathe the downstream anastomosis with a milieu that is rich in proinflammatory factors [10].

Uremia. Strong evidence suggests that uremia per se results in endothelial dysfunction [75,76] that could predispose to neointimal hyperplasia. A recent study has demonstrated pre-existing venous neointimal hyperplasia in venous samples from uremic patients before surgery for access placement, suggesting that uremia per se could predispose to venous inflammation/hypertrophy.

Surgical manipulation/vessel caliber and distensibility/surgical technique. Surgical factors are thought to play a greater role in the multifactorial pathogenesis of early AV fistula failure (failure of maturation). Attempting to create an AV fistula in patients who have an arterial diameter of less than 2 mm and a venous diameter of less than 2.5 mm generally is thought to be associated with higher rates of early AV fistula failure. Other studies have demonstrated that the skill of individual surgeon and the surgical policies at individual centers are important factors that determine access failure [77–79].

Downstream (cellular) events

All the initiating events result in the activation of endothelial cells and smooth muscle cells in the vascular intima and media; migration and proliferation of smooth muscle cells and myofibroblasts from the media into the intima results in the formation of a neointima. At the same time, the activated endothelial cell participates in the adhesion and diapedesis of inflammatory cells such as macrophages [80] and neutrophils [81] into the region of neointimal hyperplasia. A plethora of inflammatory mediators (all of which could be potential therapeutic targets) have been implicated in these processes. They include a large number of

- Signal transduction molecules (including p27 [82], p16 [83], retinoblastoma protein [84], and p38 mitogen-activated protein kinase [85])
- Cytokines (PDGF [86], bFGF [87], and tumor necrosis factor alpha [88])
- Chemokines (monocyte chemoattractant protein 1 [89,90] and the regulated on activa-

tion, normal T-cell expressed and secreted (RANTES) entity [91])
- Vasoactive molecules (nitric oxide [92] and endothelin [93])
- Adhesion molecules (intracellular adhesion molecule 1 [94] and P-selectin [95])
- Molecules such as osteopontin [96], apolipoprotein E [97], matrix metalloproteinase 2 [98], and human hepatocyte growth factor [99].

Of particular interest are studies in tumor necrosis factor alpha [88] and intracellular adhesion molecule knockout animals [94], which demonstrate a marked reduction in neointimal hyperplasia in these animals. There also has been interest in the role of genetic polymorphisms that predispose to neointimal hyperplasia. Humphries and colleagues [100] have shown that the 6A6A genotype of the matrix metalloproteinase gene is a genetic susceptibility factor for restenosis after coronary angioplasty. In the setting of dialysis access grafts, the ID polymorphism of the *ACE* gene has been linked to an increased frequency of thrombosed AV grafts [101].

The importance of the adventitia and vascular remodeling

There has recently been a great deal of interest in vascular remodeling (Fig. 9). It is postulated that the final amount of luminal stenosis depends on the magnitude of neointimal hyperplasia and on the pattern of vascular remodeling [102–104].

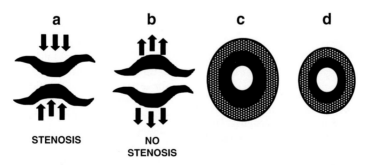

Fig. 9. Adventitial remodeling: The degree of luminal stenosis depends on both the magnitude of neointimal hyperplasia and the degree of vascular remodeling. With the same amount of neointimal hyperplasia, vascular constriction and unfavorable remodeling (*A*) results in luminal stenosis, whereas favorable remodeling (*B*) prevents the occurrence of luminal stenosis. (*C,D*) show a similar situation. The white area is the lumen. The area in black is the neointima, which is bordered on the outside by the internal elastic lamina and on the inside by the lumen. The hatched area comprises the adventitia and the media. Note that the luminal (*white*) areas are identical in C and D. The intima (*black area*) is much smaller in D, because adverse vascular remodeling has decreased the area enclosed by the internal elastic lamina. This latter parameter is a good indicator of the amount of vascular or adventitial remodeling.

Thus, in the presence of equivalent amounts of neointimal hyperplasia, vascular constriction results in a smaller luminal area, and vascular dilatation results in a larger luminal area [105]. Currently, vascular remodeling is thought to be responsible for approximately 50% of final luminal stenosis in experimental models of coronary angioplasty [103]. Although the exact pathophysiology of negative vascular remodeling remains unclear, the activation of adventitial fibroblasts could play an important role in this phenomenon by causing vascular constriction. The authors believe that vascular remodeling is a key concept, because blood flow, which is the final functional determinant of vascular stenosis, is determined by the luminal cross-sectional area rather than by the neointimal volume. Linked to the concept of vascular remodeling and the presence of an active adventitia are some elegant studies by Shi and colleagues [106], who have documented the migration of adventitial fibroblasts from the adventitia, through the media, and into the intima, where they contribute to neointimal hyperplasia after angioplasty. During the course of this migration, these alpha actin–negative adventitial fibroblasts transform into alpha actin–positive myofibroblasts [106]. Similarly, initial studies performed in the authors' laboratory [107] suggest that up to 40% of neointimal cells in dialysis patients who have venous stenosis of PTFE grafts could be alpha actin–negative, desmin-negative, vimentin-positive adventitial fibroblasts. The authors believe that an important advance in the understanding of neointimal hyperplasia is the recognition that the adventitia may not be a benign bystander but could be an important player in the pathogenesis of luminal stenosis.

Is there a role for circulating bone marrow–derived cells?

Emerging data suggest that circulating bone marrow stem cells could also contribute to neointimal hyperplasia. Sata and colleagues [108] performed femoral angioplasties in chimeric mice whose bone marrow cells expressed the LacZ marker. The mice were killed 28 days after angioplasty, and an analysis of neointimal hyperplasia at the site of balloon angioplasty revealed that up to 60% of the cells in the region of neointimal hyperplasia were modified bone marrow stem cells expressing either endothelial or smooth muscle cell markers. The same group has also demonstrated the presence of modified stem cells within neointimal lesions in a mouse model of coronary arteriolosclerosis [109]. In addition, Bayes-Genis and colleagues [110] have identified bone marrow–derived cells of a monocyte/macrophage lineage that have converted to a smooth muscle cell/myofibroblast phenotype in a pig model of coronary artery injury. Other authors have recently demonstrated that some neointimal smooth muscle cells in models of allograft arteriolosclerosis, mechanical vascular injury, and hyperlipidemia-induced atherosclerosis are derived from circulating bone marrow–derived cells [111]. These results suggest a completely new paradigm for the pathogenesis and for therapy of neointimal hyperplasia. This paradigm would explain the relative lack of efficacy of traditional interventions that have tried to target the vascular media and would also point toward the development of novel interventions aimed at preventing the adhesion of circulating bone marrow–derived cells to the site of vascular injury.

Lack of effective therapies for hemodialysis vascular access dysfunction

Despite a reasonable understanding of the pathology and pathogenesis of neointimal hyperplasia and luminal stenosis, there are still few effective therapeutic interventions for the prevention or treatment of this condition. This deficiency is particularly true for the venous stenosis and the VNH that characterizes hemodialysis vascular access dysfunction. The current standard of care for venous stenosis in the setting of hemodialysis vascular access is repeated angioplasty of the stenotic lesions. As mentioned earlier, the results of such intervention, in the setting of PTFE dialysis grafts in particular, are dismal (40% 3-month survival for a thrombosed graft and 50% 6-month survival for a patent but dysfunctional graft). In view of the tremendous advances that have been made in preventing restenosis in the setting of coronary angioplasty [112–114], it seems almost unethical to continue to perform standard angioplasties with such poor results for hemodialysis vascular access dysfunction.

The authors believe there are three main causes for the current lack of effective therapies for dialysis access dysfunction:

1. The lack of a validated large animal model of AV graft stenosis that could be used to test novel interventions.

2. An emphasis on systemic rather than local therapies.
3. An inadequate understanding of the role of adventitial or vascular remodeling and of circulating stem cells in the pathogenesis of this lesion.

The following discussion focuses on the first two issues; the potential role of adventitial/vascular remodeling and the contribution of bone marrow–derived stem cells have been discussed already.

Development of a validated large animal model of arteriovenous graft stenosis

In an attempt to test novel interventions targeted at reducing venous stenosis and VNH in PTFE dialysis grafts, the authors have developed a pig model of AV PTFE graft stenosis (Fig. 10) [115]. Detailed histologic and immuno-histochemical analyses in this pig model clearly demonstrated the development of significant venous neointimal hyperplasia at the graft–vein anastomosis as early as 14 days after surgery

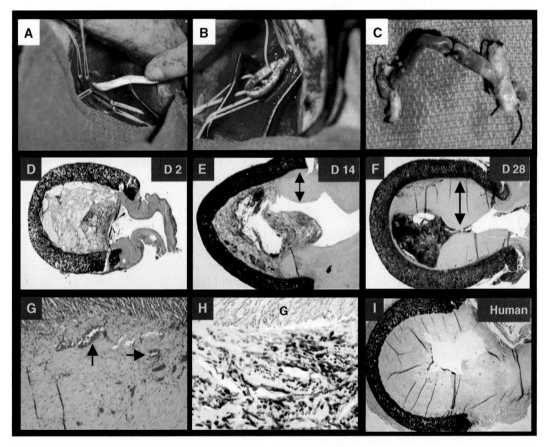

Fig 10. Neointimal hyperplasia in the pig model. (*A*) Suturing of the PTFE graft to the venous anastomosis. (*B*) The completed PTFE graft lying in its pocket. (*C*) The dissected PTFE graft before sectioning. The red dotted lines indicate the usual site where the graft is cut to obtain a Y-shaped specimen for further analysis. (*D–F*) (H&E × 50) The temporal course of venous neointimal hyperplasia in the authors' pig model. All the sections are from the site of the graft–vein anastomosis. (*D*) Two days after surgery, there is no encroachment of neointima into the graft. (*E*) Fourteen days after surgery, approximately one third of the graft–vein anastomosis is covered by venous neointima (*extent of arrow*). (*F*) Twenty-eight days after surgery, the graft–vein anastomosis is almost occluded (*extent of arrow*). (*G*) Graft–vein anastomosis, day 28. Neointima (H&E × 1000) shows prominent angiogenesis (*arrow*), together with smooth muscle cells/myofibroblasts and extracellular matrix components. (*H*) Graft–vein anastomosis (alpha SMA × 1000). The neointima in the authors' pig model is made up of a large number of smooth muscle cells/myofibroblasts. G, graft. (*I*) Low-power view (H&E × 50) of the graft–vein anastomosis from a human dialysis patient with venous stenosis. Note the remarkable similarity between the authors' 28-day pig sample (*F*) and the human sample (*I*).

(see Fig. 10E). Maximal neointimal hyperplasia occurred 28 days after surgery at the site of the graft–vein anastomosis (see Fig. 10F). The key features of neointimal hyperplasia in the pig model (see Fig. 10G) were (1) smooth muscle cell/myofibroblast proliferation (see Fig. 10H), (2) active angiogenesis (endothelial cell proliferation) within the neointima and adventitia, and (3) a prominent macrophage infiltrate (including giant cells) on both sides of the graft with significant infiltration of mononuclear cells into the actual graft material. Thus, the identifying characteristics of this pig model (see Fig. 10) are similar to those in the authors' human studies of venous neointimal hyperplasia (see Figs. 8 and 10I) and suggest that this pig model is a clinically relevant model to evaluate novel interventions for the treatment. Kohler and colleagues [116] have reported a sheep model of AV stenosis that is similar to the authors' pig model, and Lumsden and colleagues [117] have reported a canine model of AV stenosis. Thus, for the first time, there are validated large animal models of venous stenosis and venous neointimal hyperplasia at the graft–vein anastomosis that could be used for testing novel interventions aimed specifically at hemodialysis vascular access dysfunction.

Local versus systemic therapy

A second possible reason for the current lack of effective therapies for neointimal hyperplasia is that it may be difficult to achieve adequate local concentrations of a specific antiproliferative agent without causing substantial systemic toxicity. In this context, dialysis grafts and fistulae could be ideally suited to local therapeutic intervention because of their superficial location, their distance from vital organs, and the relative ease of delivering local therapy either at the time of graft placement or during subsequent dialyses (when hollow needles are placed within 3 cm of the site of lesion). It is likely that local drug delivery systems will allow potent doses of antiproliferative therapy to be targeted at the graft–vein anastomosis with minimal systemic toxicity. Compare, for example, the relative ease of local delivery in the setting of a dialysis access graft with the intricacies of a repeat cardiac catheterization in the setting of local therapy for coronary restenosis. Extensive literature in the setting of experimental coronary angioplasty models documents a variety of endovascular drug-delivery systems for use at the time of angioplasty. These

methods include double-balloon systems [118], hydrogel-coated balloon catheters, porous and microporous balloons, and coated stents [119,120]. There is a critical need to apply these drug-delivery techniques to experimental models of AV stenosis.

Clinical trials of currently available drugs

Despite the lack of effective therapies for venous neointimal hyperplasia, a large number of currently available drugs are known to inhibit smooth muscle cell and endothelial cell activation and neointimal hyperplasia in experimental models of neointimal hyperplasia. These drugs include angiotensin-converting enzyme inhibitors [121], angiotensin-receptor blockers [122], the peroxisome proliferator–activated receptor agonists such as pioglitazone and rosiglitazone [123–125], verapamil [126], 3-hydroxy-3-methylglutaryl coenzyme reductase inhibitors [127–130], and immunosuppressive agents such as mycophenolate mofetil and sirolimus [127–132]. A recent retrospective analysis of the use of angiotensin-converting enzyme inhibitors in hemodialysis patients indicates a reduction in vascular access dysfunction in patients taking these agents [133]. Prospective studies of these and other drugs to identify specific effects on venous stenosis and neointimal hyperplasia in dialysis access grafts are desperately needed. In response to this need, the National Institutes of Health has recently initiated a multicenter trial to test currently available therapies for dialysis access dysfunction. The agents chosen for the initial studies are clopidogrel for the prevention of thrombosis in AV fistulae and dipyridamole for use in the setting of PTFE grafts [134].

Novel therapies for venous neointimal hyperplasia in the setting of dialysis access

Radiation therapy

In a number of studies in animal models of balloon angioplasty–induced stenosis in coronary and peripheral arteries, external [135] or intravascular [136,137] radiation has been shown to reduce neointimal hyperplasia and restenosis following angioplasty. The beneficial effects of radiation therapy in the treatment of coronary restenosis after angioplasty and stent placement have also been confirmed in large, multicenter clinical studies [112,138]. Although the clinical use of radiation therapy in the setting of coronary artery disease has declined significantly since the introduction of drug-eluting stents, this could still be an effective therapeutic modality for hemodialysis vascular access stenosis. Thus, in the specific setting of their pig model, the authors have demonstrated that external beam radiation significantly reduces VNH [139]. In these studies, the percent of luminal stenosis at the graft–vein anastomosis was reduced by 23% on the irradiated side as compared with contralateral controls (52.7% $\pm$ 7.42% versus 40.7% $\pm$ 7.75%; $P = .039$) [139].

At a clinical level, Parikh and colleagues [140] have performed a phase I study (10 patients) in which two 6-Gy doses of external beam radiation were given after angioplasty. There were no adverse effects of radiation therapy. Cohen and colleagues [141] have conducted the only randomized study of external beam radiation in dialysis access grafts and fistulae. They were not able to demonstrate a benefit from external radiation therapy in their heterogeneous group of dialysis accesses, although there was a trend toward better results in the radiation group. More recently, a pilot study of endovascular radiation therapy in patent but dysfunctional dialysis access grafts sponsored by the Novoste Corporation (Norcross, Georgia) demonstrated a significant improvement in 6-month target lesion primary patency in the radiation treatment arm. This benefit in target lesion patency did not translate into an improvement in cumulative patency (Fig. 11) [142]. Unfortunately, a larger multicenter study of endovascular radiation therapy in patients who have thrombosed dialysis grafts was halted. Albeit not due to any major side effects from radiation therapy.

Gene therapy

Gene therapy could become an effective local therapy for neointimal hyperplasia in dialysis access grafts and fistulae, especially if improvements continue to be made in the safety and efficacy of delivery techniques [143]. Currently, inhibition of neointimal hyperplasia in experimental angioplasty models has been achieved by the gene transfer of endothelial [144] and inducible [145] nitric oxide synthase, cyclin-dependent kinase inhibitors [82,84], retinoblastoma protein [146], hepatocyte growth factor [99], and transcription factors such as E2F [147].

Coated stents

The most significant advance in the prevention and treatment of neointimal hyperplasia in recent years has been the development of intravascular stents coated with a polymer that contains an antiproliferative agent. Large, multicenter clinical trials in the setting of coronary angioplasty have demonstrated that both the sirolimus- and paclitaxel-eluting stents are extremely effective in reducing restenosis rates [113,114]. Most impressively, 2-year follow-up studies of the first patients who received the sirolimus stents demonstrate minimal neointimal hyperplasia [148].

In the specific setting of venous stenosis in hemodialysis access grafts, the placement of a bare stent following venous angioplasty has not been shown to improve survival [149,150], although there may be some role for stents in the setting of venous dissection, elastic lesions, and recurrent stenoses [151]. Whether the use of stents coated with antiproliferative agents will be effective in the setting of hemodialysis vascular access dysfunction is currently unknown.

Local perivascular drug delivery

Hemodialysis access grafts and fistulae could be ideally suited to perivascular drug delivery, because the treatment could be applied at the time of surgical placement. The validity of such an approach has been documented in a number of experimental angioplasty models using agents such as nitric oxide, paclitaxel, and tyrphostins [152–160]. In addition, the authors' group has demonstrated the complete absence of luminal stenosis in the pig model of venous neointimal hyperplasia [161]. Although most studies of perivascular delivery have used a specific drug, an alternative approach is to embed specific cell types (for example, endothelial cells) into the perivascular polymer. These cells (which may or may not be transfected with the gene of interest) could then produce a slew of mediators that, it is hoped, would promote vascular dilatation and inhibit neointimal hyperplasia [153,155–160].

Endothelial sodding/seeding

For many decades, the Holy Grail of experimental vascular surgery has been the ability to coat vascular grafts or stents with a layer of "phenotypically good" endothelial cells that would produce just the right milieu of antiadhesive and vasodilatory mediators. This technique

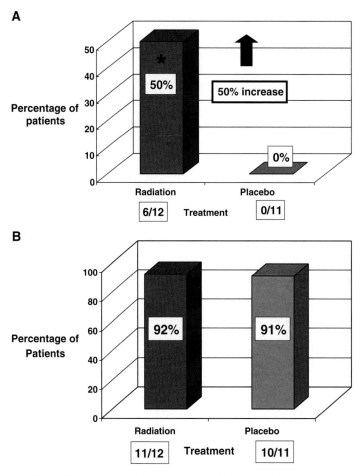

Fig. 11. Endovascular radiation therapy for dialysis access grafts. (*A*) Significant improvement in 6-month target lesion patency following a single 18-Gy dose of radiation therapy after angioplasty. (*B*) This improvement did not translate into an improved cumulative patency at 6 months.

would allow vascular grafts to function in the same manner as blood vessels. A number of different methods have been used in attempts to achieve this goal, including chronic in vitro shear stress activation of endothelial cells before seeding them onto synthetic grafts [162] and the use of electrostatic seeding techniques [163–165]. The best results in this field have come from recent work by Szmitko and colleagues [166], which has layered an antibody against CD34 (an antigen present on circulating endothelial precursor cells) onto endovascular stents, When these stents are placed in vivo, the CD34 antibody binds to circulating endothelial progenitor cells, resulting in a complete layering of the stent surface with endothelial progenitor cells. The first stent using this technology was placed in a patient with

coronary artery disease last year. A similar process has been used in the setting of vascular access grafts [167].

Other therapies

Other novel approaches that have tried to address the vexing problem of neointimal hyperplasia include photodynamic therapy [168] and intravascular sonotherapy [169].

Looking to the future

The authors believe that the last few years have laid the foundation for significant changes in the way hemodialysis vascular access dysfunction is approached. Currently, there is a clear appreciation of the magnitude of the clinical problem and an understanding that targeting venous stenosis and venous neointimal hyperplasia is an essential first step toward reducing the morbidity and cost associated with hemodialysis vascular access dysfunction. There also is a reasonable understanding of the pathology and pathogenesis of venous neointimal hyperplasia, and validated large animal models of venous stenosis are available. Novel interventions must be tested aggressively in animal models and then transferred rapidly to the clinical arena. Also necessary are clinical trials of currently available drugs that are known to block smooth muscle cell proliferation. Indeed, given the aggressiveness of the clinical lesion and the regular follow-up at the time of thrice-weekly hemodialysis, dialysis access grafts and fistulae could be the ideal clinical model for testing new therapies for neointimal hyperplasia. The results from such trials (conducted in a limited number of patients and for a limited period) then could be applied to other clinical conditions characterized by neointimal hyperplasia, such as postangioplasty restenosis, peripheral vascular disease, and coronary artery bypass graft stenosis.

In conclusion, the authors believe that the prospects for reducing dialysis access dysfunction are extremely bright. At present, the single most important intervention to reduce dialysis access morbidity remains the aggressive placement and care of native AV fistulae by a multidisciplinary vascular access team.

References

[1] US Renal Data System. USRDS 2002 Annual data report. 2002.

[2] Feldman HI, Kobrin S, Wasserstein A. Hemodialysis vascular access morbidity. J Am Soc Nephrol 1996;7:523–35.

[3] Brescia MJ, Cimino JE, Appel K, et al. Chronic hemodialysis using venipuncture and a surgically created arteriovenous fistula. N Engl J Med 1966;275:1089–92.

[4] Silva MB Jr, Hobson RW II, Pappas PJ, et al. Vein transposition in the forearm for autogenous hemodialysis access. J Vasc Surg 1997;26(6):981–6 [discussion: 7–8].

[5] Gormus N, Ozergin U, Durgut K, et al. Comparison of autologous basilic vein transpositions between forearm and upper arm regions. Ann Vasc Surg 2003;17(5):522–5.

[6] Taghizadeh A, Dasgupta P, Khan MS, et al. Long-term outcomes of brachiobasilic transposition fistula for haemodialysis. Eur J Vasc Endovasc Surg 2003;26(6):670–2.

[7] Palder SB, Kirkman RL, Whittemore AD, et al. Vascular access for hemodialysis. Patency rates and results of revision. Ann Surg 1985;202(2): 235–9.

[8] Malovrh M. Native arteriovenous fistula: preoperative evaluation. Am J Kidney Dis 2002;39(6): 1218–25.

[9] Schwab SJ, Harrington JT, Singh A, et al. Vascular access for hemodialysis [clinical conference]. Kidney Int 1999;55(5):2078–90.

[10] Albers FJ. Causes of hemodialysis access failure. Adv Ren Replace Ther 1994;1(2):107–18.

[11] Turmel-Rodrigues L, Pengloan J, Baudin S, et al. Treatment of stenosis and thrombosis in haemodialysis fistulas and grafts by interventional radiology. Nephrol Dial Transplant 2000;15(12): 2029–36.

[12] Schwab SJ, Oliver MJ, Suhocki P, et al. Hemodialysis arteriovenous access: detection of stenosis and response to treatment by vascular access blood flow. Kidney Int 2001;59(1):358–62.

[13] Beathard GA. The treatment of vascular access dysfunction: a nephrologists view and experience. Adv Ren Replace Ther 1994;1:131–47.

[14] Blankestijn PJ, Bosman PJ, Boereboom FT. Haemodialysis access without thrombosis: is it possible? [editorial]. Nephrol Dial Transplant 1996; 11(12):2394–7.

[15] Himmelfarb J, Saad T. Hemodialysis vascular access: emerging concepts. Curr Opin Nephrol Hypertens 1996;5(6):485–91.

[16] Hodges TC, Fillinger MF, Zwolak RM, et al. Longitudinal comparison of dialysis access methods: risk factors for failure. J Vasc Surg 1997;26(6): 1009–19.

[17] Schwab SJ, Weiss MA, Rushton F, et al. Multi-center clinical trial results with the LifeSite hemodialysis access system. Kidney Int 2002;62(3): 1026–33.

[18] Stevenson KB. Management of hemodialysis vascular access infections. In: Gray RJ, Sands JJ, editors. Dialysis access: a multidisciplinary approach. Philadelphia: Lippincott Williams and Wilkins; 2002. p. 98–106.

[19] Stevenson KB, Hannah EL, Lowder CA, et al. Epidemiology of hemodialysis vascular access infections from longitudinal infection surveillance data: predicting the impact of NKF-DOQI clinical practice guidelines for vascular access. Am J Kidney Dis 2002;39(3):549–55.

[20] Dialysis Outcomes Quality Initiative III. NKF-K/DOQI clinical practice guidelines for vascular access: update 2000. Am J Kidney Dis 2001;37 (1 Suppl 1):S137–81.

[21] Schanzer H. Overview of complications and management after vascular access creation. In: Gray RJ, Sands JJ, editors. Dialysis access: a multidisciplinary approach. Philadelphia: Lippincott, Williams and Wilkins; 2002. p. 93–7.

[22] MacRae JM, Pandeya S, Humen DP, et al. Arteriovenous fistula-associated high-output cardiac failure: a review of mechanisms. Am J Kidney Dis 2004;43(5):e17–22.

[23] Ori Y, Korzets A, Katz M. Hemodialysis arteriovenous access—a prospective hemodynamic evaluation. Nephrol Dial Transplant 1996;11:94–7.

[24] Iwashima Y, Horio T, Takami Y, et al. Effects of the creation of arteriovenous fistula for hemodialysis on cardiac function and natriuretic peptide levels in CRF. Am J Kidney Dis 2002;40(5):974–82.

[25] Timmis AD, McGonigle RJ, Weston MJ, et al. The influence of hemodialysis fistulas on circulatory dynamics and left ventricular function. Int J Artif Organs 1982;5(2):101–4.

[26] Unger P, Velez-Roa S, Wissing KM, et al. Regression of left ventricular hypertrophy after arteriovenous fistula closure in renal transplant recipients: a long-term follow-up. Am J Transplant 2004;4:2038.

[27] Rayner HC, Besarab A, Brown WW, et al. Vascular access results from the Dialysis Outcomes and Practice Patterns Study (DOPPS): performance against Kidney Disease Outcomes Quality Initiative (K/DOQI) clinical practice guidelines. Am J Kidney Dis 2004;44(5 Suppl 3):22–6.

[28] Polkinghorne KR, McDonald SP, Atkins RC, et al. Vascular access and all-cause mortality: a propensity score analysis. J Am Soc Nephrol 2004;15(2):477–86.

[29] Pastan S, Soucie JM, McClellan WM. Vascular access and increased risk of death among hemodialysis patients. Kidney Int 2002;62(2):620–6.

[30] Dhingra RK, Young EW, Hulbert-Shearon TE, et al. Type of vascular access and mortality in US hemodialysis patients. Kidney Int 2001;60(4):1443–51.

[31] Di Iorio BR, Bellizzi V, Cillo N, et al. Vascular access for hemodialysis: the impact on morbidity and mortality. J Nephrol 2004;17(1):19–25.

[32] Himmelfarb J, Stenvinkel P, Ikizler TA, et al. The elephant in uremia: oxidant stress as a unifying concept of cardiovascular disease in uremia. Kidney Int 2002;62(5):1524–38.

[33] Kaysen GA. The microinflammatory state in uremia: causes and potential consequences. J Am Soc Nephrol 2001;12(7):1549–57.

[34] Kaysen GA, Eiserich JP. Characteristics and effects of inflammation in end-stage renal disease. Semin Dial 2003;16(6):438–46.

[35] Elson JD, Becker GJ, Wholey MH, et al. Vena caval and central venous stenoses: management with Palmaz balloon-expandable intraluminal stents. J Vasc Interv Radiol 1991;2(2):215–23.

[36] Bornak A, Wicky S, Ris HB, et al. Endovascular treatment of stenoses in the superior vena cava syndrome caused by non-tumoral lesions. Eur Radiol 2003;13(5):950–6.

[37] Negulescu O, Coco M, Croll J, et al. Large atrial thrombus formation associated with tunneled cuffed hemodialysis catheters. Clin Nephrol 2003;59(1):40–6.

[38] Shah A, Murray M, Nzerue C. Right atrial thrombi complicating use of central venous catheters in hemodialysis. Int J Artif Organs 2004;27(9):772–8.

[39] Nassar GM, Ayus JC. Infectious complications of the hemodialysis access. Kidney Int 2001;60(1):1–13.

[40] Allon M, Ornt DB, Schwab SJ, et al. Factors associated with the prevalence of arteriovenous fistulas in hemodialysis patients in the HEMO study. Hemodialysis (HEMO) Study Group. Kidney Int 2000;58(5):2178–85.

[41] Gibson KD, Caps MT, Kohler TR, et al. Assessment of a policy to reduce placement of prosthetic hemodialysis access. Kidney Int 2001;59(6):2335–45.

[42] Sullivan KL, Besarab A, Bonn J, et al. Hemodynamics of failing dialysis grafts. Radiology 1993;186(3):867–72.

[43] Besarab A, Sullivan KL, Ross RP, et al. Utility of intra-access pressure monitoring in detecting and correcting venous outlet stenoses prior to thrombosis. Kidney Int 1995;47(5):1364–73.

[44] May RE, Himmelfarb J, Yenicesu M, et al. Predictive measures of vascular access thrombosis: a prospective study. Kidney Int 1997;52(6):1656–62.

[45] Tonelli M, Hirsch D, Clark TW, et al. Access flow monitoring of patients with native vessel arteriovenous fistulae and previous angioplasty. J Am Soc Nephrol 2002;13(12):2969–73.

[46] Tonelli M, Jindal K, Hirsch D, et al. Screening for subclinical stenosis in native vessel arteriovenous fistulae. J Am Soc Nephrol 2001;12(8):1729–33.

[47] Sands JJ, Jabyac PA, Miranda CL, et al. Intervention based on monthly monitoring decreases hemodialysis access thrombosis. ASAIO J 1999;45(3):147–50.

[48] Schwab SJ, Raymond JR, Saeed M, et al. Prevention of hemodialysis fistula thrombosis. Early detection of venous stenoses. Kidney Int 1989;36(4):707–11.

[49] McCarley P, Wingard RL, Shyr Y, et al. Vascular access blood flow monitoring reduces access morbidity and costs. Kidney Int 2001;60(3):1164–72.

[50] Ram SJ, Work J, Caldito GC, et al. A randomized controlled trial of blood flow and stenosis surveillance of hemodialysis grafts. Kidney Int 2003;64(1):272–80.

[51] Paulson WD, Ram SJ, Birk CG, et al. Accuracy of decrease in blood flow in predicting hemodialysis graft thrombosis. Am J Kidney Dis 2000;35(6):1089–95.

[52] Paulson WD, Ram SJ, Birk CG, et al. Does blood flow accurately predict thrombosis or failure of hemodialysis synthetic grafts? A meta-analysis. Am J Kidney Dis 1999;34(3):478–85.

[53] Paulson WD. Blood flow surveillance of hemodialysis grafts and the dysfunction hypothesis. Semin Dial 2001;14(3):175–80.

[54] Garland JS, Moist LM, Lindsay RM. Are hemodialysis access flow measurements by ultrasound dilution the standard of care for access surveillance? Adv Ren Replace Ther 2002;9(2):91–8.

[55] Depner TA, Krivitski NM. Clinical measurement of blood flow in hemodialysis access fistulae and grafts by ultrasound dilution. ASAIO J 1995; 41(3):M745–9.

[56] K/DOQI NKF. Clinical practice guidelines for vascular access 2000. Am J Kidney Dis 2001;37: S137–81.

[57] Stracke S, Konner K, Kostlin I, et al. Increased expression of TGF-beta1 and IGF-I in inflammatory stenotic lesions of hemodialysis fistulas. Kidney Int 2002;61(3):1011–9.

[58] Weiss MF, Scivittaro V, Anderson JM. Oxidative stress and increased expression of growth factors in lesions of failed hemodialysis access. Am J Kidney Dis 2001;37(5):970–80.

[59] Chen C, Ku DN, Kikeri D, et al. Tenascin: a potential role in human arteriovenous PTFE graft failure. J Surg Res 1996;60(2):409–16.

[60] Rekhter MD, Gordon D. Active proliferation of different cell types, including lymphocytes, in human atherosclerotic plaques. Am J Pathol 1995; 147(3):668–77.

[61] Swedberg SH, Brown BG, Sigley R, et al. Intimal fibromuscular hyperplasia at the venous anastomosis of PTFE grafts in hemodialysis patients. Clinical, immunocytochemical, light and electron microscopic assessment. Circulation 1989;80(6): 1726–36.

[62] Roy-Chaudhury P, Kelly BS, Miller MA, et al. Venous neointimal hyperplasia in polytetrafluoroethylene dialysis grafts. Kidney Int 2001;59(6): 2325–34.

[63] Abbott WM, Kwdek CJ. Aortofemoral bypass for atherosclerotic aortoiliac disease occlusive disease. In: Ernst CB, Stanley JC, editors. Current therapy in vascular surgery. St Louis (MO): Mosby Year Book; 1995. p. 355.

[64] Dalman RL, Taylor LM. Infrainguinal revascularization procedures. In: Porter JM, Taylor LM, editors. Basic data underlying clinical decision making in vascular surgery. St Louis (MO): Quality Medical Publishing; 1994. p. 141.

[65] Beathard GA. Mechanical versus pharmacomechanical thrombolysis for the treatment of thrombosed dialysis access grafts. Kidney Int 1994; 45(5):1401–6.

[66] Beathard GA. Percutaneous angioplasty for the treatment of venous stenosis: a nephrologist's view. Semin Dial 1995;8:166–70.

[67] Kanterman RY, Vesely TM, Pilgram TK, et al. Dialysis access grafts: anatomic location of venous stenosis and results of angioplasty [erratum appears in Radiology 1995;196(2):582]. Radiology 1995;195(1):135–9.

[68] Turmel-Rodrigues L, Pengloan J, Blanchier D, et al. Insufficient dialysis shunts: improved long-term patency rates with close hemodynamic monitoring, repeated percutaneous balloon angioplasty, and stent placement. Radiology 1993;187(1):273–8.

[69] Motwani JG, Topol EJ. Aortocoronary saphenous vein graft disease: pathogenesis, predisposition, and prevention. Circulation 1998;97(9):916–31.

[70] Adams LD, Geary RL, McManus B, et al. A comparison of aorta and vena cava medial message expression by cDNA array analysis identifies a set of 68 consistently differentially expressed genes, all in aortic media. Circ Res 2000;87(7):623–31.

[71] Gnasso A, Irace C, Carallo C, et al. In vivo association between low wall shear stress and plaque in subjects with asymmetrical carotid atherosclerosis. Stroke 1997;28(5):993–8.

[72] Ku DN, Giddens DP, Zarins CK, et al. Pulsatile flow and atherosclerosis in the human carotid bifurcation. Positive correlation between plaque location and low oscillating shear stress. Arteriosclerosis 1985;5(3):293–302.

[73] Meyerson SL, Skelly CL, Curi MA, et al. The effects of extremely low shear stress on cellular proliferation and neointimal thickening in the failing bypass graft. J Vasc Surg 2001;34(1):90–7.

[74] Mattsson EJ, Kohler TR, Vergel SM, et al. Increased blood flow induces regression of intimal hyperplasia. Arterioscler Thromb Vasc Biol 1997; 17(10):2245–9.

[75] Mezzano D, Pais EO, Aranda E, et al. Inflammation, not hyperhomocysteinemia, is related to oxidative stress and hemostatic and endothelial dysfunction in uremia. Kidney Int 2001;60: 1844–50.

[76] Morris ST, McMurray JJ, Spiers A, et al. Impaired endothelial function in isolated human uremic resistance arteries. Kidney Int 2001;60:1077–82.

[77] He C, Charoenkul V, Kahn T, et al. Impact of the surgeon on the prevalence of arteriovenous fistulas. ASAIO J 2002;48(1):39–40.

[78] Allon M, Robbin ML. Increasing arteriovenous fistulas in hemodialysis patients: problems and solutions. Kidney Int 2002;62(4):1109–24.

[79] O'Hare AM, Dudley RA, Hynes DM, et al. Impact of surgeon and surgical center characteristics on choice of permanent vascular access. Kidney Int 2003;64(2):681–9.

[80] Danenberg HD, Fishbein I, Gao J, et al. Macrophage depletion by clodronate containing liposomes reduces neointimal formation after balloon injury in rats and rabbits. Circulation 2002;106: 599–605.

[81] Welt FG, Edelman ER, Simon DI, et al. Neutrophil, not macrophage, infiltration precedes neointimal thickening in balloon injured arteries. Arterioscler Thromb Vasc Biol 2000;20:2553–8.

[82] Tsui LV, Camrud A, Mondesire J, et al. p27-p16 fusion gene inhibits angioplasty-induced neointimal hyperplasia and coronary artery occlusion. Circ Res 2001;89(4):323–8.

[83] McArthur JG, Qian H, Citron D, et al. p27-p16 Chimera: a superior antiproliferative for the prevention of neointimal hyperplasia. Mol Ther 2001;3(1):8–13.

[84] Chang MW, Barr E, Lu MM, et al. Adenovirus-mediated over-expression of the cyclin/cyclin-dependent kinase inhibitor, p21 inhibits vascular smooth muscle cell proliferation and neointima formation in the rat carotid artery model of balloon angioplasty. J Clin Invest 1995;96(5):2260–8.

[85] Ohashi N, Matsumori A, Furukawa Y, et al. Role of p38 mitogen-activated protein kinase in neointimal hyperplasia after vascular injury. Arterioscler Thromb Vasc Biol 2000;20(12):2521–6.

[86] Sirois MG, Simons M, Edelman ER. Antisense oligonucleotide inhibition of PDGFR-beta receptor subunit expression directs suppression of intimal thickening. Circulation 1997;95(3):669–76.

[87] Lindner V, Reidy MA. Proliferation of smooth muscle cells after vascular injury is inhibited by an antibody against basic fibroblast growth factor. Proc Natl Acad Sci U S A 1991;88(9):3739–43.

[88] Rectenwald JE, Moldawer LL, Huber TS, et al. Direct evidence for cytokine involvement in neointimal hyperplasia. Circulation 2000;102(14):1697–702.

[89] Usui M, Egashira K, Ohtani K, et al. Anti-monocyte chemoattractant protein-1 gene therapy inhibits restenotic changes (neointimal hyperplasia) after balloon injury in rats and monkeys. FASEB J 2002;16:1833–40.

[90] Egashira K, Zhao Q, Kataoka C. Importance of monocyte chemoattractant protein-1 pathway in neointimal hyperplasia after periarterial injury in mice and monkeys. Circ Res 2002;90:1167–72.

[91] Schober A, Manka D, von Hundelshausen P, et al. Deposition of platelet RANTES triggering monocyte recruitment requires P selectin and is involved in neointima formation after arterial injury. Circulation 2002;106:1523–9.

[92] Fukada J, Schena S, Tack I, et al. FK409, a spontaneous nitric oxide releaser, attenuates allograft vasculopathy in a rat aortic transplant model. Circ Res 2000;87(1):66–72.

[93] McKenna CJ, Burke SE, Opgenorth TJ, et al. Selective ET(A) receptor antagonism reduces neointimal hyperplasia in a porcine coronary stent model. Circulation 1998;97(25):2551–6.

[94] Zou Y, Hu Y, Mayr M, et al. Reduced neointima hyperplasia of vein bypass grafts in intercellular adhesion molecule-1-deficient mice. Circ Res 2000;86(4):434–40.

[95] Wang K, Zhou Z, Zhou X, et al. Prevention of intimal hyperplasia with recombinant soluble P-selectin glycoprotein ligand-immunoglobulin in the porcine coronary artery balloon injury model. J Am Coll Cardiol 2001;38(2):577–82.

[96] Isoda K, Nishikawa K, Kamezawa Y, et al. Osteopontin plays an important role in the development of medial thickening and neointimal formation. Circ Res 2002;91:77–82.

[97] Zhu B, Kuhel DG, Witte DO. Apolipoprotein E inhibits neointimal hyperplasia after arterial injury in mice. Am J Pathol 2000;157:1839–48.

[98] Hu Y, Baker AH, Zou Y, et al. Local gene transfer of tissue inhibitor of metalloproteinase-2 influences vein graft remodeling in a mouse model. Arterioscler Thromb Vasc Biol 2001;21(8):1275–80.

[99] Hayashi K, Nakamura S, Morishita R, et al. In vivo transfer of human hepatocyte growth factor gene accelerates re-endothelialization and inhibits neointimal formation after balloon injury in rat model. Gene Ther 2000;7(19):1664–71.

[100] Humphries S, Bauters C, Meirhaeghe A, et al. The 5A6A polymorphism in the promoter of the stromelysin-1 (MMP3) gene as a risk factor for restenosis. Eur Heart J 2002;23:692–4.

[101] Isbir CS, Akgun S, Yilmaz H, et al. Is there a role of angiotensin-converting enzyme gene polymorphism in the failure of arteriovenous femoral shunts for hemodialysis? Ann Vasc Surg 2001;15(4):443–6.

[102] Keren G. Compensatory enlargement, remodeling, and restenosis. Adv Exp Med Biol 1997;430:187–96.

[103] Libby P, Tanaka H. The molecular bases of restenosis. Prog Cardiovasc Dis 1997;40(2):97–106.

[104] Nakamura Y, Zhao H, Yutani C, et al. Morphometric and histologic assessment of remodeling associated with restenosis after percutaneous transluminal coronary angioplasty. Cardiology 1998;90(2):115–21.

[105] Schwartz RS, Topol EJ, Serruys PW, et al. Artery size, neointima, and remodeling: time for some standards. J Am Coll Cardiol 1998;32(7):2087–94.

[106] Shi Y, O'Brien JE, Fard A, et al. Adventitial myofibroblasts contribute to neointimal formation in injured porcine coronary arteries. Circulation 1996;94(7):1655–64.

[107] Roy-Chaudhury P, McKee L, Miller M, et al. Adventitial fibroblasts contribute to venous neointimal hyperplasia in PTFE dialysis grafts. J Am Soc Nephrol 2001;12:301A.

[108] Sata M, Saiura A, Kunisato A, et al. Hematopoietic stem cells differentiate into vascular cells that participate in the pathogenesis of atherosclerosis. Nat Med 2002;8(4):403–9.

[109] Sata M, Hirata Y, Nagai R. Circulating recipient cells contribute to graft coronary arteriolosclerosis. J Cardiol 2002;39:48–9.

[110] Bayes-Genis A, Campbell JH, Carlson PJ, et al. Macrophages, myofibroblasts and neointimal hy-

perplasia after coronary artery injury and repair. Atherosclerosis 2002;163(1):89–98.

[111] Yokote K, Take A, Nakaseko C, et al. Bone marrow-derived vascular cells in response to injury. J Atheroscler Thromb 2003;10(4):205–10.

[112] Leon MB, Teirstein PS, Moses JW, et al. Localized intracoronary gamma-radiation therapy to inhibit the recurrence of restenosis after stenting. N Engl J Med 2001;344(4):250–6.

[113] Morice MC, Serruys PW, Sousa JE, et al. A randomized comparison of a sirolimus-eluting stent with a standard stent for coronary revascularization. N Engl J Med 2002;346(23): 1773–80.

[114] Stone GW, Ellis SG, Cox DA, et al. A polymer-based, paclitaxel-eluting stent in patients with coronary artery disease. N Engl J Med 2004;350(3): 221–31.

[115] Kelly BS, Heffelfinger SC, Whiting JF, et al. Aggressive venous neointimal hyperplasia in a pig model of arteriovenous graft stenosis. Kidney Int 2002;62(6):2272–80.

[116] Kohler TR, Kirkman TR. Dialysis access failure: a sheep model of rapid stenosis. J Vasc Surg 1999; 30(4):744–51.

[117] Lumsden AB, Chen C, Coyle KA, et al. Nonporous silicone polymer coating of expanded polytetrafluoroethylene grafts reduces graft neointimal hyperplasia in dog and baboon models. J Vasc Surg 1996;24(5):825–33.

[118] Ohno T, Gordon D, San H, et al. Gene therapy for vascular smooth muscle cell proliferation after arterial injury [see comments]. Science 1994;265(5173): 781–4.

[119] Brieger D, Topol E. Local drug delivery systems and prevention of restenosis. Cardiovasc Res 1997;35:405–13.

[120] Sousa JE, Costa MA, Abizaid A, et al. Lack of neointimal proliferation after implantation of sirolimus-coated stents in human coronary arteries: a quantitative coronary angiography and three-dimensional intravascular ultrasound study. Circulation 2001;103(2):192–5.

[121] Fingerle J, Muller RM, Kuhn H, et al. Mechanism of inhibition of neointimal formation by the angiotensin-converting enzyme inhibitor cilazapril. A study in balloon catheter-injured rat carotid arteries. Arterioscler Thromb Vasc Biol 1995; 15(11):1945–50.

[122] Varty K, Allen KE, Jones L, et al. Influence of losartan, an angiotensin receptor antagonist, on neointimal proliferation in cultured human saphenous vein. Br J Surg 1994;81(6):819–22.

[123] Law RE, Meehan WP, Xi XP, et al. Troglitazone inhibits vascular smooth muscle cell growth and intimal hyperplasia. J Clin Invest 1996;98(8): 1897–905.

[124] Law RE, Goetze S, Xi XP, et al. Expression and function of PPARgamma in rat and human vascular smooth muscle cells. Circulation 2000;101(11): 1311–8.

[125] Goetze S, Xi XP, Kawano H, et al. PPAR gamma-ligands inhibit migration mediated by multiple chemoattractants in vascular smooth muscle cells. J Cardiovasc Pharmacol 1999;33(5):798–806.

[126] Huang P, Hawthorne WJ, Peng A, et al. Calcium channel antagonist verapamil inhibits neointimal formation and enhances apoptosis in a vascular graft model. Am J Surg 2001;181(6):492–8.

[127] Bellosta S, Bernini F, Ferri N, et al. Direct vascular effects of HMG-CoA reductase inhibitors. Atherosclerosis 1998;137(Suppl):S101–9.

[128] Dol F, Mares A, Herbert J. Simvastatin inhibits myointimal hyperplasia following carotid artery injury in cholesterol-fed rabbits. Blood Coagul Fibrinolysis 1996;7(8):772–8.

[129] Komukai M, Wajima YS, Tashiro J, et al. Carvastatin suppresses intimal thickening of rabbit carotid artery after balloon catheter injury probably through the inhibition of vascular smooth muscle cell proliferation and migration. Scand J Clin Lab Invest 1999;59(3):159–66.

[130] Walter DH, Rittig K, Bahlmann FH, et al. Statin therapy accelerates reendothelialization: a novel effect involving mobilization and incorporation of bone marrow-derived endothelial progenitor cells. Circulation 2002;105(25):3017–24.

[131] Gregory CR, Huang X, Pratt RE, et al. Treatment with rapamycin and mycophenolic acid reduces arterial intimal thickening produced by mechanical injury and allows endothelial replacement. Transplantation 1995;59(5):655–61.

[132] Gallo R, Padurean A, Jayaraman T, et al. Inhibition of intimal thickening after balloon angioplasty in porcine coronary arteries by targeting regulators of the cell cycle. Circulation 1999;99(16): 2164–70.

[133] Gradzki R, Dhingra RK, Port FK, et al. Use of ACE inhibitors is associated with prolonged survival of arteriovenous grafts. Am J Kidney Dis 2001;38(6):1240–4.

[134] Dialysis Access Consortium. 2002. Available at: http://www.niddk.nih.gov/patient/DAC/DAC.htm. Accessed October 10, 2002.

[135] Mayberg MR, Luo Z, London S, et al. Radiation inhibition of intimal hyperplasia after arterial injury. Radiat Res 1995;142(2):212–20.

[136] Waksman R, Robinson KA, Crocker IR, et al. Endovascular low-dose irradiation inhibits neointima formation after coronary artery balloon injury in swine. A possible role for radiation therapy in restenosis prevention. Circulation 1995;91(5): 1533–9.

[137] Wiedermann JG, Marboe C, Amols H, et al. Intracoronary irradiation markedly reduces neointimal proliferation after balloon angioplasty in swine: persistent benefit at 6-month follow-up. J Am Coll Cardiol 1995;25(6):1451–6.

[138] Raizner AE, Oesterle SN, Waksman R, et al. Inhibition of restenosis with beta-emitting radiotherapy: report of the Proliferation Reduction with Vascular Energy Trial (PREVENT). Circulation 2000;102(9):951–8.

[139] Kelly BS, Narayana A, Heffelfinger SC, et al. External beam radiation attenuates venous neointimal hyperplasia in a pig model of arteriovenous polytetrafluoroethylene (PTFE) graft stenosis. Int J Radiat Oncol Biol Phys 2002;54(1):263–9.

[140] Parikh S, Nori D, Rogers D, et al. External beam radiation therapy to prevent postangioplasty dialysis access restenosis: a feasibility study. Cardiovasc Radiat Med 1999;1(1):36–41.

[141] Cohen GS, Freeman H, Ringold MA, et al. External beam irradiation as an adjunctive treatment in failing dialysis shunts. J Vasc Interv Radiol 2000; 11(3):321–6.

[142] Roy-Chaudhury P, Zuckerman D, Duncan H, et al. Endovascular radiation therapy reduces venous stenosis in PTFE dialysis access grafts. J Am Soc Nephrol 2004;15(11).

[143] Qian HS, Channon K, Neplioueva V, et al. Improved adenoviral vector for vascular gene therapy: beneficial effects on vascular function and inflammation. Circ Res 2001;88(9):911–7.

[144] von der Leyen HE, Gibbons GH, Morishita R, et al. Gene therapy inhibiting neointimal vascular lesion: in vivo transfer of endothelial cell nitric oxide synthase gene. Proc Natl Acad Sci U S A 1995; 92(4):1137–41.

[145] Shears LL II, Kibbe MR, Murdock AD, et al. Efficient inhibition of intimal hyperplasia by adenovirus-mediated inducible nitric oxide synthase gene transfer to rats and pigs in vivo. J Am Coll Surg 1998;187(3):295–306.

[146] Chang MW, Barr E, Seltzer J, et al. Cytostatic gene therapy for vascular proliferative disorders with a constitutively active form of the retinoblastoma gene product. Science 1995;267(5197):518–22.

[147] Mann MJ, Whittemore AD, Donaldson MC, et al. Ex-vivo gene therapy of human vascular bypass grafts with E2F decoy: the PREVENT single-centre, randomised, controlled trial. Lancet 1999; 354(9189):1493–8.

[148] Degertekin M, Serruys PW, Foley DP, et al. Persistent inhibition of neointimal hyperplasia after sirolimus-eluting stent implantation: long-term (up to 2 years) clinical, angiographic, and intravascular ultrasound follow-up. Circulation 2002;106(13): 1610–3.

[149] Hoffer EK, Sultan S, Herskowitz MM, et al. Prospective randomized trial of a metallic intravascular stent in hemodialysis graft maintenance. J Vasc Interv Radiol 1997;8(6):965–73.

[150] Beathard GA. Gianturco self-expanding stent in the treatment of stenosis in dialysis access grafts. Kidney Int 1993;43(4):872–7.

[151] Turmel-Rodrigues LA, Blanchard D, Pengloan J, et al. Wallstents and Craggstents in hemodialysis grafts and fistulas: results for selective indications. J Vasc Interv Radiol 1997;8(6):975–82.

[152] Brauner R, Laks H, Drinkwater DC Jr, et al. Controlled periadventitial administration of verapamil inhibits neointimal smooth muscle cell proliferation and ameliorates vasomotor abnormalities in experimental vein bypass grafts. J Thorac Cardiovasc Surg 1997;114(1):53–63.

[153] Teomim D, Fishbien I, Golomb G, et al. Perivascular delivery of heparin for the reduction of smooth muscle cell proliferation after endothelial injury. J Control Release 1999;60(1):129–42.

[154] Villa AE, Guzman LA, Chen W, et al. Local delivery of dexamethasone for prevention of neointimal proliferation in a rat model of balloon angioplasty. J Clin Invest 1994;93(3):1243–9.

[155] Chaux A, Ruan XM, Fishbein MC, et al. Perivascular delivery of a nitric oxide donor inhibits neointimal hyperplasia in vein grafts implanted in the arterial circulation. J Thorac Cardiovasc Surg 1998;115(3):604–12 [discussion: 12–4].

[156] Edelman ER, Nugent MA, Karnovsky MJ. Perivascular and intravenous administration of basic fibroblast growth factor: vascular and solid organ deposition. Proc Natl Acad Sci U S A 1993;90(4): 1513–7.

[157] Kaul S, Cercek B, Rengstrom J, et al. Polymeric-based perivascular delivery of a nitric oxide donor inhibits intimal thickening after balloon denudation arterial injury: role of nuclear factor-kappaB. J Am Coll Cardiol 2000;35(2): 493–501.

[158] Laham RJ, Sellke FW, Edelman ER, et al. Local perivascular delivery of basic fibroblast growth factor in patients undergoing coronary bypass surgery: results of a phase I randomized, double-blind, placebo-controlled trial. Circulation 1999;100(18): 1865–71.

[159] Lopez JJ, Edelman ER, Stamler A, et al. Local perivascular administration of basic fibroblast growth factor: drug delivery and toxicological evaluation [erratum appears in Drug Metab Dispos 1996; 24(10):1166]. Drug Metab Dispos 1996;24(8): 922–4.

[160] Golomb G, Fishbein I, Banai S, et al. Controlled delivery of a tyrphostin inhibits intimal hyperplasia in a rat carotid artery injury model. Atherosclerosis 1996;125(2):171–82.

[161] Kelly B, Melhem M, Desai P, et al. Perivascular paclitaxel polymers reduce neointimal hyperplasia and venous stenosis in PTFE arteriovenous grafts: a solution for hemodialysis vascular access dysfunction? J Am Soc Nephrol 2004;15(11).

[162] Dardik A, Liu A, Ballermann BJ. Chronic in vitro shear stress stimulates endothelial cell retention on prosthetic vascular grafts and reduces subsequent

in vivo neointimal thickness. J Vasc Surg 1999; 29(1):157–67.

[163] Bowlin GL, Rittgers SE. Electrostatic endothelial cell transplantation within small-diameter (<6 mm) vascular prostheses: a prototype apparatus and procedure. Cell Transplant 1997;6(6):631–7.

[164] Bowlin GL, Rittgers SE. Electrostatic endothelial cell seeding technique for small-diameter (<6 mm) vascular prostheses: feasibility testing. Cell Transplant 1997;6(6):623–9.

[165] Bowlin GL, Rittgers SE, Milsted A, et al. In vitro evaluation of electrostatic endothelial cell transplantation onto 4 mm interior diameter expanded polytetrafluoroethylene grafts. J Vasc Surg 1998; 27(3):504–11.

[166] Szmitko PE, Fedak PW, Weisel RD, et al. Endothelial progenitor cells: new hope for a broken heart. Circulation 2003;107(24):3093–100.

[167] Shirota T, He H, Yasui H, et al. Human endothelial progenitor cell-seeded hybrid graft: proliferative and antithrombogenic potentials in vitro and fabrication processing. Tissue Eng 2003; 9(1):127–36.

[168] LaMuraglia GM, Schiereck J, Heckenkamp J, et al. Photodynamic therapy induces apoptosis in intimal hyperplastic arteries [in process citation]. Am J Pathol 2000;157(3):867–75.

[169] Oda D, Gown AM, Vande Berg JS, et al. The fibroblast-like nature of myofibroblasts. Exp Mol Pathol 1988;49(3):316–29.

ELSEVIER
SAUNDERS

Cardiol Clin 23 (2005) 275–284

CARDIOLOGY
CLINICS

Congestive Heart Failure in Chronic Kidney Disease: Disease-specific Mechanisms of Systolic and Diastolic Heart Failure and Management

Bryan M. Curtis, MD, FRCPC*, Patrick S. Parfrey, MD, FRCPC

Division of Nephrology and Clinical Epidemiology Unit Patient Research Centre, Health Sciences Centre, Memorial University of Newfoundland, 300 Prince Philip Drive, St. John's, Newfoundland A1B 3V6, Canada

In 2002, the National Kidney Foundation-sponsored Kidney Disease Outcomes Quality Initiative published evidence-based guidelines targeting earlier evaluation and intervention in patients who have chronic kidney disease (CKD) [1]. The cornerstone of the working group was the establishment of five stages of kidney disease (Table 1). Rather than using serum creatinine levels alone, the classification system focused on estimated glomerular filtration rate (GFR). Using the GFR allows correlation of severity of kidney function loss and the prevalence of comorbidities associated with the kidney disease. Furthermore, to aid in the understanding and communication of CKD, historical terms that are confusing and sometimes misleading (predialysis, progressive renal disease, progressive renal insufficiency) have been abolished.

Chronic kidney disease and the health care perspective

Kidney disease is a large and growing health care concern. The financial burden of caring for patients who have CKD far exceeds that for prostate or colorectal cancer in men and for breast cancer in black women [2]; the direct cost of caring for a patient receiving dialysis is more than US $50,000 annually [3,4]. In 2001, the incidence of the population of patients who have end-stage renal disease (ESRD) receiving dialysis was greater than 90,000 patients per United States population per year with a total prevalence greater than 290,000 patients per United States population [5]. By 2030, the number of patients who have ESRD may reach 2.24 million [5].

Although hypertension, diabetes, and cardiac disease are associated with a higher prevalence of CKD [6–8], the true prevalence of CKD has been difficult to establish, because estimates are sensitive to the definitions and methods used to identify the disease [6,9,10]. Estimates of CKD are known to be age dependent, because CKD was present in about 8% of the Framingham population at baseline and increased to 20% in the elderly [7]; this percentage, however, may be artificially increased by reliance on a single serum creatinine measurement [10]. Nonetheless, population-based studies such as the Third National Health and Nutrition Survey cross-sectional survey of 29,000 persons revealed that 3% of people over 17 years of age had serum creatinine levels above the ninety-ninth percentile for men and women aged 20 to 39 years without diabetes or hypertension [8]. Furthermore, it is estimated that approximately 8 million people in the United States have kidney disease stage III or higher [11].

Chronic kidney disease and the patient perspective

Morbidity and mortality in the dialysis population remain unacceptable despite the many advances made in the technical aspects of dialysis care. A recent analysis of data from the United States indicates that ESRD leads to more lost life-years than prostate cancer in men and almost as

* Corresponding author.

E-mail address: bcurtis@mun.ca (B.M. Curtis).

Table 1
Five stages of chronic kidney disease

GFR[a] (mL/min/1.73m^2)	Stage
>90[b]	I
60–89	II
30–59	III
15–29	IV
<15 (or dialysis)	V

Abbreviation: GFR, glomerular filtration rate.

[a] GFR: Estimated GFR from any one of several prediction equations using data in addition to serum creatinine alone.

[b] Documented kidney damage with normal or increased GFR.

Adapted from National Kidney Foundation. K/DOQI clinical practice guidelines for chronic kidney disease: evaluation, classification, and stratification. Kidney Disease Outcome Quality Initiative. Am J Kidney Dis 2002;39(2 Suppl 2):S19.

many as breast cancer in black women [2]. The largest contributor to this mortality continues to be cardiac disease [12] as originally reported in the first cohorts of patients commencing chronic dialysis in the 1960s [13]. Furthermore, although the mortality in elderly patients who have kidney disease is a little greater than in the normal population, the cardiovascular mortality in patients who are 25 to 34 years old is several orders of magnitude higher than in normal individuals of the same age [14].

Pathophysiology

Cardiomyopathy and ischemic heart disease

Although cardiovascular disease (CVD) may be clinically generally classified into two disease entities, cardiomyopathy and ischemic heart disease, the presence of these disorders varies from patient to patient, and they frequently overlap (Fig. 1) [15]. Ischemic symptoms may result from coronary artery disease or nonatherosclerotic ischemic disease, with coronary artery disease predisposing to diastolic dysfunction and to systolic failure. Left ventricular hypertrophy (LVH) is usually present in dilated cardiomyopathy but also causes diastolic dysfunction in patients with or without normal systolic function. In a recent longitudinal study of kidney transplant recipients, a model of CKD, the rate of ischemic cardiac events was similar to that seen in the Framingham study, whereas the rate of heart failure events was substantially higher. This finding suggests that

CKD may not be simply a state predisposing to atherosclerosis but may be a milieu predisposing to cardiomyopathy [16].

Cardiomyopathy

The most common symptom of cardiomyopathy in CKD patients, as in the general population, is pulmonary edema, but cardiomyopathy may also manifest as severe exercise intolerance or, in the setting of dialysis, as sudden intradialysis hypotension. These clinical manifestations of pump failure may result from systolic dysfunction, diastolic dysfunction, or a combination of both. Echocardiography [17] may reveal the cardiomyopathy to be a consequence of

1. LVH with diastolic dysfunction: concentric LVH with normal chamber volume and impaired filling, arising from left ventricular (LV) pressure overload, such as from hypertension, arteriosclerosis and aortic stenosis.
2. Dilated cardiomyopathy and systolic failure: eccentric LV dilation with impaired wall motion resulting from left ventricular volume overload. This may occur especially in CKD patients in response to salt and water overload, anemia, and arteriovenous fistula.

Thus, hemodialysis with its associated hemodynamic stresses is the quintessential model for overload cardiomyopathy, for which the end stage is systolic dysfunction.

Because LV growth starts before the initiation of dialysis, its prevalence is inversely related to the level of declining kidney function; anemia, hypertension, and diabetes mellitus are also risk factors for progressive LV growth [18,19]. In kidney transplant recipients, there is evidence that systolic dysfunction, LV dilatation, and concentric hypertrophy present during dialysis improve after transplantation, with concomitant improvement in uremic milieu. In renal transplant recipients, however, hypertension is a risk factor for LV growth, de novo heart failure, and de novo ischemic heart disease [16,20]. Anemia and hypoalbuminemia further predispose patients to de novo heart failure [16].

Ischemic heart disease

Ischemia presents as myocardial infarction or angina resulting from decreased perfusion of the myocardium. Although symptoms of ischemic heart disease are usually attributable to critical coronary artery disease, in about one quarter of

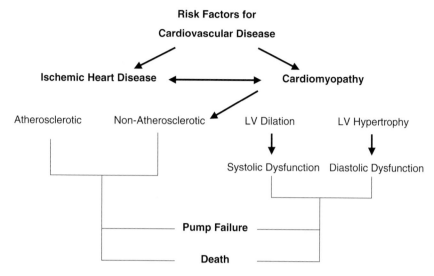

Fig. 1. The relationship of risk factors and cardiovascular disease in patients with chronic kidney disease.

the hemodialysis population these symptoms may also result from nonatherosclerotic disease, caused by small vessel disease and LV hypertrophy [21]. Symptomatic ischemic heart disease is not a significant mortality risk factor independent of congestive heart failure (CHF) [22]. Thus, the underlying cardiomyopathy predisposing the patient to heart failure is probably more prognostically important than coronary perfusion disorders, particularly in nondiabetic persons [23].

Arterial disease

Arteriosclerosis alters the structure of arteries by mechanisms other than atherogenesis. Hemodynamic overload and hypertension, common in CKD, cause intramural vascular remodeling with hypertrophy of the media and subintimal fibrosis. As a result, noncompliant vessels develop with increased stiffness and diameter. If persistent and longstanding, arteriosclerosis may adversely affect LV structure and function by increasing cardiac workload and predisposing the patient to sub-endocardial ischemia [24].

Epidemiology

The prevalence of cardiomyopathy is high in incident dialysis patients, as is the presence of ischemic heart disease and heart failure. In fact, Canadian echocardiographic data revealed only 16% of new dialysis patients have normal hearts, with LV hypertrophy present in 75%, concentric

LVH in 41%, and systolic failure in 16% [17,25]. Clinically, symptomatic ischemic heart disease was present in 38% and heart failure in 35% at first dialysis [26]. The high prevalence of CVD in patients starting dialysis suggests that the predialysis phase of CKD is a state of high cardiac risk. Indeed, earlier in the course of disease LV hypertrophy is already evident in 40% of patients who have moderate CKD [27], and admission rates for CHF are seven times greater in CKD patients than in those without CKD [5].

Risk factors

Because CVD is already well established at the onset of ESRD [28,29], it is vital to understand the interrelationship of CVD and early CKD and to recognize the importance of early intervention. Although the there are limited data on the natural history of CKD in unselected populations, most patients reach ESRD secondary to chronic progressive disease (in North America, largely caused by diabetes and hypertension [5]). Most patients who have CKD do not progress to ESRD, however, either because the CKD is not progressive [30,31] or because they die first-the major contributor of mortality being CVD [7].

In 1997 The National Kidney Foundation convened a task force to examine the epidemic of CVD in chronic kidney disease [32], focusing on decreasing death rates by developing strategies to prevent disease. Specifically, the task force considered whether strategies learned from the general population are applicable to patients who have CKD. Fortunately, interventions that retard the progression of CKD are similar to measures that reduce CVD risk. Thus, cardiac risk factor intervention in the early phases of CKD should reduce the rate of cardiac death and slow the progression of kidney disease. It is currently unknown how much of the increased prevalence of ESRD is caused by the increased prevalence of CKD [33] rather than by a reduction in mortality resulting from improved CVD management [34].

As CKD progresses, the nature of the risk factors evolves from traditional risk factors to those characteristic of chronic uremia. Recognized traditional risk factors identified in the general population include diabetes, hypertension, history of smoking, family history of coronary disease, male gender, older age, high low-density lipoprotein cholesterol, low high-density lipoprotein cholesterol, physical inactivity, menopause, and psychologic stress (Table 2). CKD imparts added cardiac risk through the increased prevalence of coexisting diseases such as hypertension, atherosclerosis, diabetes, and dyslipidemia. Additional excess cardiac risk may also be caused by hemodynamic and metabolic perturbations associated with CKD, including hemodynamic overload, anemia, malnutrition, hypoalbuminemia, inflammation, dyslipidemia, prothrombotic

factors, hyperhomocysteinemia, divalent ion abnormalities, vascular calcification, and hyperparathyroidism and other putative risk factors, including oxidative stress [22,35]. As CKD progresses, it is likely that the prevalence and severity of several risk factors change [36,37].

Although epidemiologic evidence indicates that CKD is a marker of high cardiovascular risk, it is not known whether CKD independently contributes to the risk of cardiovascular mortality [38,39]. It remains unclear how much of the association between kidney and vascular disease results from (1) vascular disease causing kidney disease, (2) kidney disease causing vascular disease, or (3) common underlying factors promoting the progression of both. It is likely that each of these mechanisms contributes.

Management

Hypertension

Hypertension is common in CKD, affecting about three quarters of the patients, and the prevalence of hypertension increases as the GFR declines. Treatment reduces mortality in those at risk for cardiovascular events [40–43], and achieving a target blood pressure lower than 130/80 mm Hg in patients who have CKD also slows progression of kidney disease [30,40,44–48]. Patients

Table 2
The spectrum of risk factors for cardiovascular disease

Traditional	Increased prevalence of coexisting diseases	Uremia-related
Age	Diabetes	Hemodynamic overload
Gender	Hypertension	Anemia
Race	Dyslipidemia	Electrolyte abnormalities
History of smoking	Atherosclerosis	Hyperparathyroidism
Family history	Proteinuria	Calcium/phosphate abnormalities
Physical inactivity	Left ventricular hypertrophy	Vascular calcification
Body mass index		Malnutrition
Menopause		Hypoalbuminemia
Psychologic stress		Inflammation
Fibrinogen		C-reactive protein
		Prothrombotic factors
		Hyperhomocysteinemia
		Increased oxidative stress
		Endothelial activation
		Prothrombotic factors
		Cytokines
		Advanced glycation end products
		Dialysis modality
		Acute rejection after transplantation
		Transplant immunosuppressives

who have proteinuria greater than 1 g/24 hours benefit from even lower blood pressure (<125/75) [30]. Three or four different medications are often required to reach these goals.

Interruption of the renin-angiotensin system

Angiotensin-converting enzyme (ACE) inhibitors clearly improve symptoms, morbidity, and survival in nonuremic individuals who have heart failure [49] and in patients who have CKD [50]. ACE inhibition is beneficial to those who have diastolic and systolic dysfunction [51,52]. Furthermore, the use of ACE inhibition reduces the progression of CKD, reduces proteinuria, and regresses LVH [53–55]. ACE inhibitors should also be used to prevent CHF in asymptomatic patients whose LV ejection fraction is less than 35% [56] and in postmyocardial infarction patients who have an ejection fraction of 40% or less [57]. Angiotensin-receptor blockers also reduce ESRD [58,59] and may benefit patients who have diastolic dysfunction [51,60]. ACE inhibitors and angiotensin-receptor blockers are relatively contraindicated in patients who have renovascular disease and volume depletion, and hyperkalemia in the later stages of CKD can make interruption of the renin-angiotensin system problematic.

Beta-blockers

Beta-blockade reduces morbidity and mortality in patients who have heart failure [61,62] and after myocardial infarction [63] and seems to be equally efficacious in patients who have CKD [64]. Patients who have CKD, however, and particularly in the later stages, often have conditions (sinus-node dysfunction, hypotension, and cardiac conduction abnormalities) that are contraindications to the use of bets-blockers.

Diuretics

Aside from their use as antihypertensives, diuretics have been a cornerstone of acute and chronic therapy in all patients who have cardiac failure, including those with CKD. The effects of loop diuretics are attenuated as the GFR declines, but the effects are not reduced as severely as those of thiazides. The synergistic effect of loop diuretics and thiazides on salt and water excretion and blood pressure persists, even at relatively advanced stages of CKD. Acutely, intravenous loop diuretics such as furosemide have a short-term benefit for symptomatic treatment of heart failure even in the presence of minimal or no

glomerular filtration because of their vasodilating properties. The effects of aldosterone antagonists are unpredictable in patients who have CKD. They are weak diuretics, but they are reported to be of benefit in cardiac disease or in reducing proteinuria in patients who have CKD [65,66].

Digoxin

Digoxin improves symptoms in non-CKD patients who have heart failure, and clinical deterioration may occur when it is discontinued [51,67]. There is a theoretical concern that digoxin may aggravate isolated diastolic dysfunction, because increased contractility induced by digoxin could worsen diastolic function by impairing myocardial relaxation [51]. Nonetheless, evidence suggests that patients who have heart failure and preserved ejection fraction treated with digoxin had fewer hospitalizations and improved symptoms [67]. Therefore, digoxin is recommended for use in patients who have CKD and heart failure and who have systolic dysfunction with or without atrial fibrillation. It should be used with caution in patients who have diastolic dysfunction and atrial fibrillation and if atrial fibrillation with a rapid ventricular response is present.

Diabetes management

Diabetes in patients who have moderate to severe CKD is a risk factor for cardiovascular deterioration [68]. Furthermore, in kidney transplant recipients, diabetes is an independent risk factor for ischemic heart disease [16,69,70] and heart failure [16]. Controlling diabetes has beneficial effects for early microvascular disease [71,72]. Metformin has shown benefit for macrovascular disease in obese type 2 diabetics [73] but is contraindicated in the later stages of CKD.

Smoking

Smoking status is associated independently with cardiac disease, peripheral vascular disease, and mortality but has received little attention in the CKD population [74]. Approximately 25% of patients who have CKD and more than 50% of dialysis and transplant patients have a history of cigarette use [74]. In 2003, 14% of dialysis patients in the United States continued to smoke [74]. Smoking is a potentially modifiable risk factor. Cessation reduces cardiovascular outcomes [75], may slow CKD progression [76–78], and improves quality of life [79] but may require intense intervention for maximal effect [80].

Statin therapy

Statin therapy in patients who have CKD seems to have an efficacy similar to that in patients who have CVD but do not have CKD [81–83]. The role of statin therapy, independent of lipid lowering, includes endothelial stabilization and antithrombogenic and anti-inflammatory mechanisms that may modulate its effectiveness. Patients who have CKD, particularly those receiving dialysis, have increased markers of inflammation such as C-reactive protein. This inflammatory state is deemed to confer an independent increased risk of CVD through oxidative stress and resultant atherosclerosis [83]. Although statins have been shown to reduce C-reactive protein levels in patients who have normal kidney function, it is not known whether this reduction translates into clinical benefit independent of lipid reduction.

Erythropoietin

There is increasing awareness of the role of anemia in the investigation and management of CHF [84]. The combination of CKD and anemia is independently associated with an increased risk of coronary heart disease and stroke in middle-aged patients [85,86] and, in patients who have CKD stage III or greater, anemia is associated with LV growth [87]. In kidney transplant recipients, anemia is an independent risk factor for the development of electrocardiographically diagnosed LV hypertrophy [16] and of symptomatic heart failure [20]. Current CKD guidelines recommend treating anemia to achieve a hemoglobin level of 110 to 120 g/L to improve quality of life, decrease hospitalization, and potentially improve LVH [88–93]. No randomized, controlled trials have shown that normalization of anemia with erythropoietin improves cardiac disease [94–98].

Nephrology referral

Late referral to nephrology before dialysis has been recognized as a problem for many years. It is associated with increased cost and morbidity [98–101]. Published recommendations emphasize timely referral to maximize potential gains from involvement of specialized nephrology teams [102]. A minimal recommendation would be referral at GFR levels greater than 60 mL/min if the primary medical care provider cannot identify the cause of the kidney disease or requires help in the management of disease. All potential dialysis patients who have GFR levels less than 30 mL/min should be seen by a nephrology team to ensure adequate clinical and psychologic preparation for kidney replacement therapy [102,103].

Dialysis

Ultrafiltration of extracellular fluid by dialysis is the ideal treatment for patients who have stage V CKD and acutely symptomatic CHF. In the patient receiving chronic dialysis, the goal is to use fluid removal to control both volume status and blood pressure. Unfortunately, this treatment may cause dialysis-associated hypotension that complicates the use of oral antihypertensives required for other indications (eg, beta-blockers for angina). Hemodialysis usually requires intradialysis anticoagulation, which may increase the bleeding risk of other cardiac medications such as acetyl salicyclic acid.

Summary

There is a high burden of cardiac disease in the CKD population. Severe LVH, dilated cardiomyopathy, and coronary artery disease occur frequently and result in the manifestations of CHF, which is probably more important with respect to prognosis than symptomatic. Multiple risk factors for CVD include traditional risk factors and those unique to the CKD population. Furthermore, the distinctive aspects of CKD patients sometimes warrant special consideration in making management decisions. Nonetheless, interventions such as controlling hypertension, specific pharmacologic options, lifestyle modification, anemia management, and early nephrology referral are recommended when appropriate.

References

[1] National Kidney Foundation K/DOQI clinical practice guidelines for chronic kidney disease: evaluation, classification, and stratification. Am J Kidney Dis 2002;39(2 Suppl 2):S1–266.
[2] Kiberd BA, Clase CM. Kidney Disease Outcome Quality Initiative. J Am Soc Nephrol 2002;13:1635–44.
[3] Goeree R, Manalich J, Grootendorst P, et al. Cost analysis of dialysis treatments for end-stage renal disease (ESRD). Clin Invest Med 1995;18(6):455–64.
[4] Lee H, Manns B, Taub K, et al. Cost analysis of ongoing care of patients with end-stage renal disease: the impact of dialysis modality and dialysis access. Am J Kidney Dis 2002;40(3):611–22.

[5] US Renal Data System. USRDS 2003 Annual Data Report: Atlas of End-Stage Renal Disease in the United States. Bethesda (MD): National Institutes of Health, National Institute of Diabetes and Digestive and Kidney Diseases; 2003.

[6] Nissenson AR, Periera BJ, Collins AJ, et al. Prevalence and characteristics of individuals with chronic kidney disease in a large health maintenance organization. Am J Kidney Dis 2001;37:1177–83.

[7] Culleton BF, Larson MG, Evans JC, et al. Prevalence and correlates of elevated serum creatinine levels. Arch Intern Med 1999;159:1785–90.

[8] Coresh J, Wei GL, McQuillan G, et al. Prevalence of high blood pressure and elevated serum creatinine level in the United States: findings from the Third National Health and Nutrition Examination Survey (1988–1994). Arch Intern Med 2001;161:1207–16.

[9] Clase CM, Garg AX, Kiberd BA. Prevalence of low glomerular filtration rate in nondiabetic Americans: Third National Health and Nutrition Survey (NHANES III). J Am Soc Nephrol 2002;13:1338–49.

[10] Hsu C-Y, Chertow GM, Curhan GC. Methodological issues in studying the epidemiology of mild to moderate chronic renal insufficiency. Kidney Int 2002;61:1567–76.

[11] Coresh J, Astor BC, Greene T, et al. Prevalence of chronic kidney disease and decreased kidney function in the adult US population: Third National Health and Nutrition Examination Survey. Am J Kidney Dis 2003;41(1):1–12.

[12] Culleton BF, Larson MG, Wilson PWF, et al. Cardiovascular disease and mortality in a community-based cohort with mild renal insufficiency. Kidney Int 1999;56:2214–9.

[13] Lazarus JM, Lowrie EG, Hampers CL, et al. Cardiovascular disease in uremic patients on hemodialysis. Kidney Int Suppl 1975;(2):167–75.

[14] Foley RN, Parfrey PS, Sarnak MJ. Epidemiology of cardiovascular disease in chronic renal disease. J Am Soc Nephrol 1998;9(12 Suppl):S16–23.

[15] London G, Parfrey PS. Cardiac disease in chronic uremia: pathogenesis. Adv Ren Replace Ther 1997;4:194–211.

[16] Rigatto C, Parfrey P, Foley R, et al. Congestive heart failure in renal transplant recipients: risk factors, outcomes, and relationship with ischemic heart disease. J Am Soc Nephrol 2002;13(4):1084–90.

[17] Parfrey PS, Foley RN, Harnett JD, et al. Outcome and risk factors for left ventricular disorders in chronic uremia. Nephrol Dial Transplant 1996;11:1277–85.

[18] Foley RN, Parfrey PS, Kent GM, et al. Longterm evolution of cardiomyopathy in dialysis patients. Kidney Int 1998;54:1720–5.

[19] Levin A, Thompson CR, Ethier J, et al. Left ventricular mass index increase in early renal disease: impact of decline in hemoglobin. Am J Kidney Dis 1999;34:125–34.

[20] Rigatto C, Foley RN, Kent GM, et al. Long-term changes in left ventricular hypertrophy after renal transplantation. Transplantation 2000;27;70(4):570–5.

[21] Rostand RG, Kirk KA, Rutsky EA. Dialysis ischemic heart disease: insights from coronary angiography. Kidney Int 1984;25:653–9.

[22] Parfrey PS. Pathogenesis of cardiac disease in dialysis patients. Semin Dial 1999;12:62–8.

[23] Foley RN, Culleton BF, Parfrey PS, et al. Cardiac disease in diabetic end-stage renal disease. Diabetologia 1997;40(11):1307–12.

[24] London GM, Guerin AP, Marchais SJ. Hemodynamic overload in end-stage renal disease patients. Semin Dial 1999;12:77–83.

[25] Foley RN, Parfrey PS, Harnett JD, et al. Clinical and echocardiographic disease in patients starting end-stage renal disease therapy. Kidney Int 1995;47(1):186–92.

[26] Barrett BJ, Parfrey PS, Morgan J, et al. Prediction of early death in end-stage renal disease patients starting dialysis. Am J Kidney Dis 1997;29:214–22.

[27] Levin A, Singer J, Thompson CR, et al. Prevalent left ventricular hypertrophy in the predialysis population: identifying opportunities for intervention. Am J Kidney Dis 1996;27(3):347–54.

[28] Dialysis and renal transplantation. Canadian Organ Replacement Register 2001, Vol. 1. Ottawa (Ontario, Canada): Canadian Institute for Health Information; 2001.

[29] Sarnak MJ, Levey AS. Cardiovascular disease and chronic renal disease: a new paradigm. Am J Kidney Dis 2000;35(4 Suppl 1):S117–31.

[30] Klahr S, Levey AS, Beck GJ, et al for the Modification of Diet in Renal Disease Study Group. The effects of dietary protein restriction and blood pressure control on the progression of chronic renal disease. N Engl J Med 1994;330:877–84.

[31] Hunsicker LG, Adler S, Caggiula A, et al for the Modification of Diet in Renal Disease Study Group. Predictors of the progression of renal disease in the Modification of Diet in Renal Disease Study. Kidney Int 1997;51:1908–19.

[32] National Kidney Foundation Task Force on Cardiovascular Disease. Controlling the epidemic of cardiovascular disease in chronic renal disease. Am J Kid Dis 1998;32(Suppl 3):S1–199.

[33] Bolton WK, Kliger AS. Chronic renal insufficiency: current understandings and their implications. Am J Kidney Dis 2000;36(6 Suppl 3):S4–12.

[34] Sarnak MJ, Levey AS. Cardiovascular disease and chronic renal disease: a new paradigm. Am J Kidney Dis 2000;36(4 Suppl 1):S117–31.

[35] Foley RN, Parfrey PS, Sarnak MJ. Clinical epidemiology of cardiovascular disease in chronic renal disease. Am J Kid Dis 1998;32(Suppl 3):112–9.

[36] Landray MJ, Thambyrajah J, McGlynn FJ, et al. Epidemiological evaluation of known and suspected cardiovascular risk factors in chronic renal impairment. Am J Kidney Dis 2001;38:537–46.

[37] Sarnak MJ, Coronado BE, Greene T, et al. Cardiovascular disease risk factors in chronic renal insufficiency. Clin Nephrol 2002;57:327–35.

[38] Muntner P, Jiang H, Hamm L, et al. Renal insufficiency and subsequent death resulting from cardiovascular disease in the United States. J Am Soc Nephrol 2002;13:745–53.

[39] Garg AX, Clark WF, Haynes B, et al. Moderate renal insufficiency and the risk of cardiovascular mortality: results from the NHANES I. Kidney Int 2002;61:1486–94.

[40] Hansson L, Zanchetti A, Carruthers SG, et al, for the HOT Study Group. Effects of intensive blood pressure lowering and low dose aspirin in patients with hypertension: principal results of the Hypertension Optimal Treatment (HOT) randomized trial. Lancet 1998;351:1755–62.

[41] Estacio RO, Gifford N, Jeffers BW, et al. Effect of blood pressure control on diabetic microvascular complications in patients with hypertension and type 2 diabetes. Diabetes Care 2000;23(Suppl 2): B54–64.

[42] UK Prospective Diabetes Study Group. Tight blood pressure control and risk of macrovascular and microvascular complications in type 2 diabetes: UKPDS 38. BMJ 1998;317:703–13.

[43] PROGRESS Collaborative Group. Randomised trial of a perindopril-based blood-pressure-lowering regimen among 6,105 individuals with previous stroke or transient ischaemic attack. Lancet 2001; 358:1033–41.

[44] Chobanian AV, Bakris GL, Black HR, et al and the National High Blood Pressure Education Program Coordinating Committee. The seventh report of the Joint National Committee on Prevention, Detection, Evaluation, and Treatment of High Blood Pressure. JAMA 2003;289:2560–71.

[45] Bakris G, Williams M, Dworkin L, et al. Preserving renal function in adults with hypertension and diabetes: a consensus approach. Am J Kidney Dis 2000;36:646–61.

[46] Toto RD, Mithell HC, Smith RD, et al. Strict blood pressure control and progression of renal disease in hypertensive nephrosclerosis. Kidney Int 1995;48:851–9.

[47] Lazarus JM, Bourgoignie JJ, Buckalew VM, et al. Achievement and safety of a low blood pressure goal in chronic renal disease. Hypertension 1997; 29:641–50.

[48] Weir MR, Dworkin LD. Antihypertensive drugs, dietary salt, and renal protection: how low should you go and with which therapy? Am J Kidney Dis 1998;32:1–22.

[49] The SOLVD Investigators. Effect of enalapril on survival in patients with reduced left ventricular ejection fractions and congestive heart failure. N Engl J Med 1991;325:293–302.

[50] Mann JFE, Gerstein HC, Pogue J, et al. Renal insufficiency as a predictor of cardiovascular outcomes and the impact of ramipril: the HOPE randomized trial. Ann Intern Med 2001;134: 629–36.

[51] Murphy SW. Diastolic dysfunction. Curr Treat Options Cardiovasc Med 2004;6(1):61–8.

[52] Lewis EJ, Hunsicker LG, Bain, et al. The effect of angiotensin-converting-enzyme inhibition on diabetic nephropathy. N Engl J Med 1993;329: 1456–61.

[53] Ravid M, Savin H, Jutrin I, et al. Long-term stabilizing effect of angiotensin-converting enzyme inhibition on plasma creatinine and on proteinuria in normotensive type II diabetic patients. Ann Intern Med 1993;118:577–81.

[54] Philipp T, Anlauf M, Distler A, et al on behalf of the HANE Trial Research Group. Randomized, double blind, multicentre comparison of hydrochlorothiazide, atenolol, nitrendipine, and enalapril in antihypertensive treatment: results of the HANE study. BMJ 1997;15:154–9.

[55] Jafar TH, Schmid CH, Landa M, et al. Angiotensin-converting enzyme inhibitors and progression of nondiabetic renal disease. A meta-analysis of patient-level data. Ann Intern Med 2001;135:73–87.

[56] The SOLVD Investigators. Effect of enalapril on mortality and the development of heart failure in asymptomatic patients with reduced left ventricular ejection fractions. N Engl J Med 1992;327:685–91.

[57] Pfeffer MA, Braunwald E, Moyé LA, et al. Effect of captopril on mortality and morbidity in patients with left ventricular dysfunction after myocardial infarction. N Engl J Med 1992;327:669–77.

[58] Brenner BM, Cooper ME, deZeeuw D, et al. Effects of losartan on renal and cardiovascular outcomes in patients with type 2 diabetes and nephropathy. N Engl J Med 2001;345:861–9.

[59] Lewis EJ, Hunsicker LG, Clarke WR, et al. Renoprotective effect of the angiotensin receptor antagonist irbesartan in patients with nephropathy due to type 2 diabetes. N Engl J Med 2001;345:851–60.

[60] Dahlof B, Devereux RB, Kjeldsen SE, et al. Cardiovascular morbidity and mortality in the Losartan Intervention For Endpoint reduction in hypertension study (LIFE): a randomised trial against atenolol. Lancet 2002;359(9311):995–1003.

[61] Bhagat K, Hakim JG. Why beta blockers should be used in heart failure. Cent Afr J Med 1999;45: 187–9.

[62] Lonn E, McKelvie R. Drug treatment in heart failure. BMJ 2000;320:1188–92.

[63] Ryan TJ, Anderson JL, Antman EM, et al. ACC/ AHA guidelines for the management of patients with acute myocardial infarction. A report of the American College of Cardiology/American Heart Association Task Force on Practice Guidelines

(Committee on Management of Acute Myocardial Infarction). J Am Coll Cardiol 1996;28:1328–428.

[64] McAlister FA, Ezekowitz J, Tonelli M, et al. Renal insufficiency and heart failure: prognostic and therapeutic implications from a prospective cohort study. Circulation 2004;109(8):1004–9.

[65] Chrysostomou A, Becker G. Spironolactone in addition to ACE inhibition to reduce proteinuria in patients with chronic renal disease. N Engl J Med 2001;345:925–6.

[66] Pitt B, Zannad F, Remme WJ, et al. The effect of spironolactone on morbidity and mortality in patients with severe heart failure. N Engl J Med 1999;341:709–17.

[67] The Digitalis Investigation Group. The effect of digoxin on mortality and morbidity in patients with heart failure. N Engl J Med 1997;336:525–33.

[68] Levin A, Djurdjev O, Barrett B, et al. Cardiovascular disease in patients with chronic kidney disease: getting to the heart of the matter. Am J Kidney Dis 2001;38(6):1398–407.

[69] London GM, Pannier B, Marchais SJ, et al. Calcification of the aortic valve in the dialyzed patient. J Am Soc Nephrol 2000;11:778–83.

[70] McLenachan JM, Henderson E, Dargie HJ. A possible mechanism of sudden death in hypertensive left ventricular hypertrophy. J Hypertens 1997; 5(Suppl 5):630.

[71] The Diabetes Control and Complications Trial/ Epidemiology of Diabetes Interventions and Complications Research Group. Retinopathy and nephropathy in patients with type I diabetes four years after a trial of intensive therapy. N Engl J Med 2000;342:381–9.

[72] Prospective Diabetes Study UK. (UKPDS) Group. Intensive blood-glucose control with sulphonylureas or insulin compared with conventional treatment and risk of complications in patients with type 2 diabetes (UKPDS 33). Lancet 1998;352: 837–53.

[73] Prospective Diabetes Study UK (UKPDS) Group. Effect of intensive blood-glucose control with metformin on complications in overweight patients with type 2 diabetes (UKPDS 34). Lancet 1998; 352:854–65.

[74] Foley RN, Herzog CA, Collins AJ. Smoking and cardiovascular outcomes in dialysis patients: the United States Renal Data System Wave 2 study. Kidney Int 2003;63(4):1462–7.

[75] Wilson K, Gibson N, Willan A, et al. Effect of smoking cessation on mortality after myocardial infarction: meta-analysis of cohort studies. Arch Intern Med 2000;160:939–44.

[76] Regalado M, Yang S, Wesson DE. Cigarette smoking is associated with augmented progression of renal insufficiency in severe essential hypertension. Am J Kidney Dis 2000;35:687–94.

[77] Orth SR, Stockmann A, Conradt C, et al. Smoking as a risk factor for end-stage renal failure in men with primary renal disease. Kidney Int 1998;54: 926–31.

[78] Orth SR. Smoking and the kidney. J Am Soc Nephrol 2002;13:1663–72.

[79] Mulder I, Tijhuis M, Smit HA, et al. Smoking cessation and quality of life: the effect of amount of smoking and time since quitting. Prev Med 2001; 33:653–60.

[80] Feeney GF, McPherson A, Connor JP, et al. Randomized controlled trial of two cigarette quit programmes in coronary care patients after acute myocardial infarction. Intern Med J 2001;31: 470–5.

[81] Tonelli M, Moye L, Sacks FM, et al. Cholesterol and Recurrent Events (CARE) Trial Investigators. Pravastatin for secondary prevention of cardiovascular events in persons with mild chronic renal insufficiency. Ann Intern Med 2003;138(2):98–104.

[82] Collins R, Armitage J, Parish S, et al for the Heart Protection Study Collaborative Group. MRC/ BHF heart protection study of cholesterol-lowering with simvastatin in 5963 people with diabetes: a randomised placebo-controlled trial. Lancet 2003;14;361(9374):2005–16.

[83] Moore R. Therapeutic considerations for the use of statin therapy in chronic renal disease. Nephron Clin Pract 2003;95(4):c107–15.

[84] Foley RN. Anaemia and the heart: what's new in 2003? Nephrol Dial Transplant 2003;18(Suppl 8):viii, 13–6.

[85] Jurkovitz CT, Abramson JL, Vaccarino LV, et al. Association of high serum creatinine and anemia increases the risk of coronary events: results from the prospective community-based atherosclerosis risk in communities (ARIC) study. J Am Soc Nephrol 2003;14(11):2919–25.

[86] Abramson JL, Jurkovitz CT, Vaccarino V, et al. Chronic kidney disease, anemia, and incident stroke in a middle-aged, community-based population: the ARIC Study. Kidney Int 2003;64(2): 610–5.

[87] Levin A, Singer J, Thompson CR, Ross H, et al. Prevalent left ventricular hypertrophy in the predialysis population: identifying opportunities for intervention. Am J Kidney Dis 1996;27(3):347–54.

[88] Canadian Erythropoietin Study Group. Association between recombinant human erythropoietin and quality of life and exercise capacity of patients receiving haemodialysis. BMJ 1990;300:573–8.

[89] Collins AJ, Ma JZ, Xia A, et al. Trends in anemia treatment with erythropoietin usage and patients outcomes. Am J Kidney Dis 1998;32(6 Suppl 4): S133–41.

[90] Sheingold S, Churchill D, Muirhead N, et al. The impact of recombinant human erythropoietin on medical care costs for hemodialysis patients in Canada. Soc Sci Med 1992;34:983–91.

[91] Powe N, Griffiths RI, Watson AJ, et al. Effect of recombinant erythropoietin on hospital admission,

readmission, length of stay and costs in dialysis patients. J Am Soc Nephrol 1994;4:1455–65.

[92] Martinez-Vea A, Bardaji A, Garcia C, et al. Long term myocardial effects of correction of anemia with recombinant human erythropoietin in aged patients on hemodialysis. Am J Kidney Dis 1992; 19:353–7.

[93] Revicki DA, Brown RE, Feeny DH, et al. Health-related quality of life associated with recombinant human erythropoietin therapy for predialysis chronic renal disease patients. Am J Kidney Dis 1995;25:548–54.

[94] Besarab A, Bolton WK, Browne JK, et al. The effects of normal as compared with low hematocrit values in patients with cardiac disease who are receiving hemodialysis and epoetin. N Engl J Med 1998;339:584–90.

[95] Foley RN, Parfrey PS, Morgan J, et al. Effect of hemoglobin levels in hemodialysis patients with asymptomatic cardiomyopathy. Kidney Int 2000; 58(3):1325–35.

[96] Roger SD, McMahon LP, Clarkson A, et al. Effects of early and late intervention with epoetin alpha on left ventricular mass among patients with chronic kidney disease (stage 3 or 4): results of a randomized clinical trial. J Am Soc Nephrol 2004;15(1):148–56.

[97] Foley RN, Parfrey PS, Wittreich BH, et al. The effect of higher haemoglobin levels on left ventricular cavity volume in patients starting haemodialysis: a blinded, randomised, controlled trial in 596 patients without symptomatic cardiac disease (abstract MO12 presented at the European Renal Association-European Dialysis Transplant Association), Lisbon, Portugal. 2004. Available at: http://www.abstracts2view.com/era/authorindex.php. Accessed January 26, 2005.

[98] Levin A. Consequences of late referral on patient outcomes. Nephrol Dial Transplant 2000;15(Suppl 3):8–13.

[99] Stack AG. Impact of timing of nephrology referral and pre-ESRD care on mortality risk among new ESRD patients in the United States. Am J Kidney Dis 2003;41(2):310–8.

[100] Kinchen KS, Sadler J, Fink N, et al. The timing of specialist evaluation in chronic kidney disease and mortality. Ann Intern Med 2002;137(6): 479–86.

[101] McLaughlin K, Manns B, Culleton B, et al. An economic evaluation of early versus late referral of patients with progressive renal insufficiency. Am J Kidney Dis 2001;38(5):1122–8.

[102] Mendelssohn DC, Barrett BJ, Brownscombe LM, et al. Elevated levels of serum creatinine: recommendations for management and referral. Can Med Assoc J 1999;161(4):413–7.

[103] McClellan WM, Knight DF, Karp H, et al. Early detection and treatment of renal disease in hospitalized diabetic and hypertensive patients: important differences between practice and published guidelines. Am J Kidney Dis 1997;29(3):368–75.

ELSEVIER
SAUNDERS

Cardiol Clin 23 (2005) 285–298

CARDIOLOGY
CLINICS

Coronary Artery Disease and Peripheral Vascular Disease in Chronic Kidney Disease: An Epidemiological Perspective

Austin G. Stack, MD, MSc, MRCPI, FASN[a,b,*]

[a]Regional Kidney Centre, Department of Medicine, Floor D, Letterkenny General Hospital, County Donegal, Ireland
[b]Internal Medicine, University of Texas Health Science Center, 6431 Fanin Street, Houston, TX 77030, USA

Since Lindner's sentinel observation in 1974 highlighting the substantial burden of cardiac disease among patients receiving chronic dialysis, it has become increasingly apparent that accelerated atherosclerosis is an inevitable consequence of progressive loss in kidney function, resulting in significant morbidity and mortality [1–3]. Although there is consensus that chronic kidney disease (CKD) represents a state of accelerated atherosclerosis, and there is accumulating epidemiologic evidence linking worsening kidney function with increased cardiovascular event rates, direct evidence demonstrating a causal relationship has been lacking [4–12]. The critical nature of these relationships has resulted in the establishment of national task forces with support from national agencies to assist in describing the extent of the problem, to define better the contribution of known risk factors and potential novel risk factors to disease occurrence, and finally to develop therapeutic strategies for prevention [3].

This article describes the epidemiology of coronary artery disease (CAD) and peripheral vascular disease (PVD) among patients who have CKD. Special emphasis is given to studies that have described the natural history of these vascular conditions at different stages of CKD in accordance with current recommendations from the National Kidney Disease Outcomes Quality Initiative [13].

Assessing the burden of disease

Coronary artery disease

During the last decade, population-based and center-specific studies have provided estimates of the prevalence of CAD and PVD, but much of these data is limited to patients who have advanced kidney failure requiring renal replacement therapy [14–16]. In general, defining the prevalence of a condition requires accurate, reliable, and validated methods of disease ascertainment. Moreover, for comparison of disease prevalence among groups and throughout calendar periods, a standardized approach offers the best strategy for recognizing changing trends. Unfortunately, definitions used to define the presence of these conditions have varied widely, and the lack of a standardized approach in CAD and PVD ascertainment may have resulted in some variation.

The prevalence of clinical CAD among patients with newly diagnosed end-stage renal disease (ESRD) is between 38% and 40% [16]. In an analysis of 4025 patients from the Dialysis and Mortality and Morbidity Study (DMMS) Wave 2, Stack and colleagues [16] found that clinical CAD was present in 38% of patients who have new ESRD. In this study, CAD was defined as being present if patients had a history of coronary disease, myocardial infarction, or angina, prior angiography for CAD, abnormal angiogram or angioplasty, or coronary artery bypass grafting. Myocardial infarction was present in 14% and suspected in an additional 3%. Nineteen percent patients had a history of angina pectoris, and an additional 4% had suspected angina. Data from

* Regional Kidney Centre, Department of Medicine, Letterkenny General Hospital, Ireland.
  E-mail address: Austin.Stack@mailb.hse.ie

the Choices for Healthy Outcomes in Caring for ESRD (CHOICE) study found CAD present in 41.6% and myocardial infarction present in 18% [17]. Despite the lack of a standardized definition of CAD between these two separately administered studies, the similarity in prevalence rates is remarkable. Moreover, these values are also similar in magnitude to estimates derived from the Canadian Organ Replacement Registry (CORR) [18] and the Australian and New Zealand Organ Replacement Registries (ANZDATA) [15]. In general, rates are higher in older persons, diabetics, and those with coexisting cardiovascular conditions. An increasing prevalence of CAD at ESRD onset may be expected if current trends in ESRD incidence and prevalence prevail, but comprehensive analysis of longitudinal trends has not been performed. A preliminary comparison of CAD prevalence in the subjects enrolled in the Case Mix Severity Study (who had new ESRD at the study inception in 1986 and 1987) and those enrolled in DMMS Wave 2 found strikingly similar CAD rates (40% versus 38%), suggesting that burden of CAD has remained relatively stable at dialysis inception despite an aging dialysis population.

Despite the high prevalence of clinical CAD, the true estimate of CAD in this high-risk population, although undetermined, is probably substantially larger than estimates obtained from registry data or chart review. The average patient who reaches ESRD in the United States has a 42% probability of having diabetes, a 30% probability of having hypertension, and has an average age of 61 years, characteristics that are associated with silent coronary ischemia [19]. As a result, underestimation rather than overestimation of CAD prevalence using registry data is highly likely, and the true prevalence of CAD is almost certainly higher than estimates reported from these data. Indeed, a recent retrospective cohort by Gradaus and colleagues [20] found a strikingly high prevalence of angiographic CAD among 26 patients receiving maintenance dialysis. Of the entire cohort (n = 26), 65% had angiographic CAD, and 34% had at least two-vessel involvement. Even more alarming, 50% of the cohort demonstrated significant progression in disease, defined as the development of a hemodynamically significant stenosis of more than 50%. The availability of novel coronary screening methods such as electron beam CT may push this estimate even higher. Preliminary observations demonstrate a direct relationship between calcium scores and the prevalence of atherosclerotic vascular disease [21]. Whether these scores are related to angiographically significant disease remains undetermined, however.

Peripheral vascular disease

PVD is increasingly recognized as an important contributor to adverse outcomes in patients who have advanced CKD [22–24]. Unfortunately, unlike CAD, epidemiologic studies describing the natural history of PVD are limited. Precise estimates of disease prevalence, again, are influenced by the underlying definition of PVD, which varies according to its clinical presentation. Defining patients who have PVD as those who had a prior diagnosis of PVD, amputation, intermittent claudication, or absent peripheral pulses, we have shown that 21% of newly diagnosed ESRD patients in the United States have clinical significant PVD using data from the DMMS Wave 2 study [16]. Among established hemodialysis patients, O'Hare and colleagues [22] reported similar prevalence (24%) using the same case-based definition. As before, a concern with these clinical definitions is the potential for the underestimation of true disease prevalence. Leskinen and colleagues [23] recently demonstrated that the prevalence of PVD might be as high as 30.6% among patients receiving maintenance dialysis when the ankle-brachial or toe brachial index measurements are included along with the standard clinical definitions as PVD indicators [23]. These estimates demonstrate the nontrivial magnitude of clinical PVD among patients who have advanced CKD and highlight the need for greater awareness, diagnostic strategies, and effective interventions.

Risk factors for coronary artery disease in patients who have chronic kidney disease receiving dialysis

Traditional Framingham-type risk factors do not explain the high prevalence of CAD among new dialysis patients (Table 1) [25–27]. These traditional factors typically include age, male gender, hypertension, diabetes, high total and low-density lipoprotein cholesterol, tobacco use, physical inactivity, and a family history of premature cardiovascular disease. Several studies have demonstrated that risk prediction equations derived from the Framingham study underestimate the burden of CAD disease in patients who have

Table 1
Traditional and nontraditional risk factors for coronary
artery disease in chronic kidney disease

Traditional risk factors	Nontraditional (novel) risk factors
Nonmodifiable	Hyperhomocysteinemia
Advancing age	Elevated lipoprotein (a)
Male gender	Elevated fibrinogen
Modifiable	Low apolipoprotein A
Hypertension	Elevated inflammatory mediators
	C-reactive protein
Diabetes mellitus	Interleukin 6
Elevated total serum cholesterol	
Elevated low-density lipoprotein cholesterol	Oxidative stress
Low high-density lipoprotein cholesterol	Abnormal calcium/ phosphate homeostasis
Tobacco use	Elevated calcium– phosphate product
Physical inactivity	Hyperphosphatemia
Family history of premature coronary disease	Malnutrition
	Albuminuria
	Dialysis modality

CKD [25–27]. These revelations have led to the
development of several theories that may explain
the large burden of CAD in these patients. First,
traditional risk factors may not exert the same
impact on coronary risk in the setting of CKD
as they do in persons who have normal kidney
function. Second, the presence of CKD may
contribute additional atherogenic toxins or mediators that augment CAD risk above that imposed
by traditional risk factors. These hypotheses currently are being explored by several investigators
using data from large, community-based cohorts
and from secondary analysis of large, randomized
clinical trials [4,6,8,10].

Although many would agree that most of the
Framingham risk factors increase the risk of CAD
in the setting of CKD, conclusive evidence demonstrating these relationships is lacking. Cross-
sectional analysis of data from the DMMS Wave
2 found strong associations between age, diabetes,
and tobacco use with clinical CAD at ESRD
initiation but failed to find any relationship
between hypertension and serum cholesterol [16].
Similar findings were reported by the hemodialysis study group, raising the possibility that the
patterns of association of known coronary disease
risk factors with CAD may not be the same in
CKD as in the general population [25]. At present,
there is no conclusive explanation for these

findings, but confounding and effect modification
of these relationships by other concurrent comorbid conditions present in advanced kidney failure
is a strong possibility. More definitive studies
using prospectively assembled cohorts to explain
these associations are lacking. One particular
study that has extended our understanding of
these complex relationships in patients receiving
dialysis is that by Parfrey and colleagues [28]. In
addition to advancing age, diabetes, and diastolic
blood pressure, these investigators found that
echocardiographic abnormalities were strong independent predictors of de nova ischemic heart
disease in a longitudinal cohort of 432 hemodialysis patients.

Of potential concern in many of the published
studies is the lack of a significant association
between serum cholesterol and hypertension and
the clinical coronary disease outcomes [16,28].
More surprisingly, several published studies have
demonstrated a reverse association between these
well-established factors and coronary disease
events, prompting a reassessment of the clinical
importance of these factors in the setting of CKD
[29,30]. An excellent illustration of these associations is that of serum cholesterol and mortality.
Lowrie and colleagues [30] found that serum
cholesterol levels varied inversely with mortality
risk in a cohort of 12,000 hemodialysis patients.
A step-wise increase in relative risk of death was
seen for serum cholesterol levels lower than
200 mg/dL. These findings have prompted the
search for alternative explanations, such as com-
petitive risk from malnutrition, confounding, and
effect modification by coexisting medical conditions, that might help explain these so-called
"paradoxical relationships."

Risk factors for coronary artery disease in the nondialysis chronic kidney disease population

Teasing out the independent contributions of
established coronary risk factors and CAD in
patients who reach ESRD is a difficult task.
Unlike the general population that has normal
kidney function, patients with ESRD represent
highly selected populations, experience high rates
of comorbid events, and undergo dialysis therapies that vary in technique and survival [14,31,32].
This constellation of factors makes it difficult, if
not impossible, to elucidate the true association of
known traditional risk factors with clinical CAD
using standard epidemiologic approaches. More
recently, studies have focused on patient groups

who have CKD but are not yet receiving dialysis, (potentially more homogeneous populations) to explore these relationships further.

Association of renal impairment with cardiovascular outcomes: a quantitative measure of traditional risk factor burden?

On of the most robust and consistent observations from several of the recently published studies is the strong, graded, independent association of elevated serum creatinine level or lower glomerular filtration rate with increased cardiovascular mortality [4–12]. These associations are arguably most evident in populations at high risk for cardiovascular events and are least evident in populations who have the least risk. In several of these studies, the associations of elevated serum creatinine levels with cardiovascular outcomes are independent of established traditional risk factors, suggesting that the observed relationships may be mediated entirely by novel or nontraditional factors. This conceptual framework may be flawed, however. Although worsening kidney function no doubt involves potential nontraditional risk factors, it may also involve components of traditional risk factors (severity or duration) that are not completely accounted for in the current definitions. For example, an elevated serum creatinine level may be more likely to indicate cumulative exposures of traditional risk factors such as hypertension and tobacco use and as a result provide a more quantitative measurement of these exposures than do single measurements. Accordingly, the strong association of elevated serum creatinine level and cardiovascular outcome may represent an indirect estimate of the cumulative effect of these traditional exposures on cardiovascular outcomes.

Contribution of traditional Framingham risk factors

Studies to date have not evaluated the simultaneous relative contributions of the so-called "traditional Framingham risk factors" and the nontraditional risk factors associated with clinical CAD in the setting of CKD. Defining and quantifying the contribution of each individual risk factor with vascular disease outcomes is a prerequisite for developing targeted interventional strategies and guiding public policy. For example, the claim that traditional risk factors impart the greatest risk in the CKD setting would be strengthened if it were shown (1) that the prevalence of these factors increases with progressive decline in kidney function, (2) that each factor contributes independently to increased cardiovascular risk, and (3) that the magnitude of cardiovascular risk is greatest for those with the worst kidney function. Analysis of cross-sectional data at the population level has revealed that hypertension, impaired glucose tolerance, and tobacco use increase with declining kidney function, supporting the notion that these factors may contribute to the excess burden of CAD [33–35]. For example, Ejerblad and colleagues [33] have recently demonstrated a strong association between tobacco use and the likelihood of CKD in a population-based, case-control study involving 1924 subjects. The odds of CKD, defined as a serum creatinine level higher than 3.4 mg/dL on as least two consecutive occasions, was increased in subjects who had smoked more than 20 cigarettes/d for at least 40 years' duration or who had a 20 pack-year history, as compared with controls. It is unclear, however, whether the same association exists between other traditional risk factors (such as hypercholesterolemia and its associated conditions, physical inactivity and obesity) and the likelihood of CKD. Second, although an increasing prevalence of traditional risk factors with declining kidney function suggests an augmentation of overall cardiovascular risk, it is by no means conclusive. The evidence would be stronger if independent associations were demonstrated between each traditional risk factor and coronary disease in patients who have reduced kidney function. Finally, definitive evidence linking traditional risk factors with CAD would require prospectively designed studies that illustrate an independent association of each factor with CAD and show that the associated risks increase in magnitude with worsening kidney function.

Contribution of nontraditional risk factors

The enormous burden of CAD among patients who have CKD is a perplexing observation that has led many to believe that nontraditional factors, accumulating in the setting of declining kidney function, exert a sizable impact [2,36]. Several inflammatory, thrombotic, and metabolic cardiovascular risk factors have been implicated as important contributors to the excess CAD burden in the CKD setting [37–43]. To date, however, no single study has demonstrated beyond doubt that any one or any combination of these risk factors is causally involved in the acceleration of coronary disease in the CKD setting. Nonetheless, emerging data from several cross-sectional and prospective cohorts, regional or national in scope, have provided supportive evidence linking nontraditional factors with vascular disease in CKD.

Muntner and colleagues [37] have recently reported on the relationship of several inflammatory and novel cardiovascular risk factors with CKD (defined as a glomerular filtration rate of less than 60 mL/min/1.73m^2 based on the modified Modification of Diet in Renal Disease Study Formula equation) using data from the third National Health and Nutrition Examination Survey. As renal function decreased, levels of homocysteine, lipoprotein (a), fibrinogen, and C-reactive protein increased, while levels of apolipoprotein (a) decreased. Their findings are in agreement with several other smaller-center cohorts that have shown abnormally increased levels of these nontraditional factors in persons with CKD [38–40]. Similarly, Shlipak and colleagues [41] found strong independent correlations between several inflammatory and procoagulant markers and decline in renal function using baseline data from the Cardiovascular Health Study. In this study, higher levels of C-reactive protein, fibrinogen, interleukin-6, factor VII-c, factor VIII-c, plasmin–antiplasmin complex, and D-dimer were significantly associated with worsening kidney disease among individuals aged 65 years and older. These findings have been reproduced by other investigators and add to a growing body of literature demonstrating the presence of increased inflammation, oxidant stress, and impaired hemostatic function in persons who have CKD [42,43].

Although the cross-sectional data are interesting and suggestive, they are no substitute for prospectively designed epidemiologic studies. In fact, few published studies have investigated associations of nontraditional factors with coronary events in longitudinal cohorts. By far the most widely studied nontraditional factor is homocysteine, a sulfur-containing amino acid with putative thrombotic properties [44–51]. The increased thrombotic risk conferred by increased homocysteine levels in persons with homozygous genetic traits is undisputed, and pooled analysis of observational cohorts in the general population has suggested elevated homocysteine levels also confer increased cardiovascular risk [45–47]. Despite these observations, a reduction in coronary events with homocysteine lowering has not been confirmed in clinical trials, although the results from several large-scale, randomized clinical trials are awaited [48]. Homocysteine levels increase in a dose-dependent fashion with declining kidney function, however. Furthermore, prospective studies of persons with CKD of varying degrees have identified an elevated homocysteine level as an independent risk factor for future coronary events [49–52]. Some have interpreted these findings as suggesting a more pathogenetic role for homocysteine among persons who have reduced kidney function as compared with those who have normal kidney function. Whether this hypothesis can be confirmed in randomized clinical trials remains to be seen. The currently funded NIH FAVORIT trial in transplant recipients is a first step in answering this question (www.clinicaltrials.gov/ct/show/NCT00064753).

Risk factors for peripheral vascular disease in the general population

The epidemiology of PVD in CKD patients has received far less attention than that of CAD, and consequently the ability to develop risk factor profiles is reduced. Nevertheless, given the pathophysiologic similarities between PVD and CAD, it is likely that factors operating in one disease process are also important in the other. Risk factor profiles generated from longitudinal cohorts in the general population suggest that many, if not all, of the traditional coronary risk factor are also risk factors for development of PVD [53–56]. A recent review by Belch and colleagues [53] acknowledges the importance of several of these factors including advancing age, male gender, diabetes, hypertension, smoking, and hyperlipidemia. The relative importance of several novel risk factors such as lipoprotein (a), von Willebrand's factor, tissue plasminogen activator, and fibrin D-dimer has been demonstrated by investigators from the Edinburgh Artery Study [54,55]. Ridker and colleagues [56,57] demonstrated the independent predictive values of C-reactive protein and apolipoprotein-B 100 in the Physicians' Health Study, a prospective, randomized trial of aspirin and beta-carotene in the primary prevention of cardiovascular disease and cancer.

Risk factors for peripheral vascular disease in the chronic kidney disease population

Whether factors that predict PVD development in the general population are also predictive in patients who have CKD is not fully understood. O'Hare and colleagues [58] found that advancing age, diabetes, and elevated systolic blood pressure were significantly associated with the risk for future amputations, as was a prior history of PVD in an analysis of 8633 patients receiving maintenance dialysis. Moreover, she demonstrated a gradient of risk with increasing serum phosphorus concentration, suggesting a further role for abnormal mineral metabolism in vascular disease development or progression. Taken together, population studies of CAD and PVD in patients receiving dialysis suggest that these vascular conditions have a similar natural history, with contributions from both traditional and nontraditional coronary risk factors.

To our knowledge, the contribution of novel cardiovascular risk factors to PVD development has not been evaluated in patients who have CKD but are not undergoing dialysis; however, a further study from the O'Hare group has provided useful insights [59]. Using data from the Heart and Estrogen\Progestin Replacement Study, they demonstrated a strong, graded, independent association of reduced kidney function with the risk of lower extremity vascular disease among postmenopausal women who have established CAD. The similarities between this study and those that have evaluated associations of reduced kidney function with other cardiovascular disease outcomes highlight the tremendous impact of reduced kidney

function on vascular outcomes, irrespective of location.

Outcomes of coronary artery disease and peripheral vascular disease in persons who have chronic kidney disease

Peripheral vascular disease

The impact of PVD on morbidity and mortality has been well described in persons who have ESRD and are receiving maintenance dialysis and, to a lesser degree, in persons who have varying levels of CLKD not requiring dialysis [60–63]. Multivariable analyses of incident dialysis cohorts from the United States Renal Data System (USRDS) have repeatedly demonstrated the independent predictive value of PVD on all-cause mortality [14,31,32]. Patients who present for dialysis because of new ESRD and who have a diagnosis of PVD from medical records experience a 66% higher crude mortality risk compared with those without PVD [31]. Moreover, with adjustment for established mortality predictors, PVD still carries a 37% higher adjusted mortality risk (Fig. 1). A more focused study by Eggers and colleagues [60] based on Medicare data from the USRDS database has permitted a quantitative assessment of the outcomes after lower extremity amputations in this high-risk population. In an analysis of 24,886 patients who experienced

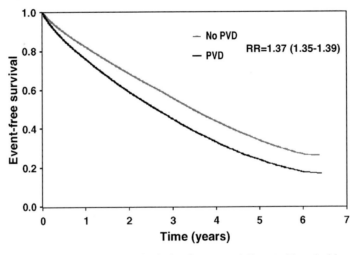

Fig. 1. Adjusted survival curves for new patients who had end-stage renal disease with and without peripheral vascular disease (PVD) in the United States who began dialysis between 5/1995 and 12/2000 and were followed until 2001. Relative risk (RR) is adjusted for age, gender, and race. (*Adapted from* Stack AG, Molony DA, Rahman SN, et al. Impact of dialysis modality on survival of new ESRD patients with congestive heart failure in the United States. Kidney Int 2003;64:1071–9.)

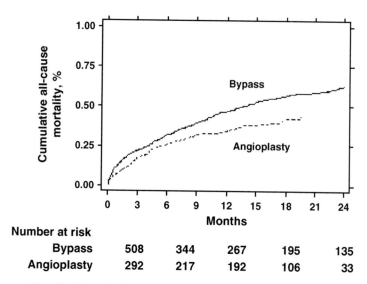

Fig. 2. Cumulative mortality of patients who have peripheral vascular disease after undergoing initial surgical bypass or percutaneous transluminal angioplasty (*From* Jaar BG, Astor BC, Berns JS, et al. Predictors of amputation and survival following lower extremity revascularization in hemodialysis patients. Kidney Int 2004;65:617; with permission.)

35,898 first amputations between 1991 and 1994, the overall survival at 2 years was 32.7%, compared with a survival of 63.2% for the entire ESRD dialysis population. For patients who experienced a toe-level amputation, the survival rates at 30 days, 90 days, and 2 years were 95.2%, 85.4%, and 44.8% respectively. For those with a below-knee amputation, survival rates were 89.6%, 75.2%, and 31.7%, respectively. For

patients who underwent an above-knee amputation, rates were lowest, at 76.3%, 52.7%, and 15.2%, respectively. The mortality risks were 37% higher for patients who underwent a below-knee procedure and more than twofold higher for those who underwent an above-knee amputation compared with those who had a toe-level procedure.

Although the prognostic impact of peripheral arterial disease (PAD) on mortality is well

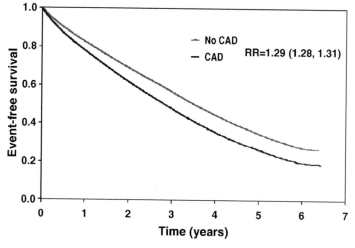

Fig. 3. Adjusted survival curves for new patients who have end-stage renal disease with and without coronary artery disease (CAD) in the United States who began dialysis between 5/1995 and 12/2000 and were followed until 2001. Relative risk (RR) is adjusted for age, gender, and race. (*Adapted from* Stack AG, Molony DA, Rahman SN, et al. Impact of dialysis modality on survival of new ESRD patients with congestive heart failure in the United States. Kidney Int 2003;64:1071–9.)

A

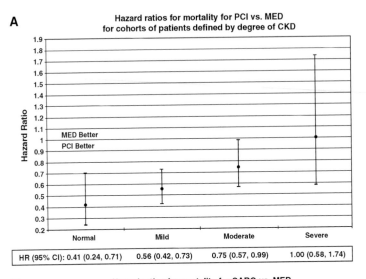

Hazard ratios for mortality for PCI vs. MED
for cohorts of patients defined by degree of CKD

HR (95% CI):	0.41 (0.24, 0.71)	0.56 (0.42, 0.73)	0.75 (0.57, 0.99)	1.00 (0.58, 1.74)

B

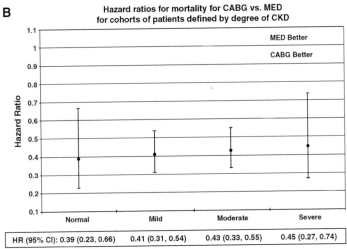

Hazard ratios for mortality for CABG vs. MED
for cohorts of patients defined by degree of CKD

HR (95% CI):	0.39 (0.23, 0.66)	0.41 (0.31, 0.54)	0.43 (0.33, 0.55)	0.45 (0.27, 0.74)

C

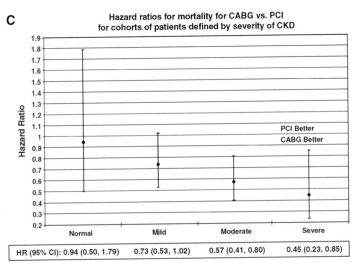

Hazard ratios for mortality for CABG vs. PCI
for cohorts of patients defined by severity of CKD

HR (95% CI):	0.94 (0.50, 1.79)	0.73 (0.53, 1.02)	0.57 (0.41, 0.80)	0.45 (0.23, 0.85)

established, the relative benefits of different therapeutic interventions in these patients are less well studied. For example, one key question might be whether in patients who have severe lower extremity PAD outcomes after arterial bypass procedures are better than after angioplasty. Unfortunately, clinical trial data comparing these therapies in patients who have ESRD are not available, even in the general non-ESRD population. The recent work of Jaar and colleagues [64], however, has provided useful insights into the outcomes of patients who have ESRD and who have PAD requiring revascularization intervention. In a comparative analysis of 508 bypass surgeries and 292 angioplasties from the USRDS database, they found that the mortality risks of patients who underwent a first lower extremity bypass were more than fourfold higher than those of patients who underwent angioplasty, a difference that persisted after adjusting for case mix (Fig. 2). As the authors acknowledge, unmeasured baseline differences between the groups, such as severity of angiographic disease or duration of disease, could have accounted for these results given the observational, nonrandomized study design. The clinical benefits of other pharmacologic and nonpharmacologic measures for PAD management are yet to be tested in this population. The high prevalence of traditional cardiovascular risk factors in this population almost certainly contributes to the development and progression of PAD, suggesting that targeted efforts should be directed to the optimal management of these factors in patients who have ESRD, as in the general population. Furthermore, the accumulating body of evidence linking hyperphosphatemia, elevated calcium–phosphate product, and hyperparathyroidism with increased vascular disease burden and vascular-related mortality cannot be ignored; the mortality benefits of specific therapies to control these derangements need further evaluation [65–67]. Given the high prevalence of PAD, with its attendant morbidity

and mortality, in this population, it is perplexing that clinical trials are sparse.

Coronary artery disease

The optimal strategies for the management of CAD in patients who have CKD are yet to be defined. The clinical evidence favoring one or more treatment strategies has been gleaned thus far from analysis of observational cohorts with additional supportive evidence coming from secondary analysis of existing clinical trials. It has not been demonstrated that pharmacologic treatments or interventional cardiovascular procedures with proven efficacy in the general population are also effective in CKD cohorts, and such extrapolation must be viewed with caution. For many established therapies with established efficacy in the general population, it is unclear whether the therapeutic effect on outcomes is modified by the presence of renal impairment and, if so, to what degree.

Most clinical trials to date evaluating treatments for acute coronary syndromes (ACS) have excluded patients who have renal impairment at study entry [68–74]. Accordingly, it is unclear whether treatment strategies used in the management of ST segment elevation myocardial infraction (STEMI) or non-STEMI ACS are equally effective in CKD cohorts. Several major trials have demonstrated the clinical efficacy of thrombolytic agents, such as streptokinase and altepase, and of platelet glycoprotein IIb/IIIa inhibitors, including abciximab, eptifibatide, and tirofiban, in the management of ACS in the general population. Unfortunately, in most studies subgroup analyses to evaluate therapeutic potential in persons with reduced renal function were not performed. Recent post hoc analyses of two large, randomized clinical trials, however, did not demonstrate any interaction between the level of renal impairment and glycoprotein IIb/IIIa inhibitors with respect to the primary end point, suggesting

Fig. 4. (A) Hazard ratios for mortality for medical (MED) management versus percutaneous coronary artery intervention (PCI) for cohorts of patients defined by severity of chronic kidney disease (CKD) (adjusted). (B) Hazard ratios for mortality for medical management (MED) versus coronary artery bypass grafting (CABG) for cohorts of patients defined by severity of chronic kidney disease (CKD) (adjusted). (C) Hazard ratios for mortality for coronary artery bypass grafting (CABG) versus percutaneous coronary artery intervention (PCI) for cohorts of patients defined by severity of chronic kidney disease (CKD) (adjusted). (From Reddan DN, Szczech LA, Tuttle RH, et al. Chronic kidney disease, mortality, and treatment strategies among patients who have clinically significant coronary artery disease. J Am Soc Nephrol 2003;14:2378; with permission.)

that the efficacy of these agents in patients who have CKD is equivalent to that of the general population [74,75]. An additional consideration in the use of these agents in persons who have ACS and renal impairment is whether the increased risk of bleeding is offset by therapeutic benefit in reducing ACS complications. What is clear from existing studies is that patients who present with ACS and who have coexisting renal impairment at baseline experience significantly higher mortality rates than those without renal impairment [76].

Whether the therapeutic benefits of aspirin, beta-adrenergic blockers, and statins in preventing cardiovascular events in the general population extend to patients who have CKD has not been firmly established [77–79]. Although results are conflicting, prospective cohorts and secondary analyses of clinical trials suggest that the clinical benefit of these agents in reducing cardiovascular events among patients who have ACS or prior CAD may be similar to that seen in the general population [78–80]. The limited availability of clinical trial data on secondary prevention of coronary events in advanced CKD patients has led to increased mining of large registries to assess cardioprotective associations. From these efforts, three points are worth noting. First, the use of known cardioprotective medications among new dialysis patients is abysmally low and warrants investigation. Second, calcium-channel blockers and 3-hydroxy-3-methyl-glutaryl coenzyme-A inhibitors seem to offer cardioprotection in new dialysis patients who have pre-existing cardiovascular disease [81,82]. Third, analysis of cohort data to evaluate an association between the use of cardioprotective medication and cardiovascular outcomes may be flawed, because the indication for medication use is likely to confound observed associations [83].

A diagnosis of CAD at dialysis initiation predicts significantly reduced patient survival (Fig. 3). During the past decade, controversy has existed as to the optimal revascularization strategy for patients who have CKD [84–89]. A recent study by Herzog and colleagues [90] in more than 15,784 dialysis patients found significantly better overall survival among those who were treated with coronary artery bypass surgery (CABG) as compared with percutaneous transluminal angioplasty (PTCA) or stent placement. Overall all-cause mortality was 20% lower, and cardiovascular mortality was 28% lower among patients in the CABG group versus those treated with PTCA. The mortality risks of stent placement were also better than for PTCA; however; this benefit was mainly confined to nondiabetics. These findings have confirmed and have extended the observations of several other groups in demonstrating the benefit of CABG over PTCA and stent placement, at least in observational studies [84–89]. The question of confounding by selection bias will always remain, because patients who undergo CABG are likely to have more severe disease and to have higher overall cardiovascular risk than those treated with PTCA.

An equally interesting question is whether the advantage of CABG observed in ESRD cohorts extends to those with less severe renal impairment. The recent observations of Reddan and colleagues [91] from the Duke Cardiovascular Database have provided useful insights in this area. Comparisons of CABG with percutaneous coronary intervention or medical therapy alone yielded significant benefits in favor of CABG (Fig. 4). This benefit was observed in almost all stages of CKD, with one exception. Patients who have angiographic CAD who were classified as having normal kidney function had similar survival with either CABG or medical therapy. Furthermore, those who underwent percutaneous coronary intervention experienced significantly better survival than those who received medical therapy alone, except for those who had severe CKD. Again, although the potential for selection bias and indication bias exists in mortality comparisons of this nature, some messages are clear. First, the survival advantage of CABG over PTCA is consistent from several studies. Second, the impact of percutaneous coronary interventions and medical therapies on outcomes varies by level of renal function and highlights the need for randomized comparisons of these therapies.

Summary

The enormous burden of CAD and PVD in patients who have CKD contributes substantially to increased morbidity and mortality. The increased risk of vascular disease observed in CKD patients is likely to be multifactorial, with contributions from traditional and nontraditional cardiovascular factors. Given the overwhelming evidence on the known benefits of cardioprotective medications, their underuse remains puzzling in a population at enormous risk. During the past 5 years, the research community and national interest groups have made significant progress in organizing a concerted approach to improve the management of patients who have CKD and vascular disease. Much work remains to be done. The development of national guidelines in the management of these patients at high risk for future cardiovascular events will be a welcome step. The evaluation of multitargeted interventions for reduction of cardiovascular risk through randomized clinical trials is desperately needed. Finally, the low use of known cardioprotective strategies in this high-risk group is a serious issue and warrants immediate attention at local and national levels.

References

[1] Lindner A, Charra B, Sherrard DJ, et al. Accelerated atherosclerosis in prolonged maintenance hemodialysis. N Engl J Med 1974;290:697–701.

[2] Levey AS, Beto JA, Coronado BE, et al. Controlling the epidemic of cardiovascular disease in chronic renal disease: What do we know? What do we need to know? Where do we go from here? Am J Kidney Dis 1998;32:853–905.

[3] Foley RN, Parfrey PS, Sarnak MJ. Clinical epidemiology of cardiovascular disease in chronic renal disease. Am J Kidney Dis 1998;32:S112–9.

[4] Culleton BF, Larson MG, Wilson PW, et al. Cardiovascular disease and mortality in a community-based cohort with mild renal insufficiency. Kidney Int 1999;56:2214–9.

[5] Mann JF, Gerstein HC, Pogue J, et al. Renal insufficiency as a predictor of cardiovascular outcomes and the impact of ramipril: the HOPE randomized trial. Ann Intern Med 2001;134:629–36.

[6] Manjunath G, Tighiouart H, Ibrahim H, et al. Level of kidney function as a risk factor for atherosclerotic cardiovascular disease in the community. J Am Coll Cardiol 2003;41:47–55.

[7] Ruilope LM, Salvetti A, Jamerson K, et al. Renal function and intensive lowering of blood pressure in hypertensive participants of the hypertension optimal treatment (HOT) study. J Am Soc Nephrol 2001;12:218–25.

[8] Shlipak MG, Fried LF, Crump C, et al. Cardiovascular disease risk status in elderly persons with renal insufficiency. Kidney Int 2002;62:997–1004.

[9] Reis SE, Olson MB, Fried L, et al. Mild renal insufficiency is associated with angiographic coronary artery disease in women. Circulation 2002;105:2826–9.

[10] Manjunath G, Tighiouart H, Coresh J, et al. Level of kidney function as a risk factor for cardiovascular outcomes in the elderly. Kidney Int 2003;63:1121–9.

[11] Friedman PJ. Serum creatinine: an independent predictor of survival after stroke. J Intern Med 1991; 229:175–9.

[12] McCullough PA, Soman SS, Shah SS, et al. Risks associated with renal dysfunction in patients in the coronary care unit. J Am Coll Cardiol 2000;36:679–84.

[13] Levey AS, Coresh J, Balk E, et al, for the National Kidney Foundation. National Kidney Foundation practice guidelines for chronic kidney disease: evaluation, classification, and stratification. Ann Intern Med 2002;139:137–47.

[14] US Renal Data System. Comorbid conditions and correlations with mortality risk among 3,399 incident hemodialysis patients. Am J Kidney Dis 1992; 20:32–8.

[15] Disney APS, editor. ANZDATA Report 1998. Australia and New Zealand Dialysis and Transplantation Registry. Adelaide (Australia): Australia and New Zealand Dialysis and Transplant Registry; 1999.

[16] Stack AG, Bloembergen WE. Prevalence and clinical correlates of coronary artery disease among new dialysis patients in the United States: a crosssectional study. J Am Soc Nephrol 2000;12:1516–23.

[17] Longnecker JC, Coresh J, Powe NR, et al. Traditional cardiovascular disease risk factors in dialysis patients compared with the general population. The CHOICE Study. J Am Soc Nephrol 2002;13: 1918–27.

[18] Canadian Organ Replacement Register 1998 annual report. Don Mills (Ontario, Canada): Canadian Institute for Health Information; 1998.

[19] United States Renal Data System. Patient characteristics at the start of ESRD: data from the HCFA Medical Evidence Form. Am J Kidney Dis 1999; 34:S63–73.

[20] Gradaus F, Ivens K, Peters AJ, et al. Angiographic progression of coronary artery disease in patients with end-stage renal disease. Nephrol Dial Transplant 2001;16:1198–202.

[21] Raggi P, Boulay A, Chasan-Taber S, et al. Cardiac calcification in adult hemodialysis patients. A link between end-stage renal disease and cardiovascular disease? J Am Coll Cardiol 2002;39:695–701.

[22] O'Hare AM, Hsu CY, Bacchetti P, et al. Peripheral vascular disease risk factors among patients undergoing hemodialysis. J Am Soc Nephrol 2002;13: 497–503.

[23] Leskinen Y, Salenius JP, Lehtimaki T, et al. The prevalence of peripheral arterial disease and medial arterial calcification in patients with chronic renal failure: requirements for diagnostics. Am J Kidney Dis 2002;40:472–9.

[24] Reddan DN, Marcus RJ, Owen WF Jr, et al. Long-term outcomes of revascularization for peripheral vascular disease in end-stage renal disease patients. Am J Kidney Dis 2001;38:57–63.

[25] Cheung AK, Sarnak MJ, Yan G, et al. Atherosclerotic cardiovascular disease risks in chronic hemodialysis patients. Kidney Int 2000;58:353–62.

[26] Longenecker JC, Coresh J, Powe NR, et al. Traditional cardiovascular disease risk factors in dialysis

patients compared with the general population: the CHOICE Study. J Am Soc Nephrol 2002;13: 1918–27.

[27] Sarnak MJ, Coronado BE, Greene T, et al. Cardiovascular disease risk factors in chronic renal insufficiency. Clin Nephrol 2002;57:327–35.

[28] Parfrey PS, Foley RN, Harnett JD, et al. Outcome and risk factors of ischemic heart disease in chronic uremia. Kidney Int 1996;49:1428–34.

[29] Kalantar-Zadeh K, Block G, Humphreys MH, et al. Reverse epidemiology of cardiovascular risk factors in maintenance dialysis patients. Kidney Int 2003;63: 793–808.

[30] Lowrie EG, Lew NL. Death risk in hemodialysis patients: the predictive value of commonly measured variables and an evaluation of death rate differences between facilities. Am J Kidney Dis 1990; 15:458–82.

[31] Ganesh SK, Hulbert-Shearon T, Eagle K, et al. Mortality differences by treatment modality among incident ESRD patients with and without coronary artery disease. J Am Soc Nephrol 2003;14:415–24.

[32] Stack AG, Molony DA, Rahman SN, et al. Impact of dialysis modality on survival of new ESRD patients with congestive heart failure in the United States. Kidney Int 2003;64:1071–9.

[33] Ejerblad E, Fored MC, Lindblad P, et al. Association between smoking and chronic renal failure in a nationwide population-based case-control study. J Am Soc Nephrol 2004;15:2178–85.

[34] Haroun MK, Jaar BG, Hoffman SC, et al. Risk factors for chronic kidney disease: a prospective study of 23,534 men and women in Washington county, Maryland. J Am Soc Nephrol 2003;14:2934–41.

[35] Pinto-Sietsma SJ, Mulder J, Janssen WM, et al. Smoking is related to albuminuria and abnormal renal function in nondiabetic persons. Ann Intern Med 2000;133:585–91.

[36] Madore F. Uremia-related metabolic cardiac risk factors in chronic kidney disease. Semin Dial 2003; 16:148–56.

[37] Muntner P, Hamm LL, Kusek JW, et al. The prevalence of nontraditional risk factors for coronary heart disease in patients with chronic kidney disease. Ann Intern Med 2004;140:9–17.

[38] Haffner SM, Gruber KK, Aldrete G Jr, et al. Increased lipoprotein (a) concentrations in chronic renal failure. J Am Soc Nephrol 1992;3:1156–62.

[39] Stenvinkel P, Heimburger O, Tuck CH, et al. Apo(a)-isoform size, nutritional status and inflammatory markers in chronic renal failure. Kidney Int 1998;53:1336–42.

[40] Bostom AG, Shemin D, Lapane KL, et al. Hyperhomocysteinemia, hyperfibrinogenemia, and lipoprotein (a) excess in maintenance dialysis patients: a matched case-control study. Atherosclerosis 1996; 125:91–101.

[41] Shlipak MG, Fried LF, Crump C, et al. Elevations of inflammatory and procoagulant biomarkers in elderly persons with renal insufficiency. Circulation 2003;107:87–92.

[42] Oberg BP, McMenamin E, Lucas FL, et al. Increased prevalence of oxidant stress and inflammation in patients with moderate to severe chronic kidney disease. Kidney Int 2004;65:1009–16.

[43] Koch M, Kutkuhn B, Trenkwalder E, et al. Apolipoprotein B, fibrinogen, HDL cholesterol, and apolipoprotein (a) phenotypes predict coronary artery disease in hemodialysis patients. J Am Soc Nephrol 1997;8:1889–98.

[44] Mudd SH, Skovby F, Levy HL, et al. The natural history of homocystinuria due to cystathionine betasynthase deficiency. Am J Hum Genet 1985; 37:1–31.

[45] Omenn GS, Beresford SA, Motulsky AG. Preventing coronary heart disease: B vitamins and homocysteine. Circulation 1998;97:421–4.

[46] Boushey CJ, Beresford SA, Omenn GS, et al. A quantitative assessment of plasma homocysteine as a risk factor for vascular disease: Probable benefits of increasing folic acid intakes. JAMA 1995;274: 1049–57.

[47] Beresford SA, Boushey CJ. Homocysteine, folic acid, and cardiovascular disease risk. In: Bendich A, Deckelbaum RJ, editors. Preventive nutrition: the comprehensive guide for health professionals. Totowa (NJ): Humana Press; 1997. p. 193–224.

[48] Bostom AG, Selhub J, Jacques PF, et al. Power shortage: clinical trials testing the "homocysteine hypothesis" against a background of folic acid-fortified cereal grain flour. Ann Intern Med 2001;135: 133–7.

[49] Moustapha A, Naso A, Nahlawi M, et al. Prospective study of hyperhomocysteinemia as an adverse cardiovascular risk factor in end-stage renal disease. Circulation 1998;97:138–41.

[50] Bostom AG, Shemin D, Verhoef P, et al. Elevated fasting total plasma homocysteine levels and cardiovascular disease outcomes in maintenance dialysis patients: a prospective study. Arterioscler Thromb Vasc Biol 1997;17:2554–8.

[51] Jungers P, Chauveau P, Bandin O, et al. Hyperhomocysteinemia is associated with atherosclerotic occlusive arterial accidents in predialysis chronic renal failure patients. Miner Electrolyte Metab 1997;23:170–3.

[52] Massy ZA, Chadefaux-Vekemans B, Chevalier A, et al. Hyperhomocysteinemia: a significant risk factor for cardiovascular disease in renal transplant recipients. Nephrol Dial Transplant 1994;9:1103–8.

[53] Belch JF. Metabolic, endocrine and hemodynamic risk factors in the patient with peripheral arterial disease. Diabetes Obes Metab 2002;4:S2–7.

[54] Price JF, Mowbray PI, Lee AJ, et al. Relationship between smoking and cardiovascular risk factors in the development of peripheral arterial disease and coronary artery disease. Edinburgh Artery Study. Eur Heart J 1999;20:344–53.

[55] Lee AJ, MacGregor AS, Hau CM, et al. The role of haematological factors in diabetic peripheral arterial disease: the Edinburgh artery study. British Journal of Haematology 1999;105(3):648–54.

[56] Price JF, Lee AJ, Fowkes FG. Hyperinsulinaemia: a risk factor for peripheral arterial disease in the non-diabetic general population. J Cardiovasc Risk 1996;3:501–5.

[57] Ridker PM, Stampfer MJ, Rifai N. Novel risk factors for systemic atherosclerosis: a comparison of C-reactive protein, fibrinogen, homocysteine, lipoprotein (a), and standard cholesterol screening as predictors of peripheral arterial disease. JAMA 2001;285:2481–5.

[58] O'Hare AM, Bacchetti P, Segal M, et al. Dialysis Morbidity and Mortality Study Waves. Factors associated with future amputation among patients undergoing hemodialysis: results from the Dialysis Morbidity and Mortality Study Waves 3 and 4. Am J Kidney Dis 2003;41:162–70.

[59] O'Hare AM, Vittinghoff E, Hsia J, et al. Renal insufficiency and the risk of lower extremity peripheral arterial disease: results from the Heart and Estrogen/progestin Replacement Study (HERS). J Am Soc Nephrol 2004;15:1046–51.

[60] Eggers PW, Gohdes D, Pugh J. Nontraumatic lower extremity amputations in the Medicare end-stage renal disease population. Kidney Int 1999;56:1524–33.

[61] Fleming LW, Stewart CP, Henderson IS, et al. Limb amputation on renal replacement therapy. Prosthet Orthot Int 2000;24:7–12.

[62] McGrath NM, Curran BA. Recent commencement of dialysis is a risk factor for lower-extremity amputation in a high-risk diabetic population. Diabetes Care 2000;23:432–3.

[63] Morbach S, Quante C, Ochs HR, et al. Increased risk of lower-extremity amputation among Caucasian diabetic patients on dialysis. Diabetes Care 2001;24:1689–90.

[64] Jaar BG, Astor BC, Berns JS, et al. Predictors of amputation and survival following lower extremity revascularization in hemodialysis patients. Kidney Int 2004;65:613–20.

[65] Block GA, Hulbert-Shearon TE, Levin NW, et al. Association of serum phosphorus and calcium x phosphate product with mortality risk in chronic hemodialysis patients: a national study. Am J Kidney Dis 1998;31:601–17.

[66] Ganesh SK, Stack AG, Levin NW, et al. Association of elevated serum PO_4, $Ca \times PO_4$ product, and parathyroid hormone with cardiac mortality risk in chronic hemodialysis patients. J Am Soc Nephrol 2001;12:2131–8.

[67] Chertow GM, Burke SK, Raggi P. Treat to Goal Working Group. Sevelamer attenuates the progression of coronary and aortic calcification in hemodialysis patients. Kidney Int 2002;62:245–52.

[68] Fernandez JS, Sadaniantz BT, Sadaniantz A. Review of antithrombotic agents used for acute coronary syndromes in renal patients. Am J Kidney Dis 2003;42:446–55.

[69] ISIS-2 (Second International Study of Infarct Survival) Collaborative Group. Randomized trial of intravenous streptokinase, oral aspirin, both, or neither among 17,187 cases of suspected acute myocardial infarction: ISIS-2. Lancet 1988;2:349–60.

[70] Gruppo Italiano per lo Studio della Sopravvivenza nell'Infarto Miocardico (GISSI-2). A factorial randomized trial of alteplase versus streptokinase and heparin versus no heparin among 12,490 patients with acute myocardial infarction. Lancet 1990;336:65–71.

[71] International Study Group. In-hospital mortality and clinical course of 20,891 patients with suspected acute myocardial infarction randomized between alteplase and streptokinase with or without heparin. Lancet 1990;336:71–5.

[72] ISIS-3 (Third International Study of Infarct Survival) Collaborative Group. A randomized comparison of streptokinase vs tissue plasminogen activator vs anistreplase and of aspirin plus heparin vs aspirin alone among 41,299 cases of suspected acute myocardial infarction. Lancet 1993;339:753–70.

[73] GUSTO Investigators. An international randomized trial comparing four thrombolytic strategies for acute myocardial infarction. N Engl J Med 1993;329:673–82.

[74] Januzzi JL, Snapinn SM, DiBattiste PM, et al. Benefits and safety of tirofiban among acute coronary syndrome patients with mild to moderate renal insufficiency: results from the Platelet Receptor Inhibition in Ischemic Syndrome Management in Patients Limited by Unstable Signs and Symptoms (PRISM-PLUS) trial. Circulation 2002;105:2361–6.

[75] Reddan DN, O'Shea JC, Sarembock IJ, et al. Treatment effects of eptifibatide in planned coronary stent implantation in patients with chronic kidney disease (ESPRIT Trial). Am J Cardiol 2003;91:17–21.

[76] Al Suwaidi J, Reddan DN, Williams K, et al. GUSTO-IIb, GUSTO-III, PURSUIT. Global Use of Strategies to Open Occluded Coronary Arteries. Platelet Glycoprotein IIb/IIIa in Unstable Angina: Receptor Suppression Using Integrilin Therapy. PARAGON-A Investigators. Platelet IIb/IIIa Antagonism for the Reduction of Acute coronary syndrome events in a Global Organization Network. Prognostic implications of abnormalities in renal function in patients with acute coronary syndromes. Circulation 2002;106:974–80.

[77] Gum PA, Thamilarasan M, Watanabe J, et al. Aspirin use and all-cause mortality among patients being evaluated for known or suspected coronary artery disease: a propensity analysis. JAMA 2001;286:1187–94.

[78] Trespalacios FC, Taylor AJ, Agodoa LY, et al. Incident acute coronary syndromes in chronic dialysis patients in the United States. Kidney Int 2002;62:1799–805.

[79] McCullough PA, Sandberg KR, Borzak S, et al. Benefits of aspirin and beta-blockade after myocardial infarction in patients with chronic kidney disease. Am Heart J 2002;144(2):226–32.

[80] Tonelli M, Moye L, Sacks FM, et al. Cholesterol and Recurrent Events (CARE) Trial Investigators. Pravastatin for secondary prevention of cardiovascular events in persons with mild chronic renal insufficiency. Ann Intern Med 2003;138:98–104.

[81] Kestenbaum B, Gillen DL, Sherrard DJ, et al. Calcium channel blocker use and mortality among patients with end-stage renal disease. Kidney Int 2002;61:2157–64.

[82] Seliger SL, Weiss NS, Gillen DL, et al. HMG-CoA reductase inhibitors are associated with reduced mortality in ESRD patients. Kidney Int 2002;61: 297–304.

[83] Ishani A, Herzog CA, Collins AJ, et al. Cardiac medications and their association with cardiovascular events in incident dialysis patients: cause or effect? Kidney Int 2004;65:1017–25.

[84] Reusser LM, Osborn LA, White HJ, et al. Increased morbidity after coronary angioplasty in patients on chronic hemodialysis. Am J Cardiol 1994;73:965–7.

[85] Marso SP, Gimple LW, Philbrick JT, et al. Effectiveness of percutaneous coronary interventions to prevent recurrent coronary events in patients on chronic hemodialysis. Am J Cardiol 1998;82:378–80.

[86] Simsir SA, Kohlman-Trigoboff D, Flood R, et al. A comparison of coronary artery bypass grafting and percutaneous transluminal coronary angioplasty in patients on hemodialysis. Cardiovasc Surg 1998;6: 500–5.

[87] Herzog CA, Ma JZ, Collins AJ. Long-term outcome of dialysis patients in the United States with coronary revascularization procedures. Kidney Int 1999;56: 324–32.

[88] Agirbasli M, Weintraub WS, Chang GL, et al. Outcome of coronary revascularization in patients on renal dialysis. Am J Cardiol 2000;86:395–9.

[89] Szczech L, Reddan D, Owen W Jr, et al. Differential survival after coronary revascularization procedures among patients with renal insufficiency. Kidney Int 2001;60:292–9.

[90] Herzog CA, Ma JZ, Collins AJ. Comparative survival of dialysis patients in the United States after coronary angioplasty, coronary artery stenting, and coronary artery bypass surgery and impact of diabetes. Circulation 2002;106:2207–11.

[91] Reddan DN, Szczech LA, Tuttle RH, et al. Chronic kidney disease, mortality, and treatment strategies among patients with clinically significant coronary artery disease. J Am Soc Nephrol 2003;14:2373–80.

ELSEVIER
SAUNDERS

Cardiol Clin 23 (2005) 299–310

CARDIOLOGY
CLINICS

Percutaneous Coronary Interventions in the High-Risk Renal Patient: Strategies for Renal Protection and Vascular Protection

Peter A. McCullough, MD, MPH, FACC, FACP, FCCP, FAHA*,
Aaron D. Berman, MD, FACC

*Divisions of Cardiology, Nutrition and Preventive Medicine, Department of Medicine,
William Beaumont Hospital, 4949 Coolidge, Royal Oak, MI 48073, USA*

The worldwide pandemic of obesity is threatening to erase considerable progress made in the primary and secondary prevention of coronary artery disease (CAD). Obesity has a direct and colinear relationship to the increasing prevalence of the metabolic syndrome and type 2 diabetes. Recent data suggest that chronic kidney disease (CKD) and CAD have the same conventional risk factors, including the metabolic syndrome, dyslipidemia, smoking, hypertension, and, very importantly, diabetes [1]. Approximately 50% of patients with diabetes develop CKD after 20 years of the disease [2]. With type 2 diabetes now occurring in early adulthood in large numbers of overweight and obese individuals, in future decades one can expect increasing numbers of individuals with CKD to develop CAD and require percutaneous coronary intervention (PCI). In the last 10 years sufficient data have accumulated for major guidelines committees to consider CKD a major, independent CAD risk factor [3].

Chronic kidney disease and cardiovascular risk

CKD is defined through a range of estimated glomerular filtration rate (eGFR) values by the National Kidney Foundation Kidney Disease Outcomes Quality Initiative (K/DOQI) as depicted in Fig. 1 [4]. Most studies of cardiovascular outcomes have found that a breakpoint for the development of contrast-induced nephropathy (CIN), later restenosis, recurrent myocardial infarction, diastolic/systolic congestive heart failure, and cardiovascular death occurs below an eGFR of 60 mL/min/1.73 m^2, which roughly corresponds to a serum creatinine level higher than 1.5 mg/dL in the general population [5–8]. Because creatinine level is a crude indicator of renal function and often underestimates renal dysfunction in women and elderly persons, calculated measures of eGFR or creatinine clearance by the Cockroft-Gault equation or by the Modification of Diet in Renal Disease (MDRD) equations, now available on personal digital assistants, are the preferred methods of estimating renal function [4]. The four-variable MDRD equation for creatinine clearance is ideal for the catheterization laboratory because it does not rely on body weight [4]:

$$(186.3^*[\text{serum creatinine}^{-1.154}]^*[\text{age}^{-.203}])$$

Calculated values are multiplied by 0.742 for women and by 1.21 for African Americans.

In addition, microalbuminuria at any level of eGFR is considered to represent CKD and has been thought to occur as the result of endothelial dysfunction in the glomeruli [9]. A simple definition for microalbuminuria is a random urine albumin/creatinine ratio (ACR) of 30/300 mg/g. An ACR higher than 300 mg/g is usually considered gross proteinuria. It is critical to understand that the risk of CIN is related in a curvilinear fashion to the eGFR as shown in Fig. 2 [10].

---

* Corresponding author.
E-mail address: pmc975@yahoo.com
(P.A. McCullough).

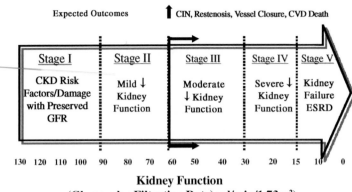

Kidney Function
(Glomerular Filtration Rate) ml/min/1.73m²)

Fig. 1. The classification of chronic kidney disease (CKD) according to the National Kidney Foundation KDOQI. Increased rates of adverse events are generally seen below an estimated glomerular filtration rate of 60 mL/min/1.73 m². CIN, contrast-induced nephropathy; ESRD, end-stage real disease; GFR, glomerular filtration rate. (*Adapted from* McCullough PA. Beyond serum creatine: defining the patient with renal insufficiency and why? Rev Cardiovasc Med 2003;4(Suppl 1):S3.)

There are several leading explanations for why CKD is such a potent risk factor for adverse outcomes, including CIN, after cardiovascular events [11]:

1. Excess comorbidities in CKD patients, including older age and diabetes
2. Underused end-organ protective strategies in CKD patients, or therapeutic nihilism
3. Excess toxicities from conventional therapies used including radiocontrast material and antithrombotic agents
4. The unique pathobiology of the CKD state, which includes intrarenal vasoconstriction when exposed to iodinated contrast agents

Small rises in creatinine level following percutaneous coronary intervention are linked to poor outcomes

CIN, defined as a transient rise in creatinine level of more than 25% above the baseline, occurs in approximately 13% of nondiabetics and 20% of diabetics undergoing PCI (Fig. 2) [12]. Fortunately, rates of CIN leading to dialysis are low (0.5%–2.0%), but, when they occur, they are related to catastrophic outcomes including a 36% in-hospital mortality rate and a 2-year survival of only 19% [12]. Transient rises in creatinine level are directly related to longer ICU and hospital-ward stays (3 and 4 more

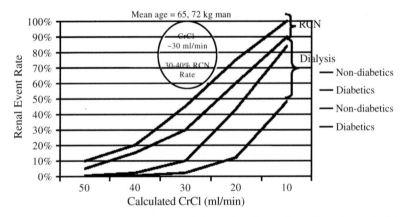

Fig. 2. Validated risk of acute renal failure requiring dialysis after diagnostic angiography and ad hoc angioplasty (assumes a mean contrast dose of 250 mL and a mean age of 65 years). CrCl, creatinine clearance; RCN, radio-contrast nephropathy. (*From* McCullough PA, Sandberg KR. Epidemiology of contrast-induced nephropathy. Rev Cardiovasc Med 2003;4(Suppl 5):S5; with permission.)

days, respectively) after bypass surgery [13]. Recently, it has been shown that even transient rises in creatinine level translate to differences in adjusted long-term outcomes after PCI (Fig. 3) [14]. This finding suggests that when renal function declines, atherosclerosis accelerates, and hence CAD progresses at a higher rate. An additional explanation is that even reversible CIN may be a marker of endothelial dysfunction and limited microvascular reserve, conferring a poor prognosis. This possibility raises the intriguing issue of whether renal protection might influence long-term CAD outcomes [11].

Rationale for renal protection for intervention patients

End-organ protection for CKD patients at risk (eGFR < 60 mL/min/1.73 m^2) can be thought of in two realms: renal protection and vascular protection. Long-term cardiorenal protection involves two important concepts. The first is blood pressure control in CKD to an ideal systolic blood pressure lower than 120 mm Hg [3]. The second is use of an agent that blocks the renin–angiotensin system, such as an angiotensin-converting enzyme (ACE) inhibitor or an angiotensin-receptor blocker (ARB) as the base of therapy [15]. Both agents will cause a chronic rise in creatinine level greater than 25% above the baseline in approximately 10% to 15% of elderly cardiovascular

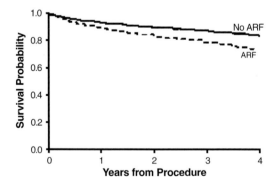

Fig. 3. Adjusted long-term outcomes in 7586 patients with and without acute renal failure after angioplasty ($P < 0.0001$). Acute renal failure is defined as a 0.5-mg/dL or greater rise in creatinine after PCI. ARF, acute renal failure; MI, myocardial infarction. (*Adapted from* Rihal CS, Textor SC, Grill DE, et al. Incidence and prognostic importance of acute renal failure after percutaneous coronary intervention. Circulation 2002;105(19): 2264; with permission.)

patients [16]. It has been shown, that despite the rise in creatinine level, ACE inhibitor/ARB agents show large benefits in reducing the number of new cases of end-stage renal disease (ESRD), congestive heart failure, or cardiovascular death [17–21]. It has been sufficiently shown that these benefits extend to nondiabetics and to African Americans with CKD [22,23]. Prevention measures done before PCI include hydration, measures to reduce the direct cellular toxicity of the contrast, and, importantly, measures to reduce the intrarenal vasoconstriction and oxidative stress that occur uniquely in CKD patients when exposed to iodinated contrast [10]. Based on the totality of evidence to date, if a patient can be carried through a cardiovascular procedure (PCI or bypass surgery) without a rise in creatinine level, one can expect a shorter hospital stay and improved long-term survival.

Pathophysiology of contrast-induced nephropathy

There are three core elements in the pathophysiology of CIN: (1) direct toxicity of iodinated contrast to nephrons, (2) microshowers of atheroemboli to the kidneys, and (3) contrast- and atheroemboli-induced intrarenal vasoconstriction [24]. Direct toxicity to nephrons with iodinated contrast has been demonstrated and seems to be related to the osmolality of the contrast [25]. Hence, low-ionic or nonionic and low-osmolar or iso-osmolar contrast agents have been shown to be less nephrotoxic in vitro. Microshowers of cholesterol emboli are thought to occur in about 50% of percutaneous interventions in which a guiding catheter is passed through the aorta [26]. Most of these showers are clinically silent. In approximately 1% of high-risk cases, however, an acute cholesterol emboli syndrome can develop manifested by acute renal failure, mesenteric ischemia, livedo reticularis, decreased microcirculation to the extremities, and in some cases, embolic stroke. Finally, intrarenal vasoconstriction as a pathologic vascular response to contrast media, and perhaps as an organ response to cholesterol emboli, is a final hypoxic/ischemic injury to the kidney during PCI caused by activation of the renal sympathetic nervous system and a reduction in renal blood flow [27]. The most important predictor of CIN is underlying renal dysfunction. The remnant nephron theory postulates that after sufficient chronic kidney damage has occurred and the eGFR is reduced to less than 60 mL/min/1.73 m^2, the remaining nephrons must pick up the remaining filtration load, have increased oxygen demands, and are more susceptible to ischemic and oxidative injury.

Prevention of contrast-induced nephropathy

For patients with significant CKD (eg, a base-line eGFR < 60 mL/min/1.73 m^2) a CIN pre-vention strategy should be employed. In general, at an eGFR of 30 mL/min/1.73 m^2, the expected rate of CIN is 30% to 40%, and the rate of acute renal failure requiring dialysis is approximately 2% to 8% (Fig. 2) [24]. There are four basic concepts in CIN prevention: (1) hydration, (2) choice and quantity of contrast, (3) pre-, intra-, and postprocedural end-organ protection with pharmacotherapy, and (4) postprocedural moni-toring and expectant care.

Hydration with intravenous normal or ½ normal saline is reasonable starting 3 to 12 hours before the procedure at a rate of 1 to 2 mL/kg/h [28]. A simple intravenous rate to remember from clinical trials of hydration is 150 mL/h. Those at risk should receive at least 300 to 500 mL of intravenous hydration before contrast is adminis-tered. If there are any concerns regarding volume overload or heart failure, a right-heart catheteri-zation is strongly recommended for management during and after the case. A urine output of 150 mL/h should be the target for hydration after the procedure. If patients have more than a 150-mL/h diuresis, extra losses should be replaced with more intravenous fluid. In general, this strategy calls for hydration orders of normal or ½ normal saline at 150 mL/h for at least 6 hours after the procedure. When adequate urine flow rates were achieved in a clinical trial setting, there was a 50% reduction in the rate of CIN observed [28].

As discussed previously, the lower the ionicity and osmolality of the contrast agent, the less renal toxicity is expected. This observation has now been confirmed in two large-scale, double-blind, randomized, controlled trials. In the Iohexol Cooperative Study (N = 1196), iohexol (Omni-paque; Amersham Health, Princeton, New Jersey) was found to be superior to the high-ionic con-trast agent (diatrizoate meglumine [Hypaque-76]; Amersham Health) in patients with diabetes and baseline CKD [29]. In the recently completed Nephrotoxicity in High-Risk Patients Study of Iso-Osmolar and Low-Osmolar Non-Ionic Contrast Media (NEPHRIC) study, iodixanol

(Visipaque; Amersham Health), a nonionic, iso-osmolar contrast agent, was proven to be superior to iohexol, with lower rates of CIN observed [30]. Iodixanol has also been demonstrated to be less thrombogenic than other contrast agents in the COURT trial with a 45% reduction in major adverse cardiac events compared with ioxaglate meglumine (Hexabrix; Mallinckrodt Inc., St. Louis, Missouri). Iodixanol is therefore the con-trast agent of choice in patients at high renal risk undergoing intervention [31]. In general, it is desirable to limit contrast to less than 100 mL for any procedure [10]. If staged procedures are planned, it is desirable to have more than 10 days between the first and second contrast exposure if CIN has occurred on the first contrast exposure.

More than 35 randomized trials have tested various strategies for the prevention of CIN [10]. Most of these trials were small, underpowered, and did not find the preventive strategy under investigation to be better than placebo. A few lessons have been learned from these trials:

1. Diuretics in the form of loop diuretics or mannitol can worsen CIN if there is inadequate volume replacement for the diuresis that follows.
2. Low-dose or renal-dose levels of dopamine cannot be achieved despite its popularity in practice, given the counterbalancing forces of intrarenal vasodilation through the dopamine-1 receptor and the vasoconstricting forces of the dopamine-2, alpha, and beta receptors.
3. Renal-toxic agents including nonsteroidal anti-inflammatory agents, aminoglycosides, and cyclosporin should not be administered in the periprocedural period.

There are currently no approved agents for the prevention of CIN. The most popular strategy at this time is optimal hydration, use of iodixanol as the contrast agent of choice, and oral or in-travenous administration of N-acetylcysteine, a cytoprotective agent against oxidative injury. A recent meta-analysis of N-acetylcysteine suggested benefit in the pooled analysis; however, a large definitive randomized trial of N-acetylcysteine in the prevention of CIN is needed (Fig. 4) [32]. Most operators believe, given the seriousness of CIN as a complication, the relative safety of the strategies used, and the evolution of clinical trials shaping current practice, that the combination of hydration and the use of iodixanol and N-acetylcysteine is a reasonable three-pronged

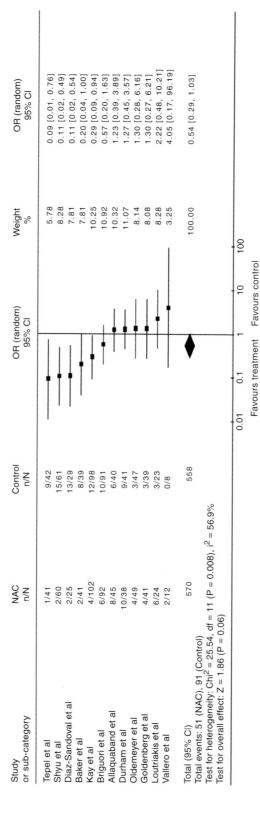

Study or sub-category	NAC n/N	Control n/N	OR (random) 95% CI	Weight %	OR (random) 95% CI
Tepel et al	1/41	9/42		5.78	0.09 [0.01, 0.76]
Shyu et al	2/60	15/61		8.28	0.11 [0.02, 0.49]
Diaz-Sandoval et al	2/25	13/29		7.81	0.11 [0.02, 0.54]
Baker et al	2/41	8/39		7.81	0.20 [0.04, 1.00]
Kay et al	4/102	12/98		10.25	0.29 [0.09, 0.94]
Briguori et al	6/92	10/91		10.92	0.57 [0.20, 1.63]
Allaquaband et al	8/45	6/40		10.32	1.23 [0.39, 3.89]
Durham et al	10/38	9/41		11.07	1.27 [0.45, 3.57]
Oldemeyer et al	4/49	3/47		8.14	1.30 [0.28, 6.16]
Goldenberg et al	4/41	3/39		8.08	1.30 [0.27, 6.21]
Loutriakis et al	6/24	3/23		8.28	2.22 [0.48, 10.21]
Vallero et al	2/12	0/8		3.25	4.05 [0.17, 96.19]
Total (95% CI)	570	558		100.00	0.54 [0.29, 1.03]

Total events: 51 (NAC), 91 (Control)
Test for heterogeneity: Chi^2 = 25.54, df = 11 (P = 0.008), I^2 = 56.9%
Test for overall effect: Z = 1.86 (P = 0.06)

0.01   0.1   1   10   100
Favours treatment   Favours control

Fig. 4. Meta-analysis of the effects of *N*-acetylcysteine versus control for the risk of contrast media–induced neuropathy in subjects with baseline renal impairment, stratified by effect size. NAC, *N*-acetylcysteine; OR, odds ratio. (*Adapted from* Fishbane S, McCullough PA, Rudnick M. Systematic review of the role of *N*-acetylcysteine in the prevention of contrast media-induced nephropathy. J Am Soc Nephrol 2003;14:1553.)

approach to minimize CIN and the risk of acute renal failure requiring dialysis.

Postprocedural monitoring is an issue in the modern era of short hospital stays and outpatient procedures. In general, in high-risk patients in the hospital hydration should start 12 hours before the procedure and continue at least 6 hours afterwards. A serum creatinine level should be measured 24 hours after the procedure. For outpatients, particularly those with eGFRs below 60 mL/hour, either an overnight hospital stay or discharge to home with 48-hour follow-up and creatinine measurement is advised. It has been demonstrated that individuals who develop severe CIN have a rise in creatinine level of more than 0.5 mg/dL in the first 24 hours after the procedure [33]. Hence, discharge to home may be considered for those who have not had this degree of

creatinine elevation and who otherwise have had uneventful courses.

In summary, for CIN risk assessment and prevention, the items in Box 1 are advised. It is important to discuss CIN risks in the consent process. For those with eGFR lower than 30 mL/min/1.73 m^2, the possibility of dialysis should be mentioned. For those with eGFR lower than 15 mL/min/1.73 m^2, nephrology consultation is advised with possible planning for dialysis after the procedure.

Coronary pathobiology in chronic kidney disease

As renal function declines, a host of abnormalities develop, including changes in coagulation, fibrinolysis, lipids, endothelial dysfunction, homocysteine, anemia, calcium–phosphorus balance, and many other factors that have been related to CVD [11]. The leading hypotheses explaining these changes include chronic hyperactivation of the renin–angiotensin system leading to adverse cardiac remodeling, accelerated atherosclerosis, and symptomatic events [11]. There are approximately 15 to 20 biologic hypotheses concerning renal dysfunction, uremia, and the acceleration of atherosclerosis [34]. At least six therapeutic approaches, including homocysteine reduction, modification of dyslipidemia with statins/ezetimibe, attenuation of vascular calcification with statins or sevelamer, use of cardiac and renal protective natriuretic peptides, and anemia correction with exogenous erythropoietin, have been investigated in prospective randomized treatment trials [34].

The decision to carry out coronary intervention in renal patients

Patients with CKD undergoing PCI also have worse short- and long-term clinical outcomes, including death, than patients with normal renal function. In the early days of PCI, the clinical outcomes with conventional balloon angioplasty alone in CKD patients were extremely poor: single-center case series evaluating small numbers of patients reported restenosis rates as high as 81%, three to four times higher than in CAD patients with normal renal function [35]. Based on these observations, coronary bypass and grafting (CABG) was considered the preferred mode of coronary revascularization for patients with CKD. The contemporary practice of deployment of intracoronary stents after balloon angioplasty has

---

Box 1. Renal protection checklist for patients at high risk undergoing percutaneous coronary intervention

1. Calculate eGFR (creatinine clearance): risk is increased if eGFR is less than 60 mL/min/1.73 m^2.
2. Check diabetic status: risk is fivefold higher in diabetic patients.
3. Discuss CIN risk in informed-consent process.
4. Discontinue nonsteroidal anti-inflammatory drugs and other renal-toxic drugs.
5. Arrange nephrology consult for eGFR less than 15 mL/min/1.73 m^2 for dialysis planning after PCI.
6. Hydration with normal saline or ½ normal saline or sodium bicarbonate, 150 mL/h 3 hours before and 6 hours after procedure [28,50,51].
7. Ensure urine flow rate greater than 150 mL/h after PCI.
8. Iodixanol is the preferred contrast agent.
9. Limit contrast volume to less than 100 mL.
10. Administer N-acetylcysteine, 600 mg in 30 cm^3 of ginger ale: two doses orally, two times/d before PCI and two doses orally, two times/d after PCI.

improved the immediate procedural success rates with PCI, nearly obviating the need for emergent CABG, and has decreased restenosis rates [35].

The emergence of new technology has also improved the ability to treat complex coronary artery lesions. Because CKD patients frequently have complex lesions, the impact of these technologies on clinical outcomes of PCI was examined in a large cohort of CKD patients. The immediate and long-term outcomes of 362 CKD patients undergoing PCI were compared with outcomes of 2972 patients with normal renal function undergoing PCI. CKD patients were older and had a greater incidence of comorbidities [36]. Strikingly, the in-hospital mortality rate of the CKD patients was 10-fold higher than that of patients with normal renal function (10.8% versus 1.1%, $P < 0.0001$). Although the use of new interventional devices, including stents, improved immediate procedural success rates, CKD patients also had higher long-term mortality rates (27.7% versus 6.1%, $P < 0.0001$) than patients with normal renal function [36].

Similar results were found in a group of patients undergoing intracoronary radiation for the treatment of in-stent restenosis [37]. In-hospital and 6-month clinical and angiographic outcomes of 118 CKD patients were compared with outcomes of 481 patients with normal renal function. Intracoronary radiation significantly reduced the rates of recurrent in-stent restenosis in patients with CKD compared with CKD patients treated without intracoronary radiation (53.8% versus 22%, $P = 0.04$). Short- and long-term major adverse events, including death, were more frequent in patients with CKD than in those with normal renal function, however. Likewise, the overall 1-year mortality rates in CKD patients undergoing saphenous vein graft interventions are higher than in persons with normal renal function [38].

The effect of varying degrees of renal dysfunction on short- and long-term mortality was assessed in 5327 patients undergoing PCI [39]. In this study, patients with lower creatinine clearance rates and those receiving dialysis were more likely to have multivessel CAD, saphenous vein graft disease, and complex coronary artery lesions and were less likely to be completely revascularized at the end of the procedure. Patients with more severe degrees of renal dysfunction and those receiving dialysis also had higher rates of in-hospital death, periprocedural myocardial infarction, and need for urgent CABG than patients with normal renal function. Renal dysfunction

was an independent predictor of adverse outcomes during and after PCI, in a dose-dependent fashion: patients with CKD had higher rates of myocardial infarction and higher short- and long-term mortality rates than patients with normal renal function. In the multivariate analysis, the relative risk of death was highest for dialysis patients (8.91; 95% confidence interval, 5.3–15.0; $P < 0.001$). In the multivariate model, the risk of death during follow-up was highest for patients with ESRD, followed by patients with moderate renal dysfunction (creatinine clearance rate < 50 mL/min). Moderate or severe renal insufficiency was associated with a greater risk of death than diabetes.

Overall, these studies demonstrate that although new interventional techniques have improved the immediate procedural outcomes in patients with CKD undergoing PCI, these patients still have worse short- and long-term outcomes than patients with normal renal function. It is not clear from the available data whether these worse outcomes are caused by the renal dysfunction itself, the extent and severity of CAD, or a greater frequency of comorbidities than seen in patients with normal renal function. Although most of the studies compare outcomes of CKD patients with those in patients with normal renal function, the more pertinent question is whether, with a given degree of CAD and comorbidities, do patients with CKD undergoing coronary revascularization fare better or worse than CKD patients treated with medical therapy alone. In a retrospective study of 4758 high-risk patients admitted with acute coronary syndromes, surgical and percutaneous revascularization conferred better outcomes in CKD patients than medical therapy alone [40]. In this study, although patients with severe CKD were disproportionately treated with medical therapy alone, coronary revascularization was associated with better long-term survival, especially in patients treated with PCI (Fig. 5). In summary, the available studies to date indicate that, despite the associated high risk, efforts to revascularize patients with CKD seem to be justified.

Primary angioplasty for acute coronary syndromes

The specific situation of acute ST-segment elevation acute myocardial infarction (STEMI) as a subset of acute coronary syndrome (ACS), poses

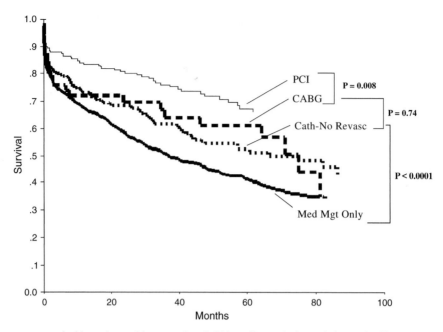

Fig. 5. Long-term survival in patients with severe chronic kidney disease (estimated glomerular filtration rate < 60 mL/min/1.73 m^2) by revascularization (Revasc) or management strategy used, adjusted for the propensity for revascularization, type of acute coronary syndrome, medical therapy received, and other significant baseline variables. CABG, coronary artery bypass grafting; Cath, catheterization; Med Mgt, medical management; PCI, percutaneous coronary intervention. (*From* Keeley EC, Kadakia R, Soman S, et al. Analysis of long-term survival after revascularization in patients with chronic kidney disease presenting with acute coronary syndromes. Am J Cardiol 2003;92:513; with permission.)

particular time-dependent issues. In STEMI, each hour that passes without reperfusion is associated with higher mortality and reduced benefit with reperfusion. CKD patients presenting with a myocardial infarction are less likely to receive aggressive therapy than those with normal renal function and are twice as likely to die in the hospital: the overall 1-year mortality rate of dialysis patients after a myocardial infarction is higher than 50% [41]. The prognostic importance of CKD in patients undergoing primary PCI for STEMI was analyzed using data from the Controlled Abciximab and Device Investigation to Lower Late Angioplasty Complications trial (CADILLAC) [42]. Although a serum creatinine level higher than 2.0 mg/dL was an exclusion criterion, baseline laboratory values were frequently not available before enrollment because of the urgency of the procedure. Of the 1933 patients with baseline creatinine values available, 350 patients had a creatinine clearance rate of 60 mL/min or less. The clinical outcomes of these patients were compared with those of the 1583 patients with creatinine clearance rates higher than 60 mL/min. Consistent

with other reports, patients with CKD were older, had more comorbidities, and were more likely to have three-vessel coronary artery disease. Procedural success rates were lower in CKD patients than in patients with normal renal function (87.2% versus 92%, $P = 0.01$), and CKD patients had a more than ninefold greater mortality at 1 month and a fivefold increase in mortality at 1 year. A key finding from the CADILLAC trial was that CKD is independently related to severe ($>70\%$) restenosis (Fig. 6) and late occlusion of coronary vessels [42]. In addition, there was a graded relationship between eGFR and mortality during the follow-up period (Fig. 7). The mechanism of restenosis in patients with CKD is not understood, and outcomes in CKD patients with drug-eluting stents have not been reported. A recently presented prospective registry in CKD non-STEMI has basically confirmed the findings of the CADILLAC trial and suggests the processes that work to create poor outcomes in STEMI are operative in non-STEMI patients as well [43].

Early series of thrombolysis in ESRD reported unacceptably high complication and mortality

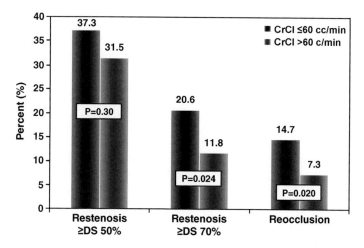

Fig. 6. Rates of restenosis after primary angioplasty for ST-segment elevation acute myocardial infarction in the Controlled Abciximab and Device Investigation to Lower Late Angioplasty Complications (CADILLAC) trial (N = 2082). CrCl, creatinine clearance; DS, diameter of stenosis. (*From* Sadeghi HM, Stone GW, Grines CL, et al. Impact of renal insufficiency in patients undergoing primary angioplasty for acute myocardial infarction. Circulation 2003;108(22):2274; with permission.)

rates [41]. In general, when available, primary angioplasty of the infarct-related vessel is the preferred approach in the ESRD patient with STEMI [41]. In a recent case series of 15 ESRD patients undergoing primary angioplasty for STEMI, however, there was a 40% incidence of cardiogenic shock on hospital admission [44]. The success rate for primary angioplasty was 80%, but the in-hospital mortality was 53%. Like all the

subtypes of ACS, there are no prospective, randomized trials of these specific approaches in ESRD.

Adjunctive medical therapy for vascular protection

Adjunctive medical therapy is key to vascular protection for CKD patients undergoing PCI. Because patients with CKD are the highest-risk

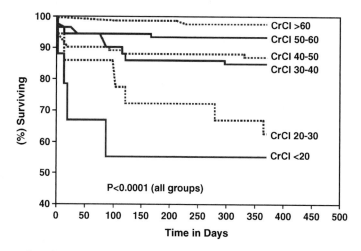

Fig. 7. All-cause mortality after primary angioplasty for ST-segment elevation acute myocardial infarction in the Controlled Abciximab and Device Investigation to Lower Late Angioplasty Complications (CADILLAC) trial (N = 2082). (*From* Sadeghi HM, Stone GW, Grines CL, et al. Impact of renal insufficiency in patients undergoing primary angioplasty for acute myocardial infarction. Circulation 2003;108(22):2272; with permission.)

subset treated by the interventionist, all the usual treatments, including aspirin, clopidogrel, ACE inhibitors or ARBs, beta blockers, and statins should be used [41]. Of interest, Khanal and coworkers [45] studied a PCI database (N = 29,409) in which pre- and postprocedure serum creatinine levels were measured. A total of 11,017 subjects (37.5%) were taking statins at baseline. Both groups (statin, no-statin) had baseline creatinine levels of 1.2 mg/dL. The rates of CIN and acute renal failure requiring dialysis were lower in the statin group. Although this study could have been confounded, the baseline characteristics were well matched, and renal protection may indeed be yet another indication for statin use.

A comprehensive discussion of intravenous antiplatelet and antithrombotic therapy is beyond the scope of this article. No large trials of abciximab have reported outcomes in patients in CKD. The small-molecule glycoprotein 2b/3a receptor antagonists (eptifibatide, tirofiban) must be given in a reduced dose when the creatine clearance level falls below 45 mL/min [46]. Retrospective studies suggest that, even though the bleeding risk is higher, the benefit of these agents outweighs the risk in CKD [41]. Both unfractionated and fractionated heparin have, in part, renal-dependent clearance mechanisms and have been linked to higher bleeding rates in patients with CKD. There are no accepted dose-reduction protocols for unfractionated heparin in CKD patients. With low molecular weight heparins, anti-factor Xa clearance begins to be reduced at creatinine clearance rates of 50 to 80 mL/min. At creatinine clearance rates below 30 mL/min, the steady-state levels of anti-factor Xa activity are increased by 65% with repeated doses of low molecular weight heparin, and bleeding events can be expected without dose adjustment [47]. Although no recommendations have been published for intravenous use in the catheterization laboratory, a reasonable approach with enoxaparin is to administer 0.5 mg intravenously and then 1 mg/kg/d subcutaneously for ACS treatment in a patient not receiving dialysis and with a creatinine clearance rate below 30 mL/min [47–48]. A recent meta-analysis of bivalirudin suggests that this agent may be the ideal antithrombotic to use during PCI in patients with CKD [49]. In this study by Chew [49], 5035 patients went PCI. Twenty-six per cent of these patients had a creatinine clearance rate below 60 mL/min, and most of them received bivalirudin for PCI at a dose of 1.0-mg/kg intravenous bolus and a 2.5-mg/kg/

hour infusion for 4 hours. Bleeding rates were considerably lower than seen in patients treated with unfractionated heparin. The absolute ischemic and bleeding benefit of bivalirudin increased with declining degrees of renal function (normal function: 2.2%; mild dysfunction: 5.8%; moderate dysfunction: 7.7%; severe dysfunction: 14.4%; P trend < 0.001).

Although patients with CKD and ESRD are at higher risks for both thrombosis and bleeding, it seems that careful, adjunctive therapy selected for these patients makes a difference in long-term outcomes. Like the decision to revascularize, the decision to use adjunctive pharmacology comes at increased risks and relative benefits.

Summary

CKD is the most important factor in predicting adverse short- and long-term outcomes after PCI. Hence, the rationale for renal end-organ protection is based on chronic renal protection, avoidance of additive renal insults, and a comprehensive CIN prophylaxis. The pathogenesis of CIN goes beyond serum creatinine and involves a unique vascular pathobiology in which interrelates renal and CVD outcomes are interrelated. Attempts at PCI in patients with CKD and ESRD are high-risk procedures, but the risks involved seem to be warranted given comparative outcomes in conservatively treated patients. The benefits of short- and long-term vascular protective therapies in CKD patients have been confirmed, and these therapies are an important component of PCI care.

References

[1] Chen J, Muntner P, Hamm LL, et al. The metabolic syndrome and chronic kidney disease in US adults. Ann Intern Med 2004;140(3):167–74.

[2] Bakris GL, Williams M, Dworkin L, et al. Preserving renal function in adults with hypertension and diabetes: a consensus approach. National Kidney Foundation Hypertension and Diabetes Executive Committees Working Group. Am J Kidney Dis 2000;36(3):646–61.

[3] Chobanian AV, Bakris GL, Black HR, for the National Heart, Lung, and Blood Institute Joint National Committee on Prevention, Detection, Evaluation, and Treatment of High Blood Pressure; National High Blood Pressure Education Program

Coordinating Committee. The seventh report of the Joint National Committee on Prevention, Detection, Evaluation, and Treatment of High Blood Pressure: the JNC 7 report. JAMA 2003;289: 2560–72.

[4] National Kidney Foundation. Clinical practice guidelines for chronic kidney disease: evaluation, classification, and stratification. Am J Kid Dis 2002;2(Suppl 1):S46–75.

[5] McCullough PA, Soman SS, Shah SS, et al. Risks associated with renal dysfunction in patients in the coronary care unit. J Am Coll Cardiol 2000;36(3): 679–84.

[6] Beattie JN, Soman SS, Sandberg KR, et al. Determinants of mortality after myocardial infarction in patients with advanced renal dysfunction. Am J Kidney Dis 2001;37(6):1191–200.

[7] Chertow GM, Lazarus JM, Christiansen CL, et al. Preoperative renal risk stratification. Circulation 1997;95:878–84.

[8] Szczech LA, Best PJ, Crowley E, et al, for the By-pass Angioplasty Revascularization Investigation (BARI) Investigators. Outcomes of patients with chronic renal insufficiency in the Bypass Angioplasty Revascularization Investigation. Circulation 2002; 14;105(19):2253–8.

[9] Keane WF, Eknoyan G. Proteinuria, albuminuria, risk, assessment, detection, elimination (PARADE): a position paper of the National Kidney Foundation. Am J Kidney Dis 1999;33(5):1004–10.

[10] McCullough PA, Manley HJ. Prediction and prevention of contrast nephropathy. J Interven Cardiol 2001;14(5):547–58.

[11] McCullough PA. Cardiorenal risk: an important clinical intersection. Rev Cardiovasc Med 2002; 3(2):71–6.

[12] McCullough PA, Wolyn R, Rocher LL, et al. Acute renal failure after coronary intervention: incidence, risk factors, and relationship to mortality. Am J Med 1997;103:368–75.

[13] Mangano CM, Diamondstone LS, Ramsay JG, et al. Renal dysfunction after myocardial revascularization: risk factors, adverse outcomes, and hospital resource utilization. The Multicenter Study of Perioperative Ischemia Research Group. Ann Intern Med 1998;128:194–203.

[14] Rihal CS, Textor SC, Grill DE, et al. Incidence and prognostic importance of acute renal failure after percutaneous coronary intervention. Circulation 2002;105(19):2259–64.

[15] Garg J, Bakris GL. Angiotensin converting enzyme inhibitors or angiotensin receptor blockers in nephropathy from type 2 diabetes. Curr Hypertens Rep 2002;4(3):185–90.

[16] Pitt B, Segal R, Martinez FA, et al. Randomised trial of losartan versus captopril in patients over 65 with heart failure (Evaluation of Losartan in the Elderly Study, ELITE). Lancet 1997;349(9054): 747–52.

[17] Toto R. Angiotensin II subtype 1 receptor blockers and renal function. Arch Intern Med 2001; 161(12):1492–9.

[18] Brenner BM, Cooper ME, de Zeeuw, D, et al, for the RENAAL Study Investigators. Effects of losartan on renal and cardiovascular outcomes in patients with type 2 diabetes and nephropathy. N Engl J Med 2001;345(12):861–9.

[19] Lewis EJ, Hunsicker LG, Clarke WR, et al, for the Collaborative Study Group. Renoprotective effect of the angiotensin-receptor antagonist irbesartan in patients with nephropathy due to type 2 diabetes. N Engl J Med 2001;345(12):851–60.

[20] Parving HH, Lehnert H, Brochner-Mortensen J, et al, for the Irbesartan in Patients with Type 2 Diabetes and Microalbuminuria Study Group. The effect of irbesartan on the development of diabetic nephropathy in patients with type 2 diabetes. N Engl J Med 2001;345(12):870–8.

[21] Dahlof B, Devereux RB, Kjeldsen SE, et al, for the LIFE Study Group. Cardiovascular morbidity and mortality in the Losartan Intervention for Endpoint reduction in hypertension study (LIFE): a randomised trial against atenolol. Lancet 2002; 359(9311):995–1003.

[22] Mann JF, Gerstein HC, Pogue J, et al. Renal insufficiency as a predictor of cardiovascular outcomes and the impact of ramipril: the HOPE randomized trial. Ann Intern Med 2001;134(8):629–36.

[23] Agodoa LY, Appel L, Bakris GL, et al, for the African American Study of Kidney Disease and Hypertension (AASK) Study Group. Effect of ramipril vs amlodipine on renal outcomes in hypertensive nephrosclerosis: a randomized controlled trial. JAMA 2001;285(21):2719–28.

[24] McCullough PA, Sandberg KR. Epidemiology of contrast-induced nephropathy. Rev Cardiovasc Med 2003;4(Suppl 5):S3–9.

[25] Andersen KJ, Christensen EI, Vik H. Effects of iodinated x-ray contrast media on renal epithelial cells in culture. Invest Radiol 1994;29(11):955–62.

[26] Keeley EC, Grines CL. Scraping of aortic debris by coronary guiding catheters: a prospective evaluation of 1,000 cases. J Am Coll Cardiol 1998; 32(7):1861–5.

[27] Denton KM, Shweta A, Anderson WP. Preglomerular and postglomerular resistance responses to different levels of sympathetic activation by hypoxia. Am Soc Nephrol J 2002;13(1):27–34.

[28] Stevens MA, McCullough PA, Tobin KJ, et al. A prospective randomized trial of prevention measures in patients at high risk for contrast nephropathy: results of the P.R.I.N.C.E. Study. Prevention of Radiocontrast Induced Nephropathy Clinical Evaluation. J Am Coll Cardiol 1999; 33(2):403–11.

[29] Rudnick MR, Goldfarb S, Wexler L, Ludbrook PA, et al. Nephrotoxicity of ionic and nonionic contrast media in 1196 patients: a randomized trial. The

Iohexol Cooperative Study. Kidney Int 1995;47(1): 254–61.

[30] Aspelin P, Aubry P, Fransson SG, et al, for the Nephrotoxicity in High-Risk Patients Study of Iso-Osmolar and Low-Osmolar Non-Ionic Contrast Media Study Investigators. Nephrotoxic effects in high-risk patients undergoing angiography. N Engl J Med 2003;348(6):491–9.

[31] Davidson CJ, Laskey WK, Hermiller JB, et al. Randomized trial of contrast media utilization in high-risk PTCA: the COURT trial. Circulation 2000;101(18):2172–7.

[32] Fishbane S, McCullough PA, Rudnick M. Systematic review of the role of N-acetylcysteine in the prevention of contrast media-induced nephropathy. J Am Soc Nephrol 2003;14:1553.

[33] Guitterez N, Diaz A, Timmis GC, et al. Determinants of serum creatinine trajectory in acute contrast nephropathy. J Interv Cardiol 2002;15(5):349–54.

[34] McCullough PA. Why is chronic kidney disease the "spoiler" for cardiovascular outcomes? J Am Coll Cardiol 2003;41(5):725–8.

[35] Keeley EC, McCullough PA. Coronary revascularization in patients with end-stage renal disease: risks, benefits, and optimal strategies. Rev Cardiovasc Med 2003;4(3):125–30.

[36] Rubenstein MH, Harrell LC, Sheynberg BV, et al. Are patients with renal failure good candidates for percutaneous coronary revascularization in the new device era? Circulation 2000;102:2966–72.

[37] Gruberg L, Waksman R, Ajani AE, et al. The effect of intracoronary radiation for the treatment of recurrent in-stent restenosis in patients with chronic renal failure. J Am Coll Cardiol 2001;38:1049–53.

[38] Gruberg L, Weissman NJ, Pichard AD, et al. Impact of renal function on morbidity and mortality after percutaneous aortocoronary saphenous vein graft intervention. Am Heart J 2003;145:529–34.

[39] Best PJ, Lennon R, Ting HH, et al. The impact of renal insufficiency on clinical outcomes in patients undergoing percutaneous coronary interventions. J Am Coll Cardiol 2002;39:1113–9.

[40] Keeley EC, Kadakia R, Soman S, et al. Analysis of long-term survival after revascularization in patients with chronic kidney disease presenting with acute coronary syndromes. Am J Cardiol 2003;92(5): 509–14.

[41] McCullough PA. Acute coronary syndromes in patients with renal failure. Curr Cardiol Rep 2003; 5:266–70.

[42] Sadeghi HM, Stone GW, Grines CL, et al. Impact of renal insufficiency in patients undergoing primary angioplasty for acute myocardial infarction. Circulation 2003;108(22):2769–75.

[43] Dumaine R, Tanguy ML, Collet JP, et al. A prospective multicenter registry evaluating renal failure in ACS patients (the SYCOMORE) [abstract 22053]. Eur Heart J 2003; (abstract Suppl).

[44] West AJ, Dixon SR, Kahn JK, et al. Effectiveness of primary angioplasty for acute myocardial infarction in patients on dialysis. Am J Cardiol 2004;93(4): 468–70.

[45] Khanal S, Attallah N, Smith DE, et al. Does statin therapy reduce contrast-induced nephropathy? An analysis from a large regional registry of contemporary percutaneous interventions. J Am Coll Cardiol 2004;45(5):420.

[46] Sica D. The implications of renal impairment among patients undergoing percutaneous coronary intervention. J Invasive Cardiol 2002;14(Suppl B): 30B–7B.

[47] Lovenox (enoxaparin sodium) [package insert]. Paris, France: Aventis Pharmaceuticals Inc; 2004.

[48] Choussat R, Montalescot G, Collet JP, et al. A unique, low dose of intravenous enoxaparin in elective percutaneous coronary intervention. J Am Coll Cardiol 2002;40(11):1943–50.

[49] Chew DP, Bhatt DL, Kimball W, et al. Bivalirudin provides increasing benefit with decreasing renal function: a meta-analysis of randomized trials. Am J Cardiol 2003;92(8):919–23.

[50] Mueller C, Buerkle G, Buettner HJ, et al. Prevention of contrast media-associated nephropathy: randomized comparison of 2 hydration regimens in 1620 patients undergoing coronary angioplasty. Arch Intern Med 2002;162(3):329–36.

[51] Merten GJ, Burgess WP, Gray LV, et al. Prevention of contrast-induced nephropathy with sodium bicarbonate: a randomized controlled trial. JAMA 2004;291(19):2328–34.

ELSEVIER
SAUNDERS

Cardiol Clin 23 (2005) 311–317

CARDIOLOGY
CLINICS

Pathophysiology of Cardiovascular Disease and Renal Failure

Ralf Dikow, MD, Martin Zeier, MD, Eberhard Ritz, MD*

Department of Nephrology, University Hospital of Heidelberg,
Bergheimer Strasse 56a 691115, Heidelberg, Germany

Observation has repeatedly confirmed the seminal observation of Lindner et al [1] on the excessive cardiovascular (CV) mortality in patients receiving renal replacement therapy. Today it is well established that in patients receiving renal replacement therapy the relative risk of dying from cardiac causes increases by a factor of 10 to 100, depending on age [2]. It has only recently been recognized, however, that even minor renal dysfunction, as reflected by an increase in urinary albumin excretion or a decrease in glomerular filtration rate, is an independent CV risk factor [3–6] in addition to the known risk factors assessed by the Framingham score. Because of the high prevalence of minor renal dysfunction in the general population, such recent insights have enormous public health relevance.

This article discusses the epidemiology of CV events in end-stage and early renal disease, summarizes the profile of classic and nonclassic CV risk factors in renal patients, highlights recent evidence documenting accelerated atherogenesis in renal disease, and closes by providing information on the central arteries and heart as target organs for CV damage in renal disease.

Cardiovascular risk in end-stage renal disease

The seminal observation of Lindner [1] of the high rate of CV events, particularly from ischemic heart disease, has been amply confirmed by numerous studies and registry reports. Fig. 1

shows early observations of the late A. Raine [7] indicating that, compared with the general population, the event rate in dialyzed patients is consistently higher by a factor of 15 to 20, irrespective of gender and country.

To interpret the underlying pathophysiology correctly, it is important appreciate that the most frequent cause of death is cardiac arrest (ie, sudden death [8]) as illustrated in Table 1.

Cardiovascular risk in incipient renal disease

It has recently been recognized that evidence of minor renal dysfunction (ie, microalbuminuria or reduced glomerular filtration rate) is associated with excessive CV risk [3–6]. In a population-based study, Hillege [9] and Borch-Johnsen [10] found that survival is significantly reduced even in nondiabetic, nonhypertensive individuals with microalbuminuria. Microalbuminuria is correlated with classic risk indicators, particularly glycemia and insulin resistance [11,12], but previous studies had documented that microalbuminuria is an independent risk predictor [10]. It is currently uncertain whether microalbuminuria is a marker of a generalized endothelial defect, evidence of minor renal dysfunction, or both. The recent finding that microalbuminuria is related to a polymorphism of podocin (NPHS2), a molecule of the glomerular filtration slit that controls the traffic of proteins into the filtrate, is consistent with the notion that it is related to podocyte dysfunction [13].

Following the observation in the Hypertension Detection and Follow-up Program [14] of a correlation between serum creatinine concentration and mortality, a number of studies confirmed [5,6] that serum creatinine or estimated glomerular filtration

* Corresponding author.
E-mail address: Prof.E.Ritz@t-online.de (E. Ritz).

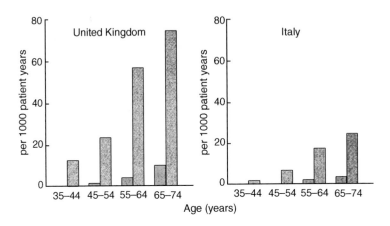

Fig. 1. Rates of ischemic events in patients receiving maintenance hemodialysis according to age and geographic origin. Note that the rate is consistently higher by a factor of 15 to 20 compared with the respective background population (*Data from* Raine AE, Margreiter R, Brunner FP, et al. Report on management of renal failure in Europe, XXII, 1991. Nephrol Dial Transplant 1992;7(Suppl 2):7–35.)

rate is a powerful predictor of CV risk in the general population [15], in hypertensive subjects [16], in patients at high CV risk [17], in patients with heart failure [18], and in patients with acute coronary events [19,20].

Risk factor profile (classic and nonclassic)

There is no doubt that the prevalence of classic risk factors is increased in renal patients [5,6], although the impact on CV events may be confounded by reverse causality. A classic example of the latter is the relationship of cholesterol to CV events. Overall, an inverse relation (the higher cholesterol, the lower the risk) or a U-shaped relationship (both high and low levels are

deleterious) is noted. The recent study of Liu [21] provided evidence that in uremic patients the relationship is confounded by microinflammation: in the absence of microinflammation, the mortality increased with increased concentrations of cholesterol, as it does in the general population.

Box 1 summarizes predictors of high CV risk including lipoprotein (a) genotype [22], low total cholesterol as an index of malnutrition, high non–HDL-cholesterol, a novel index of risk simultaneously incorporating information on low-density and very-low-density lipoprotein [23], high serum phosphate concentrations [24], and, in a complex

Table 1
Adjusted cause-specific death rates 1999 and 2001

Cause	Death per 1000 patient-years (%)
Acute myocardial infarction	19.9 (8.4%)
Cardiac arrest	51.9 (21.9%)
Cardiomyopathy	8.4 (3.6%)
Cardiac arrhythmia	11.2 (4.7%)
Heart-valve disease	1.4 (0.6%)
Cerebrovascular	12.3 (4.7%)
Total	236 ppm (100%)

Abbreviation: ppm, parts per million.
Data from USRDS. National Institutes of Health: annual data report. 1999.

Box 1. Some predictors of high cardiovascular risk in renal patients

- Lipoprotein (a) genotype (not Lipoprotein (a) concentration)
- Low total cholesterol
- High non-high-density lipoprotein cholesterol (∼low-density lipoprotein + very-low-density lipoprotein)
- High serum phosphate
- High calcium × phosphorus product
- Parathyroid hormone <65 pg/ml or >495 pg/ml
- Homocystein?
- C-reactive protein, hypoalbuminemia, fibrinogen, interleukin-6, and others

interaction, both low and high parathyroid hormone concentrations [25,26]. Although the causal role of homocysteine is still controversial, there is no doubt about the importance of inflammatory markers in both early [27] and advanced renal failure.

Apart from the indices of microinflammation/malnutrition (malnutrition, inflammation, and atherosclerosis syndrome) [28], novel markers include adiponectin, an adipocyte hormone [29]; asymmetric dimethyl-L-arginine, an inhibitor of nitric oxide synthase [30]; and fetuin, an inhibitor of vascular calcification [31].

Sympathetic overactivity is also an important factor in CV risk [32], because sudden death is the most frequent mode of death in dialyzed patients (see Table 1). Indeed, plasma norepinephrine predicts survival and incident CV events in patients with end-stage renal disease [33].

A novel risk indicator is anemia [34], which is associated with reduced survival and aggravates the risk of increasing left ventricular mass [35]. Possibly lack of erythropoietin per se may be a CV risk factor as well, because erythropoietin increases the number of endothelial cell precursors [36]. In renal failure, one finds increased numbers of endothelial cells in the circulation, possibly reflecting sloughing off of damaged cells [37], as well as reduced numbers of endothelial precursor cells [38].

Accelerated atherogenesis

Lindner [1] speculated that the high incidence of ischemic heart disease reflects accelerated atherogenesis, although later work pointed to the high prevalence of classic risk factors [39,40]. Early work by Tvedegaard [41] in the rabbit cholesterol-feeding model suggested more severe atherosclerosis in uremia, but indisputable evidence for acceleration of atherosclerosis has been presented only recently in the study by Buzello [42] in the apolipoprotein (e)–knockout mouse, a model of spontaneous rodent atherosclerosis. Even after uninephrectomy, he observed more rapid growth of atherosclerotic plaques that was associated with increased expression of nitrotyrosine (an index of oxidative stress) in non–plaque-bearing endothelial cells. Furthermore, Bro [43] recently showed increased expression of adhesion molecules only a few days after uninephrectomy or subtotal nephrectomy. These experimental studies leave no doubt that even modest impairment of renal dysfunction aggravates progression of atherosclerosis, independent of classic risk factors.

Central arteries as a target organ

In renal failure, restructuring of the aortic wall is observed [44] with reduction of elastin and increase of collagen content, similar to that seen in aging [45]. Uremia can be interpreted a state of premature and accelerated aging.

The functional consequences of remodeling of aorta and central arteries have been underestimated in the past, but recent work shows that they have a major impact on CV risk. The consequences are both functional, as reflected by impaired reactive hyperemia [46], and structural, as reflected by altered mechanical properties of the vascular wall resulting from changed intrinsic properties of the wall material [47].

An additional factor is the propensity of central arteries to undergo calcification of both the media (elastic fibers) and intima (atherosclerotic plaques) [48]. The increased stiffness of central arteries accelerates the propagation of the pulse wave and earlier return of the reflected wave (augmentation). The altered pressure–volume relationship causes increased peak systolic pressure and accelerated decrease of diastolic pressure. The net result is an increase in peak systolic wall stress and oxygen demand, on the one hand, and reduced coronary perfusion during diastole on the other. This process explains why aortic stiffness is correlated with left ventricular hypertrophy and CV events. Clinically useful indices of aortic stiffness are pulse-wave velocity [49] and central pulse pressure [50], which are predictive of CV death.

A further complication is calcification of both the central elastic arteries and the muscular conduit arteries such as coronary arteries [51]. Calcification is favored by the absence of calcification inhibitors such as fetuin [31,52] and by high phosphate concentrations, which promote expression by vascular smooth muscle cells of genes involved in osteogenesis such as *Cbfa1* [53] or osteopontin [54]. Vascular calcification of either type predicts poor survival [55], as has also been shown using quantification of coronary calcification by electron-beam CT [56].

The heart as a target organ

Although atherogenesis is undoubtedly accelerated in uremia, it is naive (as has often been done in the past) to assume that all CV problems

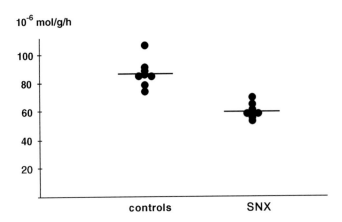

Fig. 2. Insulin-dependent glucose uptake in the isolated perfused Langendorf heart of uremic rats. (*Data from* Ritz E, Koch M. Morbidity and mortality due to hypertension in patients with renal failure. Am J Kidney Dis 1993;21:113–8.)

are explained by ischemic heart disease. In uremia oxygen delivery to the myocardium is reduced, and tolerance of ischemia is also diminished [57]. The issue is further complicated by the occurrence of interstitial fibrosis [58] and microvessel disease [59] in the heart of uremic animals and humans. Cardiac fibrosis reduces left ventricular compliance and electrical stability by favoring re-entry type arrhythmias that may contribute to the higher rates of cardiac death. The abnormalities of vessels distal to the coronary conduit artery (microvessel disease) comprise arteriolar wall thickening, limiting compensatory vasodilatation (when oxygen demand is increased), and capillary deficit with cardiomyocyte/capillary mismatch (increasing the distance for oxygen diffusion between capillary and cardiomyocyte core).

Furthermore, the frequency of heart failure is higher in uremic patients. In dialyzed patients, heart failure carries the worst prognosis of all cardiac abnormalities [60]. The factors causing heart failure have been poorly defined, but cardiomyocyte dropout has been demonstrated in experimental studies [61] and may play a major role in the genesis of heart failure.

Finally, the heart is exposed to excessive sympathetic stimulation [62]. Excess sympathetic activity is caused by stimulatory afferent signals emanating from the diseased kidney. Sympathetic overactivity is seen in renal patients even before the glomerular filtration rate decreases [63]. The causal role of sympathetic overactivity has been demonstrated by an intervention study that showed substantially reduced cardiac death when dialyzed patients were given the beta blocker carvedilol instead of placebo [64].

The results of the DIGAMI study indicate that administration of insulin and glucose substantially improves the prognosis in patients with myocardial infarction and insulin resistance [65] (although these findings apparently could not be replicated in an unpublished follow-up study). Nevertheless, we were able to document diminished insulin-dependent glucose uptake (Fig. 2) in the isolated perfused Langendorf preparation of the heart of uremic rats [66]. Improved insulin-dependent glucose uptake could be a therapeutic target. Diminished insulin-dependent glucose uptake may not be the only metabolic abnormality interfering with ischemia tolerance in uremia: Raine [67] had found instability of energy-rich nucleotides and abnormal handling of calcium during ischemia.

Given the multifactorial pathogenesis and the complexity of the underlying mechanisms, it is unlikely that there will ever be a single approach that eliminates excess cardiac risk in uremic patients.

References

[1] Lindner A, Charra B, Sherrard DJ, et al. Accelerated atherosclerosis in prolonged maintenance hemodialysis. N Engl J Med 1974;290:697–701.
[2] Parfrey PS, Foley RN. The clinical epidemiology of cardiac disease in chronic renal failure. J Am Soc Nephrol 1999;10:1606–15.

[3] Ruilope LM, van Veldhuisen DJ, Ritz E, et al. Renal function: the Cinderella of cardiovascular risk profile. J Am Coll Cardiol 2001;38:1782–7.

[4] Ritz E, McClellan WM. Overview: increased cardiovascular risk in patients with minor renal dysfunction: an emerging issue with far-reaching consequences. J Am Soc Nephrol 2004;15:513–6.

[5] Sarnak MJ, Levey AS, Schoolwerth AC, et al. Kidney disease as a risk factor for development of cardiovascular disease: a statement from the American Heart Association Councils on Kidney in Cardiovascular Disease, High Blood Pressure Research, Clinical Cardiology, and Epidemiology and Prevention. Hypertension 2003;42:1050–65.

[6] Sarnak MJ, Levey AS, Schoolwerth AC, et al. Kidney disease as a risk factor for development of cardiovascular disease: a statement from the American Heart Association Councils on Kidney in Cardiovascular Disease, High Blood Pressure Research, Clinical Cardiology, and Epidemiology and Prevention. Circulation 2003;108:2154–69.

[7] Raine AE, Margreiter R, Brunner FP, et al. Report on management of renal failure in Europe, XXII, 1991. Nephrol Dial Transplant 1992;7(Suppl 2): 7–35.

[8] US Renal Data Systems. National Institutes of Health: annual data report. 1999.

[9] Hillege HL, Fidler V, Diercks GF, et al. Urinary albumin excretion predicts cardiovascular and non-cardiovascular mortality in general population. Circulation 2002;106:1777–82.

[10] Borch-Johnsen K, Feldt-Rasmussen B, Strandgaard S, et al. Urinary albumin excretion. An independent predictor of ischemic heart disease. Arterioscler Thromb Vasc Biol 1999;19:1992–7.

[11] Verhave JC, Hillege HL, Burgerhof JG, et al. Cardiovascular risk factors are differently associated with urinary albumin excretion in men and women. J Am Soc Nephrol 2003;14:1330–5.

[12] Mykkanen L, Zaccaro DJ, Wagenknecht LE, et al. Microalbuminuria is associated with insulin resistance in nondiabetic subjects: the insulin resistance atherosclerosis study. Diabetes 1998;47: 793–800.

[13] Pereira AC, Pereira AB, Mota GF, et al. NPHS2 R229Q functional variant is associated with microalbuminuria in the general population. Kidney Int 2004;65:1026–30.

[14] Shulman NB, Ford CE, Hall WD, et al. Prognostic value of serum creatinine and effect of treatment of hypertension on renal function. Results from the hypertension detection and follow-up program. The Hypertension Detection and Follow-up Program Cooperative Group. Hypertension 1989;13:180–93.

[15] Henry RM, Kostense PJ, Bos G, et al. Mild renal insufficiency is associated with increased cardiovascular mortality: The Hoorn Study. Kidney Int 2002;62: 1402–7.

[16] Ruilope LM, Salvetti A, Jamerson K, et al. Renal function and intensive lowering of blood pressure in hypertensive participants of the hypertension optimal treatment (HOT) study. J Am Soc Nephrol 2001;12:218–25.

[17] Mann JF, Gerstein HC, Pogue J, et al. Renal insufficiency as a predictor of cardiovascular outcomes and the impact of ramipril: the HOPE randomized trial. Ann Intern Med 2001;134:629–36.

[18] Hillege HL, Girbes AR, de Kam PJ, et al. Renal function, neurohormonal activation, and survival in patients with chronic heart failure. Circulation 2000;102:203–10.

[19] Shlipak MG, Fried LF, Crump C, et al. Cardiovascular disease risk status in elderly persons with renal insufficiency. Kidney Int 2002;62:997–1004.

[20] Wright RS, Reeder GS, Herzog CA, et al. Acute myocardial infarction and renal dysfunction: a high-risk combination. Ann Intern Med 2002; 137:563–70.

[21] Liu Y, Coresh J, Eustace JA, et al. Association between cholesterol level and mortality in dialysis patients: role of inflammation and malnutrition. JAMA 2004;291:451–9.

[22] Kronenberg F, Neyer U, Lhotta K, et al. The low molecular weight apo(a) phenotype is an independent predictor for coronary artery disease in hemodialysis patients: a prospective follow-up. J Am Soc Nephrol 1999;10:1027–36.

[23] Shoji T, Nishizawa Y, Kawagishi T, et al. Intermediate-density lipoprotein as an independent risk factor for aortic atherosclerosis in hemodialysis patients. J Am Soc Nephrol 1998;9:1277–84.

[24] Block GA, Hulbert-Shearon TE, Levin NW, et al. Association of serum phosphorus and calcium x phosphate product with mortality risk in chronic hemodialysis patients: a national study. Am J Kidney Dis 1998;31:607–17.

[25] Ganesh SK, Stack AG, Levin NW, et al. Association of elevated serum PO(4), Ca x PO(4) product, and parathyroid hormone with cardiac mortality risk in chronic hemodialysis patients. J Am Soc Nephrol 2001;12:2131–8.

[26] Stevens LA, Djurdjev O, Cardew S, et al. Calcium, phosphate, and parathyroid hormone levels in combination and as a function of dialysis duration predict mortality: evidence for the complexity of the association between mineral metabolism and outcomes. J Am Soc Nephrol 2004;15:770–9.

[27] Shlipak MG, Fried LF, Crump C, et al. Elevations of inflammatory and procoagulant biomarkers in elderly persons with renal insufficiency. Circulation 2003;107:87–92.

[28] Stenvinkel P, Heimburger O, Lindholm B, et al. Are there two types of malnutrition in chronic renal failure? Evidence for relationships between malnutrition, inflammation and atherosclerosis (MIA syndrome). Nephrol Dial Transplant 2000; 15:953–60.

[29] Zoccali C, Mallamaci F, Tripepi G, et al. Adiponectin, metabolic risk factors, and cardiovascular events among patients with end-stage renal disease. J Am Soc Nephrol 2002;13:134–41.

[30] Kielstein JT, Boger RH, Bode-Boger SM, et al. Asymmetric dimethylarginine plasma concentrations differ in patients with end-stage renal disease: relationship to treatment method and atherosclerotic disease. J Am Soc Nephrol 1999;10:594–600.

[31] Ketteler M, Bongartz P, Westenfeld R, et al. Association of low fetuin-A (AHSG) concentrations in serum with cardiovascular mortality in patients on dialysis: a cross-sectional study. Lancet 2003;361: 827–33.

[32] Zuanetti G, Maggioni AP, Keane W, et al. Nephrologists neglect administration of betablockers to dialysed diabetic patients. Nephrol Dial Transplant 1997;12:2497–500.

[33] Zoccali C, Mallamaci F, Parlongo S, et al. Plasma norepinephrine predicts survival and incident cardiovascular events in patients with end-stage renal disease. Circulation 2002;105:1354–9.

[34] Ma JZ, Ebben J, Xia H, et al. Hematocrit level and associated mortality in hemodialysis patients. J Am Soc Nephrol 1999;10:610–9.

[35] Levin A, Thompson CR, Ethier J, et al. Left ventricular mass index increase in early renal disease: impact of decline in hemoglobin. Am J Kidney Dis 1999;34:125–34.

[36] Bahlmann FH, De Groot K, Spandau JM, et al. Erythropoietin regulates endothelial progenitor cells. Blood 2004;103:921–6.

[37] Koc M, Bihorac A, Segal MS. Circulating endothelial cells as potential markers of the state of the endothelium in hemodialysis patients. Am J Kidney Dis 2003;42:704–12.

[38] Bahlmann FH, DeGroot K, Duckert T, et al. Endothelial progenitor cell proliferation and differentiation is regulated by erythropoietin. Kidney Int 2003;64:1648–52.

[39] Rostand SG, Gretes JC, Kirk KA, et al. Ischemic heart disease in patients with uremia undergoing maintenance hemodialysis. Kidney Int 1979;16: 600–11.

[40] Rostand SG, Kirk KA, Rutsky EA. Relationship of coronary risk factors to hemodialysis-associated ischemic heart disease. Kidney Int 1982;22:304–8.

[41] Tvedegaard E, Kamstrup O. The effect of chronic renal failure in rabbits on plasma lipids and the concentration of cholesterol, calcium and phosphate in the aortic wall. Proc Eur Dial Transplant Assoc 1980;17:240–6.

[42] Buzello M, Tornig J, Faulhaber J, et al. The apolipoprotein e knockout mouse: a model documenting accelerated atherogenesis in uremia. J Am Soc Nephrol 2003;14:311–6.

[43] Bro S, Moeller F, Andersen CB, et al. Increased expression of adhesion molecules in uremic atherosclerosis in apolipoprotein-e-deficient mice. J Am Soc Nephrol 2004;15:1495–503.

[44] Amann K, Wolf B, Nichols C, et al. Aortic changes in experimental renal failure: hyperplasia or hypertrophy of smooth muscle cells? Hypertension 1997; 29:770–5.

[45] Amann K, Ritz E. Cardiovascular abnormalities in ageing and in uraemia—only analogy or shared pathomechanisms? Nephrol Dial Transplant 1998; 13(Suppl 7):6–11.

[46] London GM, Pannier B, Agharazii M, et al. Forearm reactive hyperemia and mortality in end-stage renal disease. Kidney Int 2004;65:700–4.

[47] Safar ME, London GM, Plante GE. Arterial stiffness and kidney function. Hypertension 2004;43: 163–8.

[48] London GM. Cardiovascular calcifications in uremic patients: clinical impact on cardiovascular function. J Am Soc Nephrol 2003;14:S305–9.

[49] Blacher J, Safar ME, Guerin AP, et al. Aortic pulse wave velocity index and mortality in end-stage renal disease. Kidney Int 2003;63: 1852–60.

[50] Safar ME, Blacher J, Pannier B, et al. Central pulse pressure and mortality in end-stage renal disease. Hypertension 2002;39:735–8.

[51] Schwarz U, Buzello M, Ritz E, et al. Morphology of coronary atherosclerotic lesions in patients with end-stage renal failure. Nephrol Dial Transplant 2000; 15:218–23.

[52] Schafer C, Heiss A, Schwarz A, et al. The serum protein alpha 2-Heremans-Schmid glycoprotein/fetuin-A is a systemically acting inhibitor of ectopic calcification. J Clin Invest 2003;112: 357–66.

[53] Moe SM, Duan D, Doehle BP, et al. Uremia induces the osteoblast differentiation factor Cbfa1 in human blood vessels. Kidney Int 2003; 63:1003–11.

[54] Chen NX, O'Neill KD, Duan D, et al. Phosphorus and uremic serum up-regulate osteopontin expression in vascular smooth muscle cells. Kidney Int 2002;62:1724–31.

[55] Blacher J, Guerin AP, Pannier B, et al. Arterial calcifications, arterial stiffness, and cardiovascular risk in end-stage renal disease. Hypertension 2001;38: 938–42.

[56] Matsuoka M, Iseki K, Tamashiro M, et al. Impact of high coronary artery calcification score (CACS) on survival in patients on chronic hemodialysis. Clin Exp Nephrol 2004;8:54–8.

[57] Dikow R, Kihm LP, Zeier M, et al. Increased infarct size in uremic rats: reduced ischemia tolerance? J Am Soc Nephrol 2004;15:1530–6.

[58] Mall G, Rambausek M, Neumeister A, et al. Myocardial interstitial fibrosis in experimental uremia–implications for cardiac compliance. Kidney Int 1988;33:804–11.

[59] Amann K, Ritz E. Microvascular disease—the Cinderella of uraemic heart disease. Nephrol Dial Transplant 2000;15:1493–503.

[60] Parfrey PS, Foley RN, Harnett JD, et al. Outcome and risk factors for left ventricular disorders in chronic uraemia. Nephrol Dial Transplant 1996;11: 1277–85.

[61] Amann K, Tyralla K, Gross ML, et al. Cardiomyocyte loss in experimental renal failure: prevention by ramipril. Kidney Int 2003;63:1708–13.

[62] Converse RL Jr, Jacobsen TN, Toto RD, et al. Sympathetic overactivity in patients with chronic renal failure. N Engl J Med 1992;327:1912–8.

[63] Klein IH, Ligtenberg G, Oey PL, et al. Sympathetic activity is increased in polycystic kidney disease and is associated with hypertension. J Am Soc Nephrol 2001;12:2427–33.

[64] Cice G, Ferrara L, D'Andrea A, et al. Carvedilol increases two-year survival in dialysis patients with dilated cardiomyopathy: a prospective, placebo-controlled trial. J Am Coll Cardiol 2003;41:1438–44.

[65] Malmberg K, Norhammar A, Ryden L. Insulin treatment post myocardial infarction: the DIGAMI study. Adv Exp Med Biol 2001;498:279–84.

[66] Ritz E, Koch M. Morbidity and Mortality due to hypertension in patients with renal failure. Am J Kidney Dis 1993;21:113–8.

[67] Raine AE, Seymour AM, Roberts AF, et al. Impairment of cardiac function and energetics in experimental renal failure. J Clin Invest 1993;92:2934–40.

ELSEVIER
SAUNDERS

Cardiol Clin 23 (2005) 319–330

CARDIOLOGY
CLINICS

Relevance of Oxidative Pathways in the Pathophysiology of Chronic Kidney Disease

Jonathan Himmelfarb, MD

Division of Nephrology and Transplantation, Maine Medical Center,
22 Bramhall Street, Portland, ME 04102, USA

The expected life span for patients with advanced chronic kidney disease (CKD) is substantially shorter than that expected for age-, gender-, and race-matched members of the general population without kidney disease. For patients with stage 5 CKD or end-stage renal disease (ESRD), the single largest cause of morbidity and mortality is cardiovascular disease, which accounts for 50% of premature deaths [1,2]. Furthermore, although the prevalence of traditional cardiovascular risk factors exemplified by the Framingham Study are high in this population, the extent and severity of ensuing cardiovascular events remains disproportionate to the underlying risk factor profile [3]. Consequently, there have been considerable recent efforts to focus on so-called "nontraditional" risk factors for cardiovascular events in this patient population. Among examined nontraditional risk factors, there is increasing interest in oxidative stress, which is postulated to contribute to the excessive uremic cardiovascular risk. Other important and emerging considerations for evaluating cardiovascular risk in uremia include inflammation, malnutrition, and endothelial dysfunction, all of which phenomena are at least partially related to the dysmetabolism that produces increased oxidative stress [4]. This article outlines the scope of the evidence linking an increased burden of uremic oxidative stress to kidney disease and describes the emerging relationship of oxidative stress with acute-phase inflammation, endothelial dysfunction, and malnutrition. It reviews data suggesting that oxidative stress biomarkers are powerful predictors of

mortality risk in kidney disease. Finally, it reviews the growing evidence concerning the potential efficacy of antioxidants in patients with kidney disease.

What is oxidative stress?

Oxidative stress is commonly viewed as a disturbance in the balance between oxidant production and antioxidant defense. A pro-oxidant imbalance can lead to the oxidation of macromolecules resulting in tissue injury. Oxygen is ubiquitous in the environment, and the prooxidant status of an organism is at least partly dependent on the state of oxygenation of the organism or cell. In eukaryotes, oxidative processes occur predominantly within the mitochondria, and the mitochondrial cytochrome oxidase enzyme complex accounts for most of the oxygen humans metabolize. The cytochrome oxidase enzyme complex transfers four electrons to oxygen in a coordinated reaction that produces two molecules of water as a byproduct. The enzyme complex contains four redox centers, each of which stores a single electron. The simultaneous reduction of the four redox centers results in no detectable reactive oxygen intermediates and thereby limits the production of reactive oxygen species. Nevertheless, mitochondrial oxygen can sometimes leak through the electron transport chain, resulting in the formation of reactive oxygen intermediates and free radicals, which can then diffuse out of the mitochondria and be a source of oxidant stress [5,6]. Recently, attention has been focused on uncoupling of the electron transport chain to ATP production in the mitochondria in disease states; this uncoupling may

E-mail address: himmej@mmc.org

alter redox balance, cell signaling, and induce apoptosis.

An additional important in vivo source of excess oxidants occurs through the action of another enzyme complex, nicotinamide adenine dinucleotide phosphate (NADPH) oxidase. NADPH oxidase is especially active within the endothelium and in leukocytes for the generation of reactive oxygen intermediates [7,8]. In particular, leukocytes use high levels of oxygen and the generation of reactive oxygen intermediates in host defense against pathogens in a process known as the respiratory burst. Leukocytes contain other enzymes, including superoxide dismutase, nitric oxide synthase, and myeloperoxidase (MPO), that contribute to the production of hydrogen peroxide, nitric oxide, peroxynitrite, and hypochlorous acid, respectively [9,10]. Recently a novel additional oxidative pathway within leukocytes has been described, whereby nitrite is converted to nitryl chloride and nitrogen dioxide through the MPO enzyme or through hypochlorous acid [11]. Ozone derived from singlet oxygen in leukocytes may also be a by-product of oxidative stress that contributes to atherosclerosis [12].

In vivo, critical oxygen intermediates are produced in minute quantities and have short biologic half-lives. The low concentrations and extreme reactivity make the in vivo detection of reactive oxygen species technically difficult. In response to these technical difficulties, a powerful strategy has emerged for understanding the underlying in vivo mechanisms of oxidative injury by detecting stable end products of oxidative chemistry produced by different reaction pathways as biomarkers. These biomarkers measure the oxidation of important macromolecules, including lipids, carbohydrates, proteins, amino acids, and DNA.

Although the concepts and pathophysiologic processes leading to an increase in oxidative stress may seem clear cut, unfortunately the use of the terms oxidative stress and oxidant stress are relatively nonspecific. Whereas oxidants are continuously being produced in living organisms, a multitude of antioxidant defense mechanisms are also constantly at work, and most biologic systems are not in redox equilibrium. In most biologic systems, reducing equivalents are constantly being generated, converted, and interconverted, indicating that a major component of antioxidant balance has to do with how extensively fed the cell or organism is at the time of measurement. This limitation on the definition of oxidative stress requires that mechanisms thought to contribute to oxidative stress be investigated in vivo with a series of detailed biochemical assays rather than relying on a single biomarker.

Oxidative stress in the pathogenesis of atherosclerosis

Conditions predisposing to atherosclerosis, including hypercholesterolemia, diabetes mellitus, tobacco use, and chronic kidney disease, are also commonly associated with increased oxidative stress, reduced vascular availability of nitric oxide, and inflammation. Steinberg and colleagues [13] first advanced the hypothesis that atherogenicity of low-density lipoproteins (LDL) is greatly increased upon oxidative modification. Oxidatively modified LDL is taken up by a family of scavenger receptors on monocytes leading to conversion into foam cells, an early step in the development of atherosclerosis (Fig. 1). Reactive oxygen species can directly promote LDL oxidation, stimulate vascular smooth muscle cell proliferation and migration, and potentiate the production of proinflammatory cytokines [14]. Reactive oxygen species can also activate several matrix metalloproteinases, which contribute to atherosclerotic plaque instability and rupture, thereby precipitating acute coronary syndromes [15].

Oxidative stress probably contributes to atherosclerosis risk by increasing the production of proinflammatory cytokines such as interleukin 6 (IL-6) and acute-phase proteins such as C-reactive protein (CRP) through activation of the transcription nuclear factor κ-B (NF-κB). NF-κB is a ubiquitous rapid-response transcription factor involved in inflammatory reactions through its action on expression of cytokines, chemokines, and cell-adhesion molecules [16,17] and has been identified in situ in human atherosclerotic plaques [18]. NF-κB activation leads to synthesis of IL-1β, tumor necrosis factor alpha, IL-6, and CRP. In addition to its role as a powerful risk marker, recent evidence suggests that CRP itself may directly contribute to the atherosclerotic process by leukocyte activation, by induction of endothelial dysfunction, and by attenuating endothelial progenitor cell survival, differentiation, and function [19–21]. CRP itself can potently increase the expression of NF-κB, thereby constituting a positive feedback loop that contributes to ongoing

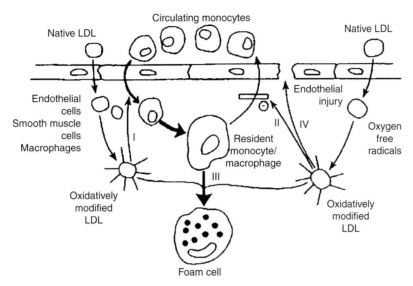

Fig. 1. Potential mechanisms for the role of oxidatively modified low-density lipoprotein (LDL) in atherosclerosis. (*From* Steinberg D, Parthasarathy S, Carew TE, et al. Beyond cholesterol: modifications of low-density lipoprotein that increase its atherogenicity. N Engl J Med 1989;320:919; with permission.)

proatherosclerotic risk [22]. NF-κB activation is controlled by the redox status of the cell, and intracellular reactive oxygen species may be common to all of the signaling pathways that lead to activation of NF-κB [23].

The vascular endothelium plays an important role in the regulation of arterial tone, local platelet aggregation, and vessel inflammation, in part through the release of nitric oxide [24]. Nitric oxide derived from endothelium has potent anti-atherogenic properties manifested through inhibition of platelet aggregation, prevention of smooth muscle cell proliferation, and reduced expression of endothelial adhesion molecules. The reactive oxygen intermediate superoxide anion produced by NADPH oxidase reacts extremely rapidly with nitric oxide, resulting in the loss of nitric oxide bioactivity. The close relationship between increased oxidative stress biomarkers, inactivation of nitric oxide, and the subsequent cardiovascular event rate has been prospectively validated [25,26]. These observations collectively suggest that oxidative stress, inflammation, and endothelial dysfunction are all causally and synergistically linked to the pathogenesis of atherosclerosis.

Recent data suggest increased oxidative stress may also contribute to the pathogenesis of congestive heart failure [27]. Studies have shown that chronic volume overload directly increases oxidative stress [28,29]. Numerous biomarkers of oxidative stress, including urinary isoprostane concentrations and plasma lipid peroxide levels, are elevated in patients with dilated cardiomyopathy and congestive heart failure in the absence of coronary atherosclerosis [30–32]. Excess myocardial NADPH oxidase activity has been detected in the myocardium of failing hearts when compared with the myocardium of explanted nonfailing hearts at the time of cardiac transplantation [33]. Many agents effective in the treatment of congestive heart failure, including carvedilol, blockers of the renin–angiotensin system, amiodarone, and probucol, are known to have antioxidative properties [34–36].

Prevalence of oxidative stress in kidney disease

Biomarkers of oxidative stress in kidney disease have been best studied in ESRD patients. In 1994, Maggi et al [37] reported that LDL isolated from uremic patients has greater susceptibility to copper-induced lipid peroxidation in vitro than LDL isolated from healthy subjects. This report was the first to suggest that oxidative stress may contribute to atherosclerosis in uremic patients. Since then, numerous studies using more direct in vivo biomarkers have shown that biomarkers of oxidative stress are altered in uremic patients (Box 1). The importance of uremic oxidative stress is emphasized by the role that lipid peroxidation

---

Box 1. Assays for in vivo detection of oxidative stress in uremia

Lipids
Malondialdehyde and other aldehydes
Lipid peroxidation
Oxidized LDL
Exhaled ethane
Advanced lipoxidation end products

Arachidonic acid derivatives
F2-isoprostanes
Isolevuglandins

Carbohydrates
Reactive aldehydes
Advanced glycosylation end products

Amino acids
Cysteine/cysteine
Homocysteine/homocysteine
Isoaspartate

Proteins
Thiol oxidation
Carbonyl formation
Advanced oxidation protein products

DNA
8 hydroxy 2′ deoxyguanine

Other
Spin traps (electron paramagnetic resonance)
Exhaled hydrogen peroxide

---

products, reactive aldehydes, and oxidized thiols play in the atherosclerotic process.

Reactive aldehydes are formed as the end products of numerous oxidative reactions, including oxidation of alcohol and amino groups and through the addition of oxygen to unsaturated double bonds. In particular, the formation of α,β-unsaturated aldehydes as oxidation products is important in that the formation of two sites of reactivity frequently leads to the formation of cyclic adducts or crosslinks with other macromolecules [38]. α,β-Unsaturated aldehydes, or dicarbonyls, are also capable of reacting with protein nucleophiles to form advanced glycation end products [39]. Several groups have demonstrated that many such reactive aldehyde compounds, including

glyoxal, methylglyoxal, malondialdehyde, acrolein, and hydroxynonenal, are detectable at concentrations up to 10-fold higher in uremic plasma than in the plasma of healthy individuals [39,40]. In uremia, reactive aldehydes accumulate because of diminished renal catabolism and increased production, largely through MPO-catalyzed leukocyte activation. The importance of increased reactive aldehyde products is evidenced by their prominent role in the pathogenesis of atherosclerosis, including the oxidative modification of LDL. A variety of aldehyde adducts can be detected in macrophages and foam cells by immunohistochemical analysis from human atherosclerotic aortic lesions [38].

Thiol groups have an important antioxidant function as redox buffers [41]. Intracellular thiols, including glutathione and thioredoxin, which are found in millimolar concentrations, are crucial for maintaining the highly reduced environment within the cell [42]. Extracellular thiols also constitute an important component of antioxidant defense [43]. The plasma protein–reduced thiols (located primarily on the albumin molecule) are depleted in hemodialysis patients and are thus not able to participate in antioxidant defense [40]. In addition, there are diminished plasma glutathione levels and a profound decrease in glutathione peroxidase function in hemodialysis patients [44]. Furthermore, although protective reduced thiols are depleted in uremia, oxidized thiols that include homocysteine and cysteine accumulate in uremia and may have proatherogenic effects [45]. Homocysteine and cysteine can promote atherogenesis by changing endothelial function and increasing vascular smooth muscle cell activation and contribute to thrombosis by increasing tissue factor expression.

In uremic patients, lipid peroxidation can also contribute to atherosclerosis through the oxidation of LDL. The nonenzymatic free radical–induced peroxidation of arachidonic acid results in the formation of F2-isoprostanes [46]. The detection of free and esterified plasma F2-isoprostanes has been used to demonstrate an increase in lipid peroxidation in uremic individuals [47,48]. In addition, another family of highly reactive electrophiles can be generated by the free radical–induced lipid oxidation of arachidonic acid with the production of isolevuglandins. Isolevuglandin adducts to plasma proteins are elevated in ESRD patients compared with healthy individuals [49]. Levels of breath ethane, which results from the scission of lipid hydroperoxides, are also higher in hemodialysis patients than in healthy individuals

[50]. An important consequence of increased lipid peroxidation in uremic patients is the increased production of minimally oxidatively modified LDL [51]. This form of LDL is extremely athero-genic and is higher in the plasma of hemodialysis patients than in that of healthy individuals. These (and other) studies conclusively demonstrate that there is increased lipid peroxidation and oxidative stress in uremic patients.

Although the ESRD population is better studied, data increasingly suggest that patients with less severe varying degrees of kidney in-sufficiency are also predisposed to accelerated atherosclerosis and cardiovascular events, even in the absence of traditional cardiovascular risk factors [1,2]. Thus, more patients with stage 3 to 5 CKD will die of cardiovascular complications than will progress to develop ESRD that requires renal replacement therapy. Analysis from ran-domized clinical trials as well as community-based studies have identified the level of kidney dys-function as an independent risk factor for adverse cardiovascular outcomes and all-cause mortality [52]. In the Chronic Renal Impairment in Bir-mingham Study, chronic kidney disease was clearly associated with low-grade inflammation, endothelial dysfunction, and platelet activation, even among patients with moderate renal impair-ment [53]. In a similar cross-sectional cohort analysis, multiple biomarkers of inflammation and oxidative stress were elevated in patients with stage 3 to 5 CKD compared with healthy subjects (Table 1) [54]. Levels of CRP and IL-6 have been found to be significantly higher in patients with renal insufficiency than in patients with normal kidney function in the Cardiovascu-lar Health Study [55]. Other investigators using different biomarkers have demonstrated that CKD patients have evidence of increased oxida-tive stress including increases in lipid peroxida-tion, advance oxidation protein products, and changes in glutathione content [56–59]. Thus, it is becoming increasingly clear that a surprisingly high prevalence of inflammation and oxidative stress, as well as a high rate of cardiovascular complications, is associated with the development of mild renal insufficiency.

Are the levels of oxidative stress and inflammation linked in kidney disease?

In numerous studies, elevations in the plasma levels of proinflammatory cytokines (especially

IL-6) and the acute-phase reactant CRP are the most powerful independent predictors of sub-sequent cardiovascular morbidity and mortality in uremic patients [60–70]. Total white blood cell count has also recently been reported as an independent biomarker of inflammation and mor-tality in dialysis patients [71]. Levels of plasmal-ogen, a phospholipid surrogate marker of oxidative stress, has also recently been associated with increased cardiovascular mortality in the dialysis population [72]. Levels of serum malon-dialdehyde, a lipid peroxidation biomarker of oxidative stress, have also been associated with cardiovascular morbidity in the dialysis popula-tion [73]. Recent studies have also used malon-dialdehyde-modified protein content and oxidized LDL content to predict mortality in uremic patients.

Although these studies show independent as-sociation between biomarkers of inflammation, oxidative stress, and subsequent cardiovascular morbidity and mortality, other investigations have also demonstrated an association between the levels of inflammatory and oxidative stress biomarkers. For instance, a positive correlation between elevated serum CRP levels and plasma thiobarbituric acid reaction substance (a bioassay measuring lipid peroxidation) have been observed in a hemodialysis patient cohort [74]. Plasma CRP levels are also correlated with plasma F2-isopros-tane content in hemodialysis patients [47,48]. Similarly, a linkage between increased oxidative stress, inflammation, and endothelial dysfunction in hemodialysis patients has also recently been described [56]. A recent study identified a higher rate of oxidative stress in hemodialysis patients with increased inflammation and hypoalbumine-mia than in normoalbuminemic hemodialysis patients [70]. These and other data suggest a bi-directional and synergistic linkage of inflam-mation and oxidative stress contributing to cardiovascular risk in uremic patients (Fig. 2).

Oxidative stress and inflammation are linked in uremic patients through myeloperoxidase

Stimulated leukocytes generate the reactive oxygen intermediate superoxide and its dismuta-tion product hydrogen peroxide and secrete the heme enzyme MPO [75]. MPO is one of the most abundant proteins in leukocytes, constituting approximately 5% of neutrophil protein and 1% of monocyte protein. MPO has the unique

Table 1
Comparison of inflammatory and oxidative stress biomarkers in patients with chronic kidney disease and healthy subjects

Biomarker	Healthy subjects median (range)	CKD patients median (range)	P
CRP (mg/L)	1.8 (0–28.6)	3.9 (0.6–28.4)	0.02
IL-6 (pg/mL)	2.1 (1.5–12.5)	6.4 (1.5–95.4)	0.001
Thiols (uM)	415 (262–497)	303 (193–435)	<0.001
Carbonyls (mmol/mg) protein	0.029 (0–0.154)	0.061 (0.020–0.134)	<0.001
F_2-isoprostanes (ng/mL)	0.036 (0.019–0.179)	0.046 (0.025–0.156)	<0.001

Abbreviations: CKD, chronic kidney disease; CRP, C-reactive protein; IL-6, interleukin-6.

Modified from Oberg BP, McMenamin E, Lucas FL, et al. Increased prevalence of oxidant stress and inflammation in patients with moderate to severe chronic kidney disease. Kidney Int 2004;65(3):1009–16; with permission.

property of converting chloride in the presence of hydrogen peroxide to hypochlorous acid:

$$H_2O_2 + Cl^- \xrightarrow{MPO} H_2O_2 + HOCl$$

MPO can also directly modulate vascular inflammatory responses by functioning as a vascular nitric oxide oxidase, thereby regulating nitric oxide availability [76]. Because MPO is released during acute inflammation, MPO-catalyzed oxidative injury and endothelial nitric oxide regulation provide a direct mechanistic linkage between inflammation, oxidative stress, and endothelial dysfunction.

A substantial body of evidence has accumulated to suggest that MPO is involved in inflammation and oxidative stress in patients with kidney disease. Catalytically active MPO can be released during the hemodialysis procedure, and 3-chlorotyrosine, an oxidative stress biomarker highly specific for MPO-catalyzed oxidation through hypochlorous acid, has been demonstrated in the plasma

proteins of dialysis patients but not in that of healthy subjects [77]. Uremic plasma containing advance oxidation protein products can induce MPO-dependent oxidation activity ex vivo in leukocytes [78]. Patterns of plasma protein oxidation observed in uremic patients (excess plasma protein carbonyl formation and oxidation of plasma protein thiol groups) can be replicated in normal plasma by the addition of hypochlorous acid, but not hydrogen peroxide and other oxidants [79]. These data strongly suggest that MPO may be a critical link between acute-phase inflammation and oxidative stress in the uremic patient population.

Use of antioxidants in uremia

Given the robust clinical and experimental data supporting the concept that an increase in oxidative stress contributes to cardiovascular disease in uremic patients, it is logical to hypothesize that antioxidant therapy may be beneficial in

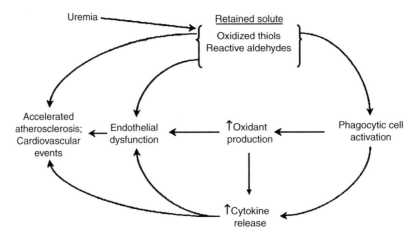

Fig. 2. Model of oxidative stress and cardiovascular complications in uremia. (*From* Himmelfarb J, Hakim RM. Oxidative stress in uremia. Curr Opin Nephrol Hypertens 2003;12:596; with permission.)

reducing these complications [80,81]. Enthusiasm for this concept, however, must be tempered by the knowledge that large, randomized clinical trials providing antioxidant therapy for either primary or secondary cardiovascular prevention in the general population have usually supported the null hypothesis. Notably, the Gruppo Italiano per lo Studio della Sopravvivenza nell'Infarto miocardico study, the Heart Outcomes Prevention Evaluation study, the Study to Evaluate Carotid Ultrasound Changes in Patients Treated with Ramapril and Vitamin E, and the Heart Protection Study were all negative trials [82–85]. A recent meta-analysis confirms a lack of demonstrated efficacy with the use of antioxidant therapy in the general population. Given the weight of these large clinical trials, a high standard of evidence for clinical efficacy should be demonstrated before antioxidants are routinely recommended as therapy for uremic patients [81].

Antioxidant studies in dialysis patients

To date, several well-conducted, well-controlled published studies have suggested that the provision of antioxidant therapy to hemodialysis patients may have clinical efficacy in reducing the cardiovascular event rate. The Secondary Prevention with Antioxidants for Cardiovascular Disease in End-stage Renal Disease (SPACE) study examined the effects of administering 800 IU of alpha tocopherol daily in a randomized, clinical trial in hemodialysis patients [86]. A clinically and statistically significant reduction in myocardial infarction and other cardiovascular events was noted in the alpha tocopherol–treated group compared with the placebo-treated group (Fig. 3). Despite the observed reduction in cardiovascular morbidity, however, overall survival between the two groups was not different. In another randomized, clinical trial, treatment of hemodialysis patients with the thiol-containing antioxidant N-acetylcysteine also significantly decreased cardiovascular events in the treated group compared with the placebo group [87]. Similar to the results of the SPACE study, this study also demonstrated no significant effect of treatment on overall mortality. These investigators have also demonstrated in a separate study that the use of N-acetylcysteine decreases plasma homocysteine concentration and improves endothelial function in dialysis patients, suggesting a direct mechanism for benefits of antioxidant therapy in this patient population [88]. Thus, there are now well-conducted published studies that suggest that providing antioxidants to dialysis patients may have some efficacy in decreasing the rate of cardiovascular events.

In addition to the above-mentioned studies with clinical end points, a number of published clinical studies of tocopherols used laboratory end points in dialysis patients. These studies have generally demonstrated either a decrease in the acute-phase inflammatory response or improved erythropoiesis. Most of these studies, however, involve small numbers of patients, are not powered to detect significant differences in clinical

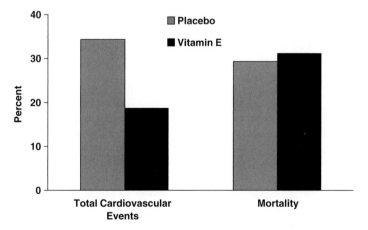

Fig. 3. Major end points of the SPACE study. (*Adapted from* Boaz M, Smetana S, Weinstein T, et al. Secondary prevention with antioxidants of cardiovascular disease in end-stage renal disease (SPACE): randomised placebo-controlled trial. Lancet 2000;356:1213–8; with permission.)

event rate, and employ antioxidant therapy for short periods. Thus, none of these studies reaches a level of evidence that would support the routine clinical use of antioxidants in dialysis patients. These studies do suggest that future randomized clinical trials should measure biomarkers of inflammation, erythropoiesis, and endothelial function in hopes of establishing a potential mechanism of beneficial effect of antioxidants and correlate with any demonstrated improved clinical outcomes.

Vitamin E–bonded hemodialyzers

Although much of the excess oxidative stress observable in hemodialysis patients seems to be caused by uremia [40,89,90], it has also been suggested that the hemodialysis procedure itself may generate excess oxidant protection through inflammatory pathways. It is well known that the contact of blood with biomaterials used during the hemodialysis can elicit an organized inflammatory response that involves the activation of the body's defense against non-self, and the term hemodialysis membrane bioincompatibility has been used to describe these interactions [91,92]. Hemodialysis membranes can elicit different degrees of leukocyte and complement activation with consequent neutropenia and leukocyte degranulation, cytokine production, and reactive oxygen species production.

Because the dialysis procedure itself may elicit excess oxidative stress, an interesting approach to alleviating excess oxidative stress during hemodialysis involves incorporating antioxidant therapy into the dialysis membrane. Alpha tocopherol has been incorporated into the coating of commercial cellulose-based hemodialysis membrane (Excebrane; Terumo Corp., Tokyo, Japan). This dialyzer has numerous modifications, all made in an attempt to improve the biocompatibility of the membrane. The cellulose material is covered with a synthetic copolymer layer to cover free hydroxyl groups. The membrane further incorporates fluororesin, which theoretically could inhibit complement activation, and oleyl alcohol, in an effort to prevent platelet aggregation. Finally, vitamin E is bonded to the oleyl alcohol component of the membrane [93]. It is unclear if a dialysis membrane is an effective mode of vitamin E delivery, or if the Excebrane modifications will truly improve biocompatibility.

A number of surrogate rather than clinical end points have been investigated in small studies with the use of vitamin E-coated hemodialysis membranes. These studies generally suggest that improvements are obtainable in serum vitamin E levels, red blood cell viscosity, endothelial dysfunction, and biomarkers of oxidative stress as compared with dialysis using untreated cellulose membranes [81]. A recent randomized, prospective, controlled study with 17 patients suggested there may be differences in the rate of progression of carotid intimal media thickness as a measure of atherosclerosis, with regression of carotid intimal thickness in the vitamin E– bonded dialyzer group [94]. Further studies using the rate of clinical cardiovascular events as primary end points will be required to determine if vitamin E–bonded hemodialyzers can decrease cardiovascular morbidity in the hemodialysis population.

Electrolyzed-reduced water treatment for hemodialysis

An alternative and intriguing approach to improving oxidative stress in hemodialysis patients is the use of electrolyte-reduced water obtained by electrolysis for dialysate. Electrolyte-reduced water can scavenge reactive oxygen species through the production of active atomic hydrogen with high reducing ability. In a preliminary study, water for dialysate production was subjected to electrolysis through a solenoid valve resulting in electrolyte-reduced water. After 1 month of therapy, the use of electrolyte-reduced water partially restored total antioxidant status and decreased plasma lipid hydroperoxide levels [95]. Further studies evaluating this novel approach to reducing oxidative stress in dialysis patients are warranted.

Summary

Patients with uremia (whether requiring renal replacement therapy or not) have a greatly increased cardiovascular risk that cannot be explained entirely by traditional cardiovascular risk factors. An increase in oxidative stress has been proposed as a nontraditional cardiovascular risk factor in this patient population. Using a wide variety of different biomarkers of increased oxidative stress status, numerous laboratories around the world have now unequivocally demonstrated that uremia is a state of increased oxidative stress. Recent data also suggest linkages between oxidative stress inflammation, endothelial dysfunction, and malnutrition in the uremic population. These factors are probably synergistic in their effects on atherogenecity and risk of a cardiovascular event. The pathophysiology of increased oxidative stress in uremia is multifactorial, but the retention of oxidized solute by the loss of kidney function is probably a major contributor. Uremic oxidative stress can be characterized biologically by an increase in lipid peroxidation products and reactive aldehyde groups as well as by increased retention of oxidized thiols. Two recently published studies have suggested that antioxidative therapy may be particularly promising in reducing cardiovascular events in this patient population. Further definitive studies of antioxidant use are greatly needed.

Acknowledgment

The author gratefully acknowledges the administrative assistance of Karen A. Kinne in the preparation of this article.

References

[1] Foley RN, Parfrey PS, Sarnak MJ. Clinical epidemiology of cardiovascular disease in chronic renal disease. Am J Kidney Dis 1998;32(5 Suppl 3):S112–9.

[2] Baigent C, Burbury K, Wheeler D. Premature cardiovascular disease in chronic renal failure. Lancet 2000;356:147–52.

[3] Cheung AK, Sarnak MJ, Yan G, et al. Atherosclerotic cardiovascular disease risks in chronic hemodialysis patients. Kidney Int 2000;58:353–62.

[4] Stenvinkel P, Pecoits-Filho R, Lindholm B. Coronary artery disease in end-stage renal disease: no longer a simple plumbing problem. J Am Soc Nephrol 2003;14(7):1927–39.

[5] Marnett LJ, Riggins JN, West JD. Endogenous generation of reactive oxidants and electrophiles and their reactions with DNA and protein. J Clin Invest 2003;111(5):583–93.

[6] Papa S, Skulachev VP. Reactive oxygen species, mitochondria, apoptosis, and aging. Mol Cell Biochem 1997;174(1–2):305–19.

[7] Babior BM. The NADPH oxidase of endothelial cells. IUBMB Life 2000;50(4–5):267–9.

[8] Babior BM. The respiratory burst oxidase. Adv Enzymol Relat Areas Mol Biol 1992;6549–95.

[9] Winterbourn CC, Vissers MC, Kettle AJ. Myeloperoxidase. Curr Opin Hematol 2000;7(1):53–8.

[10] Koppenol WH, Moreno JJ, Pryor WA, et al. Peroxynitrite, a cloaked oxidant formed by nitric oxide and superoxide. Chem Res Toxicol 1992;5(6):834–42.

[11] Eiserich JP, Hristova M, Cross CE, et al. Formation of nitric oxide-derived inflammatory oxidants by myeloperoxidase in neutrophils. Nature 1998;391:393–7.

[12] Wentworth P Jr, Nieva J, Takeuchi C, et al. Evidence for ozone formation in human atherosclerotic arteries. Science 2003;302(5647):1053–6.

[13] Steinberg D, Parthasarathy S, Carew TE, et al. Beyond cholesterol: modifications of low-density lipoprotein that increase its atherogenicity. N Engl J Med 1989;320(14):915–24.

[14] Landmesser U, Harrison DG. Oxidant stress as a marker for cardiovascular events: OX marks the spot. Circulation 2001;104:2638–40.

[15] Rajagopalan S, Meng XP, Ramasamy S, et al. Reactive oxygen species produced by macrophage-derived foam cells regulate the activity of vascular matrix metalloproteinases in vitro. Implications for atherosclerotic plaque stability. J Clin Invest 1996;98(11):2572–9.

[16] Barnes PJ, Karin M. Nuclear factor $\kappa\beta$–a pivotal transcription factor in chronic inflammatory disease. N Eng J Med 1997;336:1066–71.

[17] Collins T, Cybulsky MI. NF-kappaB: pivotal mediator or innocent bystander in atherogenesis? J Clin Invest 2001;107(3):255–64.

[18] Brand K, Page S, Rogler G, et al. Activated transcription factor nuclear factor-kappa B is present in the atherosclerotic lesion. J Clin Invest 1996;97(7):1715–22.

[19] Verma S, Wang CH, Li SH, et al. A self-fulfilling prophecy: C-reactive protein attenuates nitric oxide production and inhibits angiogenesis. Circulation 2002;106(8):913–9.

[20] Devaraj S, Xu DY, Jialal I. C-reactive protein increases plasminogen activator inhibitor-1 expression and activity in human aortic endothelial cells: implications for the metabolic syndrome and atherothrombosis. Circulation 2003;107(3):398–404.

[21] Verma S, Kuliszewski MA, Li SH, et al. C-reactive protein attenuates endothelial progenitor cell survival, differentiation, and function: further evidence of a mechanistic link between C-reactive protein and cardiovascular disease. Circulation 2004;109(17):2058–67.

[22] Verma S, Badiwala MV, Weisel RD, et al. C-reactive protein activates the nuclear factor-kappaB signal transduction pathway in saphenous vein endothelial cells: implications for atherosclerosis and restenosis. J Thorac Cardiovasc Surg 2003;126(6):1886–91.

[23] Janssen-Heininger YMW, Poynter ME, Baeuerle PA. Recent advances towards understanding redox mechanisms in the activation of nuclear factor $\kappa\beta$. Free Radic Biol Med 2000;28:1317–27.

[24] Furchgott R. Role of endothelium in response to vascular smooth muscle. Circ Res 1983;53:557–73.

[25] Heitzer T, Schlinzig T, Krohn K, et al. Endothelial dysfunction, oxidative stress, and risk of cardiovascular events in patients with coronary artery disease. Circulation 2001;104:2673–8.

[26] Cai H, Harrison DG. Endothelial dysfunction in cardiovascular diseases: the role of oxidant stress. Circ Res 2000;87:840–4.

[27] Mak S, Newton GE. The oxidative stress hypothesis of congestive heart failure: radical thoughts. Chest 2001;120(6):2035–46.

[28] Belch JJ, Chopra M, Hutchison S, et al. Free radical pathology in chronic arterial disease. Free Radic Biol Med 1989;6(4):375–8.

[29] Prasad K, Gupta JB, Kalra J, et al. Oxidative stress as a mechanism of cardiac failure in chronic volume overload in canine model. J Mol Cell Cardiol 1996; 28(2):375–85.

[30] Khaper N, Kaur K, Li T, et al. Antioxidant enzyme gene expression in congestive heart failure following myocardial infarction. Mol Cell Biochem 2003; 251(1–2):9–15.

[31] Yucel D, Aydogdu S, Senes M, et al. Evidence of increased oxidative stress by simple measurements in patients with dilated cardiomyopathy. Scand J Clin Lab Invest 2002;62(6):463–8.

[32] Nonaka-Sarukawa M, Yamamoto K, Aoki H, et al. Increased urinary 15–F2t-isoprostane concentrations in patients with non-ischaemic congestive heart failure: a marker of oxidative stress. Heart 2003; 89(8):871–4.

[33] Heymes C, Bendall JK, Ratajczak P, et al. Increased myocardial NADPH oxidase activity in human heart failure. J Am Coll Cardiol 2003;41(12): 2164–71.

[34] Chin BS, Langford NJ, Nuttall SL, et al. Anti-oxidative properties of beta-blockers and angiotensin-converting enzyme inhibitors in congestive heart failure. Eur J Heart Fail 2003;5(2):171–4.

[35] Book WM. Carvedilol: a nonselective beta blocking agent with antioxidant properties. Congest Heart Fail 2002;8(3):173–7, 190.

[36] Sia YT, Lapointe N, Parker TG, et al. Beneficial effects of long-term use of the antioxidant probucol in heart failure in the rat. Circulation 2002;105(21): 2549–55.

[37] Maggi E, Bellazzi R, Falaschi F, et al. Enhanced LDL oxidation in uremic patients: an additional mechanism for accelerated atherosclerosis? Kidney Int 1994;45:876–83.

[38] Uchida K. Role of reactive aldehyde in cardiovascular diseases. Free Radic Biol Med 2000;28(12): 1685–96.

[39] Miyata T, van Ypersele de Strihou C, Kurokawa K, et al. Alterations in nonenzymatic biochemistry in uremia: origin and significance of "carbonyl stress" in long-term uremic complications. Kidney Int 1999;55:389–99.

[40] Himmelfarb J, McMonagle E, McMenamin E. Plasma protein thiol oxidation and carbonyl formation in chronic renal failure. Kidney Int 2000;58: 2571–8.

[41] Deneke SM. Thiol-based antioxidants. Curr Top Cell Regul 2000;36:151–80.

[42] Schafer FQ, Buettner GR. Redox environment of the cell as viewed through the redox state of the glutathione disulfide/glutathione couple. Free Radic Biol Med 2001;30(11):1191–212.

[43] Ueland PM, Mansoor MA, Guttormsen AB, et al. Reduced, oxidized and protein-bound forms of homocysteine and other aminothiols in plasma comprise the redox thiol status—a possible element of the extracellular antioxidant defense system. J Nutr 1996;126(4 Suppl):1281S–4S.

[44] Ceballos-Picot I, Witko-Sarsat V, Merad-Boudia M, et al. Glutathione antioxidant system as a marker of oxidative stress in chronic renal failure. Free Radic Biol Med 1996;21(6):845–53.

[45] Bostom AG, Lathrop L. Hyperhomocysteinemia in end-stage renal disease: prevalence, etiology, and potential relationship to arteriosclerotic outcomes. Kidney Int 1997;52:10–20.

[46] Morrow JD, Hill KE, Burk RF, et al. A series of prostaglandin F2-like compounds are produced in vivo by humans by a non-cyclooxygenase, free radical-catalyzed mechanism. Proc Natl Acad Sci U S A 1990;87(23):9383–7.

[47] Handelman GJ, Walter MF, Adhikarla R, et al. Elevated plasma F2-isoprostanes in patients on long-term hemodialysis. Kidney Int 2001;59: 1960–6.

[48] Ikizler TA, Morrow JD, Roberts LJ, et al. Plasma F2-isoprostane levels are elevated in chronic hemodialysis patients. Clin Nephrol 2002;58(3): 190–7.

[49] Salomon RG, Batyreva E, Kaur K, et al. Isolevuglandin-protein adducts in humans: products of free radical-induced lipid oxidation through the isoprostane pathway. Biochim Biophys Acta 2000; 1485:225–35.

[50] Handelman GJ, Rosales LM, Barbato D, et al. Breath ethane in dialysis patients and control subjects. Free Radic Biol Med 2003;35(1):17–23.

[51] Ziouzenkova O, Asatryan L, Akmal M, et al. Oxidative cross-linking of ApoB100 and hemoglobin results in low density lipoprotein modification in blood. J Biol Chem 1999;274(27):18916–24.

[52] Weiner DE, Tighiouart H, Amin MG, et al. Chronic kidney disease as a risk factor for cardiovascular disease and all-cause mortality: a pooled analysis of community-based studies. J Am Soc Nephrol 2004; 15(5):1307–15.

[53] Landray MJ, Wheeler DC, Lip GY, et al. Inflammation, endothelial dysfunction, and platelet activation in patients with chronic kidney disease: the chronic renal impairment in Birmingham (CRIB) study. Am J Kidney Dis 2004;43(2):244–53.

[54] Oberg BP, McMenamin E, Lucas FL, et al. Increased prevalence of oxidant stress and inflammation in patients with moderate to severe chronic kidney disease. Kidney Int 2004;65(3):1009–16.

[55] Shlipak MG, Fried LF, Crump C, et al. Elevations of inflammatory and procoagulant biomarkers in

elderly persons with renal insufficiency. Circulation 2003;107:87–92.

[56] Annuk M, Zilmer M, Lind L, et al. Oxidative stress and endothelial function in chronic renal failure. J Am Soc Nephrol 2001;12:2747–52.

[57] Bolton CH, Downs LG, Victory JGG, et al. Endothelial dysfunction in chronic renal failure: roles of lipoprotein oxidation and pro-inflammatory cytokines. Nephrol Dial Transplant 2001;16:1189–97.

[58] Mezzano D, Pais EO, Aranda E, et al. Inflammation, not hyperhomocysteinemia, is related to oxidative stress and hemostatic and endothelial dysfunction in uremia. Kidney Int 2001;60:1844–50.

[59] Witko-Sarsat V, Friedlander M, Nguyen-Khoa T, et al. Advanced oxidation protein products as novel mediators of inflammation and monocyte activation in chronic renal failure. J Immunol 1998;161: 2524–32.

[60] Stenvinkel P. Inflammatory and atherosclerotic interactions in the depleted uremic patient. Blood Purif 2001;19:1053–61.

[61] Arici M, Walls J. End-stage renal disease, atherosclerosis, and cardiovascular mortality: Is C-reactive protein the missing link? Kidney Int 2001;59:407–14.

[62] Zimmermann J, Herrlinger S, Pruy A, et al. Inflammation enhances cardiovascular risk and mortality in hemodialysis patients. Kidney Int 1999;55(2): 648–58.

[63] Yeun Jy, Levine RA, Mantadilok V, et al. C-reactive protein predicts all-cause and cardiovascular mortality in hemodialysis patients. Am J Kidney Dis 2000;35:469–76.

[64] Ikizler TA, Wingard RL, Harvell J, et al. Association of morbidity with markers of nutrition and inflammation in chronic hemodialysis patients: a prospective study. Kidney Int 1999;55(5):1945–51.

[65] Stenvinkel P, Heimburger O, Jogestrand T. Elevated interleukin-6 predicts progressive carotid artery atherosclerosis in dialysis patients: association with Chlamydia pneumoniae seropositivity. Am J Kidney Dis 2002;39:274–82.

[66] Pecoits-Filho R, Bárány P, Lindholm B, et al. Interleukin-6 is an independent predictor of mortality in patients starting dialysis treatment. Nephrol Dial Transplant 2002;17:1684–8.

[67] Kimmel PL, Phillips TM, Simmens SJ, et al. Immunologic function and survival in hemodialysis patients. Kidney Int 1998;54(1):236–44.

[68] Bologa RM, Levine DM, Parker TS, et al. Interleukin-6 predicts hypoalbuminemia, hypocholesterolemia, and mortality in hemodialysis patients. Am J Kidney Dis 1998;32(1):107–14.

[69] Kimmel PL, Chawla LS, Amarasinghe A, et al. Anthropometric measures, cytokines and survival in haemodialysis patients. Nephrol Dial Transplant 2003;18(2):326–32.

[70] Danielski M, Ikizler TA, McMonagle E, et al. Linkage of hypoalbuminemia, inflammation, and oxidative stress in patients receiving maintenance hemodialysis therapy. Am J Kidney Dis 2003; 42(2):286–94.

[71] Reddan DN, Klassen PS, Szczech LA, et al. White blood cells as a novel mortality predictor in haemodialysis patients. Nephrol Dial Transplant 2003; 18(6):1167–73.

[72] Stenvinkel P, Diczfalusy U, Lindholm B, et al. Phospholipid plasmalogen, a surrogate marker of oxidative stress, is associated with increased cardiovascular mortality in patients on renal replacement therapy. Nephrol Dial Transplant 2004; 19(4):972–6.

[73] Boaz M, Mataz Z, Biro A, et al. Serum malondialdehyde and prevalent cardiovascular disease in hemodialysis. Kidney Int 1999;56:1078–83.

[74] Nguyen-Khoa T, Massy ZA, Pascal De Bandt J, et al. Oxidative stress and haemodialysis: role of inflammation and duration of dialysis treatment. Nephrol Dial Transplant 2001;16:335–40.

[75] Podrez EA, bu-Soud HM, Hazen SL. Myeloperoxidase-generated oxidants and atherosclerosis. Free Radic Biol Med 2000;28(12):1717–25.

[76] Eiserich JP, Baldus S, Brennan ML, et al. Myeloperoxidase, a leukocyte-derived vascular NO oxidase. Science 2002;296(5577):2391–4.

[77] Himmelfarb J, McMenamin E, Loseto G, et al. Myeloperoxidase-catalyzed 3-chlorotyrosine formation in dialysis patients. Free Radic Biol Med 2001; 31(10):1163–9.

[78] Witko-Sarsat V, Gausson V, Nguyen AT, et al. AOPP-induced activation of human neutrophil and monocyte oxidative metabolism: a potential target for N-acetylcysteine treatment in dialysis patients. Kidney Int 2003;64(1):82–91.

[79] Himmelfarb J, McMonagle E. Manifestations of oxidant stress in uremia. Blood Purif 2001;19:200–5.

[80] Galle J, Seibold S. Has the time come to use antioxidant therapy in uraemic patients? Nephrol Dial Transplant 2003;18(8):1452–5.

[81] Gordon CA, Himmelfarb J. Antioxidant therapy in uremia—evidence-based medicine? Semin Dial 2004;17:327–32.

[82] Gruppo Italiano per lo Studio della Sopravvivenza nell'Infarto miocardico. Dietary supplementation with n-3 polyunsaturated fatty acids and vitamin E after myocardial infarction: results of the GISSI-Prevenzione trial. Lancet 1999;354(9177):447–55.

[83] Lonn EM, Yusuf S, Dzavik V, et al. Effects of ramipril and vitamin E on atherosclerosis: a study to evaluate carotid ultrasound changes in patients treated with ramipril and vitamin E (SECURE). Circulation 2001;103:919–25.

[84] Yusuf S, Dagenais G, Pogue J, et al. Vitamin E supplementation and cardiovascular events in high-risk patients. The Heart Outcomes Prevention Evaluation Study Investigators. N Engl J Med 2000; 342(3):154–60.

[85] MRC/BHF Heart Protection Study of antioxidant vitamin supplementation in 20,536 high-risk

individuals: a randomised placebo-controlled trial. Lancet 2002;360(9326):23–33.

[86] Boaz M, Smetana S, Weinstein T, et al. Secondary prevention with antioxidants of cardiovascular disease in end-stage renal disease (SPACE): randomised placebo-controlled trial. Lancet 2000;356:1213–8.

[87] Tepel M, van der Giet M, Statz M, et al. The antioxidant acetylcysteine reduces cardiovascular events in patients with end-stage renal failure: a controlled trial. Circulation 2003;107:992–5.

[88] Scholze A, Rinder C, Beige J, et al. Acetylcysteine reduces plasma homocysteine concentration and improves pulse pressure and endothelial function in patients with end-stage renal failure. Circulation 2004;109(3):369–74.

[89] Himmelfarb J, McMenamin E, McMonagle E. Plasma aminothiol oxidation in chronic renal failure. Kidney Int 2002;61(2):705–16.

[90] Roselaar SE, Nazhat JB, Winyard PG, et al. Detection of oxidants in uremic plasma by electron spin resonance spectroscopy. Kidney Int 1995;48:199–206.

[91] Cheung AK. Biocompatibility of dialysis membranes. J Am Soc Nephrol 1990;1:150–61.

[92] Klinkmann H, Wolf H, Schmitt E. Definition of biocompatibility. Contrib Nephrol 1984;37:70–7.

[93] Sasaki M, Hosoya N, Saruhashi M. Development of vitamin E-modified membrane. Contrib Nephrol 1999;127:49–70.

[94] Kobayashi S, Moriya H, Aso K, et al. Vitamin E-bonded hemodialyzer improves atherosclerosis associated with a rheological improvement of circulating red blood cells. Kidney Int 2003;63(5):1881–7.

[95] Huang KC, Yang CC, Lee KT, et al. Reduced hemodialysis-induced oxidative stress in end-stage renal disease patients by electrolyzed reduced water. Kidney Int 2003;64(2):704–14.

ELSEVIER
SAUNDERS

Cardiol Clin 23 (2005) 331–342

Management of Cardiovascular Disease in the Renal Transplant Recipient

Claudio Rigatto, MD[a,b,*]

[a]Department of Medicine, University of Manitoba, 97 Dafoe Road, Winnipeg, Manitoba R3T 2N2, Canada
[b]Manitoba Renal Program, Winnipeg, Manitoba R2H 2A6, Canada

Cardiovascular disease is the major cause of death among renal transplant recipients (RTRs). Between 17% and 50% of deaths on transplantation are caused by cardiovascular disease [1,2], and the incidence of cardiovascular disease among RTRs seems to be increased threefold to fourfold over that observed in age-matched control populations [1].

The optimum management of cardiovascular disease in transplant patients is not as clear as it should be. The large corpus of cardiovascular trials virtually excludes patients with advanced renal disease. Concern has been expressed that the risk factors associated with cardiovascular disease in RTRs may differ from those in the traditional Framingham model, and that the traditional cardiac pharmacopeia may have an unfavorable therapeutic index. For example, until very recently, nephrologists have been tentative in using angiotensin-converting enzyme (ACE) inhibitors and statins in transplant patients.

Although the concerns regarding the generalizability of data derived from non-RTR populations are legitimately raised, on balance the literature suggests that the following assumptions hold:

1. The major risk factors for cardiovascular disease in RTRs are similar to those in the general population.
2. The risk-modification strategies proven in the general population are likely to be effective in RTRs.

* Section of Nephrology, Rm BG007, St. Boniface General Hospital, 409 Tachí Avenue, Winnipeg, Manitoba R2H 2A6, Canada.
   E-mail address: crigatto@sbgh.mb.ca

3. The rates of adverse effects are manageable, and the therapeutic index of most interventions is favorable.

This article reviews the causes of and major risk factors for cardiovascular disease in RTRs, followed by an appraisal of the evidence for specific risk-factor interventions for cardiovascular disease in RTRs.

Etiology of cardiac disease in renal transplant recipients

The term cardiac disease is frequently taken to mean ischemic heart disease (IHD). This implied identity is unfortunate, because cardiac disease in RTRs frequently results not from coronary disease but from disordered ventricular geometry and function, a condition that can be called cardiomyopathy of overload (Fig. 1). Cardiomyopathy may present as asymptomatic left ventricular hypertrophy (LVH) or manifest clinically as congestive heart failure (CHF). This distinction is perhaps moot in the general population, in which most left ventricular disorders are closely associated with underlying coronary artery disease, the two disorders developing pari passu. In RTRs, however, as in dialysis and chronic renal insufficiency, left ventricular disorders are commonly caused by ventricular remodeling in response to hemodynamic stresses from anemia and hypertension in the absence of clinically overt IHD [3–8]. Although IHD and cardiomyopathy have several risk factors in common, they are distinct entities and diverge with respect to the importance of hemodynamic factors, particularly the role of chronic anemia, which is predictive of CHF but not of IHD [8].

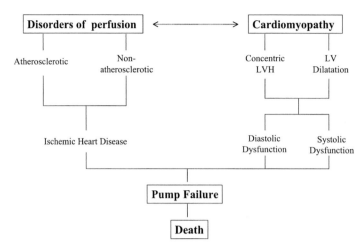

Fig. 1. Causes of cardiac death. LV, left ventricular; LVH, left ventricular hypertrophy.

Burden of disease

Left ventricular abnormalities

Several studies confirm the high prevalence of left ventricular abnormalities in RTRs and in aggregate suggest that elevated left ventricular mass is present in 40% to 60% of RTRs. Parfrey et al [9] examined an inception cohort of 102 renal transplant patients and found that only 17% had normal ventricles, whereas concentric LVH was found in 41%, eccentric LVH in 32%, and systolic dysfunction in 12% [9]. Regression of LVH does occur after transplantation but is incomplete: approximately 39% of patients still have an elevated left ventricular mass index (>132 g/m^2 in men, >102 g/m^2 in women) at 4 years, indicating that renal transplantation only partially reverses the stimulus to hypertrophy [10].

Clinical disease: congestive heart failure versus ischemic heart disease

Prevalence

Approximately 15% of transplanted patients have a history of IHD before transplantation. In a cohort of 1021 RTRs in Manitoba and Newfoundland, 10% had a documented history of IHD, and 11% had a documented history of CHF. IHD and CHF were almost mutually exclusive: only 2% of recipients had clinical evidence of both disorders, supporting the notion that these syndromes show less overlap in renal failure than in the general population.

Incidence

Among patients free of cardiac disease in the first year after transplantation, the subsequent incidence of a major ischemic event (de novo IHD) is 1.2% to 1.5% per year [1,9,11], similar to the incidence observed in the Framingham Study [12] (Table 1). At 1.2% per year, the incidence of de novo CHF is two to three times higher in RTRs than in the general population, suggesting that renal transplantation may represent a state of accelerated heart failure [13,14]. As in other populations, the development of IHD or CHF predicts poor patient outcome. Compared with patients who remain free of cardiac events, RTRs who develop de novo CHF or IHD have a 1.5-fold to twofold higher risk of death, independently of age, gender, and diabetes (relative risk [RR], for CHF 1.8, 95% confidence interval [CI], 1.2–2.6; RR, for IHD 1.5; CI, 1.05–2.1) [7].

Risk factors for cardiomyopathy

Left ventricular hypertrophy

Long-term cohort studies of cardiac hypertrophy in RTRs are rare. Most studies have shown that LVH regresses but does not normalize following transplantation [10,11,15–22]. In a 4-year follow-up study, the major predictors of nonregression of LVH were age, duration of hypertension, and severity of hypertension as measured by the number of antihypertensive medications used [11]. The impact of EKG LVH was examined in a large retrolective cohort of RTRs in Manitoba [9]. Fourteen percent of patients had LVH by Cornell EKG criteria in the first year after transplantation. LVH was a risk factor for death (RR, 1.9; CI, 1.22–3.22) and CHF (RR, 2.27; CI, 1.08–4.81) independent of other major prognostic variables. Persistent or de novo LVH 5 years after

Table 1
Studies of risk factors for vascular disease

Study	N	Inception cohort?	Free of cardiac disease?	Posttransplantion risk factors	Endpoints	Incidence Events/ 100 patient-years
Aker	427	N	No	No	CV events	4.9
Ducloux	207	Y	No	Yes	CV events	8.8
Kasiske	706	Y	No	Yes	IHD	1.53
					CVA	1.00
					PVD	1.00
Kasiske	1124	Y	Yes	Yes	IHD	Not given
Lindholm	1347	Y	No	Yes	CV death	Not given
Rigatto	638	Y	Yes	Yes	IHD	1.23
					CVA	1.26
					Death	2.5

Abbreviations: CV, cardiovascular; CVA, cerebrovascular accident; IHD, ischemic heart disease; PVD, peripheral vascular disease.

transplantation also predicted CHF (RR, 2.71; CI, 1.17–6.3) and subsequent death (RR, 2.15; CI, 1.14–4.01). Anemia and diastolic blood pressure were the only independent risk factors for increasing Cornell voltage (a marker of left ventricular mass) between the first and fifth years.

Congestive heart failure

Rigatto et al [8] examined the development of CHF in a cohort of 638 RTRs in Canada. Only de novo events in patients free of cardiac disease at 1 year after transplantation were examined to minimize confounding by pretransplant disease and risk factors. The independent risk factors identified are summarized in Table 2.

As expected, age and diabetes were identified as major risk factors for CHF. These variables have long been shown to predict CHF in the general population.

Table 2
Risk factors for de novo congestive heart failure in 638 adult renal transplant recipients

Variable	Relative risk (95% confidence interval); P value*
Age (decade)	1.43 (1.16, 1.77); 0.001
Diabetes	2.30 (1.43, 3.69); 0.001
Hemoglobin (per 10-g/L decrease)	1.24 (1.10, 1.39); 0.001
Systolic blood pressure (per 10 mm Hg)	1.29 (1.10, 1.50); 0.001
Serum albumin (per 10-g/L decrease)	2.10 (1.08, 4.07); 0.03
Cadaveric donor	3.18 (1.24, 8.18); 0.02

* Results of a multivariate Cox regression model.

The major modifiable risk factors identified were anemia and hypertension. The relationship between hemoglobin and risk of CHF was smoothly progressive for any hemoglobin level below normal. Risk was highest for patients in the lower hemoglobin quartiles (hemoglobin < 126), suggesting that even modest reductions in hemoglobin may be associated with cardiac morbidity (Fig. 2). Similar trends were observed for blood pressure. No threshold of risk was identified for either variable.

Several direct and indirect observations support a causal association between these hemodynamic factors and CHF. Both anemia and hypertension were documented to occur well before the development of CHF [8]. The monotonic increasing risk of CHF observed with worsening hypertension and anemia is consistent with causality. Moreover, studies in renal transplantation and in related populations (with chronic renal insufficiency or undergoing dialysis) have consistently shown an association between hypertension/anemia, and left ventricular growth [11,23]. Finally, a direct link has been documented between EKG LVH, hemodynamic factors, and CHF in RTR [9]. It is therefore likely that anemia and hypertension promote ventricular growth and remodeling, leading to CHF.

De novo IHD preceded or occurred simultaneously with CHF in only one-third of the cases in this cohort. Although IHD was a significant risk factor for CHF, it was not implicated in the majority of cases. Anemia and hypertension remained highly significant risk factors even after adjustment for IHD, suggesting that most CHF develops independently of coronary artery disease,

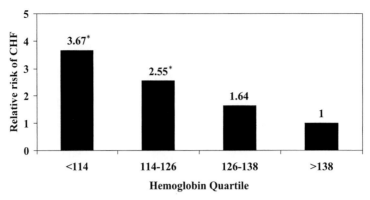

*p<0.03 with respect to reference quartile

Fig. 2. Adjusted RR of de novo congestive heart failure according to hemoglobin quartile in 638 renal transplant recipients. *, $P < .03$ with respect to reference quartile.

because of hemodynamic stress from anemia and hypertension.

Cadaveric donation is probably a marker for unmeasured patient-selection biases, because cadaveric donation is preferred for marginal recipients. Hypoalbuminemia has been associated with CHF and progressive left ventricular cavity enlargement in dialysis patients [24]. It may be a marker of malnutrition or chronic inflammation, either of which could promote cardiomyocyte attrition, cardiomyopathy, and CHF [25].

Ischemic heart disease

Several large cohort studies have examined risk factors for IHD in RTR (see Tables 1 and 3) [1,2,8,26–28]. The occurrence of IHD was measured differently in each study (eg, all-cause mortality, cardiovascular mortality, myocardial infarction, coronary revascularization), so a formal meta-analysis is impossible. Despite this heterogeneity, several important patterns emerge. Most studies have corroborated the importance of age, gender, and diabetes in the development of IHD. The modifiable risk factors smoking and hyperlipidemia have been identified repeatedly.

Blood pressure has not been implicated in many studies. Two considerations deserve mention in this regard. First, hypertension is predictive of graft failure, which is a censoring end point in almost all studies [29]. If the impact on the graft occurs more rapidly than the impact on the heart, a true relationship between blood pressure and IHD events will be obscured by the phenomenon of competing outcomes (ie, patients are censored before they experience a cardiac event). Second, and perhaps more importantly,

most cohorts examined recurrent and de novo disease together. This aggregation may obscure the relationship with blood pressure as measured after transplantation, because recurrent events are probably related to risk factors existing before transplantation. The methodology used by Rigatto et al [8] minimized the latter source of confounding by studying de novo disease occurring after 1 year in patients free of cardiac disease in the first year after transplantation. Consequently, the expected relationship between blood pressure and IHD was seen in that study. A more recent study by Kasiske et al [30] has confirmed an independent association between systolic blood pressure and graft failure.

In contrast to its close association with cardiomyopathy, anemia has not been associated with IHD in renal transplant cohorts. This lack of association may result from opposing physiologic effects. On the one hand, anemia may promote cardiac ischemia by decreased oxygen delivery to myocardium and increased cardiac work; on the other, it may lower blood viscosity, enhancing flow and perfusion pressure distal to a coronary stenosis, thus compensating for a decrease in oxygen-carrying capacity. Moreover, most major ischemic events (eg, unstable angina, myocardial infarction) occur because of thrombosis over nonstenotic, unstable, lipid-rich atherosclerotic plaques. Anemia might weakly inhibit plaque thrombosis by lowering blood viscosity and increasing flow. It is likely that anemia has a neutral, or at most a weak protective effect on the incidence of major IHD events.

Acute rejection has been identified frequently as an independent risk factor for IHD. It is not merely a marker for hypertension, donor status, steroid use, cadaveric donation, renal function, or delayed graft function, because it seems to be independent of these variables [8,12]. Repeated episodes of acute rejection may cause a state of chronic inflammation. Atherosclerosis is widely considered an inflammatory disorder, and markers of inflammation such as C-reactive protein have been independently associated with IHD in the general population [31]. Hypoalbuminemia is a crude marker of chronic inflammation and has been associated with IHD in several renal transplantation cohorts as well. In RTR, acute rejection and hypoalbuminemia may therefore reflect a state of chronic inflammation, which in turn may promote atherosclerosis.

Much debate has taken place regarding the relative cardiac toxicity of immunosuppressive agents. Different agents clearly have different cardiovascular risk profiles (eg, tacrolimus is associated with posttransplant diabetes mellitus [PTDM], and sirolimus is associated with hyperlipidemia). The impact of these differences on the patient is unclear, however. For example, one observational study showed that although tacrolimus is associated with higher risk of PTDM, and PTDM is associated with lower graft and patient survival, tacrolimus use nevertheless was associated with better patient outcomes overall [32]. Such results suggest that the impact of antirejection drugs on cardiovascular disease and survival is probably very complex, mediated by both direct vascular effects and by indirect effects on multiple risk factors. Effects on known cardiovascular risk factors cannot easily or simply predict the overall impact of these drugs on patient survival. In the absence of randomized clinical trial data showing a clear superiority of one regimen over another, the author and colleagues prefer to base antirejection therapy primarily on the patient's risk of allograft rejection and to manage cardiovascular risk with other medications as necessary.

The role of homocysteine elevations in the genesis of IHD in RTRs is unclear. Limited observational data in RTRs suggest an association. To date, the evidence linking homocysteine with cardiac disease in the general population is purely observational [33–35]. The causal inference is thus less robust than for risk factors such as blood pressure and hyperlipidemia, for which extensive clinical trial evidence exists. A randomized clinical trial of homocysteine lowering in RTRs is currently under way and may settle the issue.

Treatment

With rare exceptions, few clinical trials in RTRs exist to help guide therapeutic decisions for prevention and treatment of cardiovascular disease. In the absence of direct evidence, recommendations must be based on observational data and on extrapolation of data from other populations. The recommendations made in the following section conform to these necessities

Risk-factor modification

Lifestyle modifications

As with nontransplant patients, all RTRs should be advised to stop smoking and to exercise, achieve ideal body weight, and eat a balanced diet.

Cholesterol reduction with statins

In several studies (Table 3), high cholesterol has been shown to be a risk factor for

Table 3
Studies of risk factors for vascular disease

Study	Endpoints	Risk factors						
		Age	Male Gender	DM	BP	Lipids	Rejection	Other
Aker	CV events	Y		Y		Y		Smoking, BMI urate
Ducloux	CV events	Y	Y					HCY, GFR
Kasiske	IHD	Y	Y	Y		Y	Y	Splenectomy
Kasiske	IHD	Y		Y		Y	Y	Albumin, proteinuria
Lindholm	CV death	Y	Y	Y			Y	Delayed function, transfusion
Rigatto	IHD	Y	Y	Y	Y		Y	

Abbreviations: BMI, body mass index; CV, cardiovascular; DM, diabetes mellitus; GFR, glomerular filtration rate; HCY, homocysteine; IHD, ischemic heart disease; Y, yes.

cardiovascular disease in RTRs. Specific lipid targets for RTRs have not been developed, so treatment targets for the highest-risk groups of the general population are recommended by the American National Kidney Foundation [36]. A recent randomized, controlled trial of fluvastatin in RTRs with low-density lipoprotein (LDL) levels between 4 and 9 mmol/L demonstrated a statistically significant reduction in the secondary end point of nonfatal myocardial infarction and cardiovascular death [37]. Subgroup analyses using this end point showed similar efficacy in younger and older RTRs, men and women, diabetics and nondiabetics, and persons with low and high LDL levels at entry [38]. Because the primary composite outcome, death or myocardial infarction or coronary revascularization, did not achieve statistical significance, the results are not definitive. Taken in context, however, the results are strikingly consistent with the larger body of statin trials in the general population and strongly support the aggressive and liberal use of statins in RTRs.

The risk of adverse events with fluvastatin, particularly musculoskeletal complaints, was not higher than with placebo. Unlike fluvastatin, however, most other statins are metabolized through the same microsomal cytochrome as the calcineurin inhibitors tacrolimus and cyclosporine. Concomitant use of statins and calcineurin inhibitors may lead to higher levels and higher toxicities of both drugs. In practice, toxicities can be avoided by starting at half of the usual statin dose, titrating carefully, and monitoring calcineurin inhibitor levels and markers of myositis at each dose change. Combinations of statins, calcineurin inhibitors, and fibrates are not recommended.

Blood pressure targets

Hypertension is a risk factor for CHF, IHD, and graft failure in RTRs, but randomized, controlled trials of blood pressure lowering in RTRs are rare, and none have examined clinical end points (death, cardiovascular events, graft failure). Thus, recommendations must be extrapolated from the general population and nontransplant chronic kidney disease. Hypertension is a long-established risk factor for death, IHD, CHF, and LVH and for the progression of renal disease in the general population and in patients with chronic kidney disease [39–46]. Clinical trials in type 1 diabetes have established the benefit on proteinuria

and glomerular filtration rate of reducing blood pressure below 140/90. The relationship between achieved blood pressure and outcome in these studies suggests continued accrual of benefit at blood pressures lower than 140/90. The Modification of Diet in Renal Disease study, conducted in nondiabetic patients with renal failure, demonstrated that the impact on renal failure progression of an age-specific, lower-than-usual blood pressure target (< 125/75 mm Hg in patients < 65 years; < 130/85 in patients > 65 years) was dependent on the degree of proteinuria. Patients with protein excretion exceeding 1 g/d benefited more than those with protein excretion of less than 1 g/d [47,48]. The Hypertension Optimal Treatment study demonstrated a survival benefit for a lower-than-usual diastolic blood pressure (<80 mm Hg) in diabetics [49]. There was no evidence of increased mortality in patients with very low achieved blood pressures, supporting the safety of lower-than-usual blood pressure targets. Based on these data, the clinical practice guidelines promulgated in the seventh report of the Joint National Committee on Prevention, Detection, Evaluation, and Treatment of High Blood Pressure recommend a blood pressure target of less than 130/80 mm Hg in patients with chronic kidney disease or diabetes [50]. Given the similarities between RTRs and patients with chronic kidney disease, a target of 130/80 mm Hg or lower seems appropriate for all RTRs.

Renin-angiotensin antagonists

Again, direct evidence of benefit in RTR is lacking for renin-angiotensin antagonists (RAAs). Numerous large, randomized controlled trials, however, have shown that ACE inhibitors are superior to non-RAAs in reducing progression of renal disease, ischemic and CHF event rates, and mortality [51–59]. Angiotensin-receptor blockers (ARBs) also reduce renal and cardiovascular events in type 2 diabetics, in patients with CHF with and without low ejection fraction, and after myocardial infarction [60–67]. The reduction in event rates seems to be similar to those achieved with ACE inhibitors in most settings. Direct comparisons with ACE inhibitors suggest ARBs are not superior [68,69], but one trial established that valsartan is at least 87% as effective as captopril after myocardial infarction [66]. The combination of ACE inhibitors and ARBs seems to reduce further the risk of cardiac and renal events in nondiabetic renal disease and heart failure [70,71]. The benefit of ACE inhibitors on cardiovascular disease seems to extend to patients with mild-to-moderate renal failure [72].

There is no compelling biologic reason to believe RAAs would not be of benefit in RTRs. There are no important interactions between RAAs and immunosuppressive medications. RTRs are at higher risk of acute renal failure and hyperkalemia, but these risks are also elevated in chronic renal insufficiency and severe heart failure, where the overall benefit of these agents has been clearly demonstrated. ACE inhibitors may be associated with worse anemia, possibly because of reduced erythropoietin production, although the impact of this effect is not clear [73,74]. It would seem reasonable to recommend RAAs to any transplant patient with diabetes, chronic allograft nephropathy, or cardiovascular disease. Whether treatment of all transplant recipients with RAAs would prolong graft and patient survival, reduce cardiovascular events, and reduce PTDM is a compelling question that should be addressed in a randomized, controlled trial.

Antiplatelet therapy

It is well established that antiplatelet therapy is effective for secondary prophylaxis of cardiovascular events in patients with known atherosclerotic disease (ischemic stroke, peripheral vascular disease, ischemic heart disease, after myocardial infarction) and for primary prophylaxis in diabetes [37,75,76]. A large observational study of outcomes following myocardial infarction in patients with chronic kidney disease showed that acetylsalicylic acid (ASA) use is associated with improved survival after myocardial infarction across a broad spectrum of renal function, as would be expected in this high-risk population [77]. Compared with high-dose ASA (> 650 mg/d), low-dose ASA is less likely to cause renal dysfunction or gastric ulceration and probably has similar clinical efficacy [78]. Overall, the use of ASA for prophylaxis of cardiovascular events seems appropriate in RTRs with known atherosclerotic disease or diabetes.

Should all RTRs receive ASA for primary prophylaxis? This is a much harder question to answer, and, as usual, direct trial evidence is lacking. A large meta-analysis of ASA use for primary prevention in the general population showed a 28% reduction in the odds ratio for myocardial infarction but a very much smaller impact (odds ratio, 0.93; CI, 0.84–1.02) on overall mortality, largely because of fatal gastrointestinal

bleeding and hemorrhagic strokes attributed to ASA [79]. It was estimated that ASA treatment would result in clinical benefit for patient groups having an annual risk for cardiovascular disease greater than 1%, assuming a similar bleed rate across risk groups. The fact that the overall benefit of antiplatelet agents in primary prophylaxis is highly dependent on the bleeding rate is of concern to nephrologists, because the risk of bleeding in renal populations is much higher. The rate of gastrointestinal bleeds in RTRs, for example, may be as much as 10 times higher than in the general population [80]. Thus, the risk/benefit ratio of primary prophylaxis with antiplatelet therapy in RTRs is unclear, and recommendations cannot be made.

Beta blockers

Several large randomized, controlled trials have shown improved short- and long-term survival with beta blockade in patients with myocardial infarction [81–84]. A large meta-analysis of several randomized, controlled trials estimated the odds ratio for death following myocardial infarction in patients given beta blockers versus placebo to be 0.81 (CI, 0.75–0.87) [85]. More recently, several trials have demonstrated improved survival and less frequent hospitalization for CHF with beta blockade in patients with moderate and severe CHF or left ventricular dysfunction [86–90]. The beneficial effect is seen in both ischemic and nonischemic heart disease and over a wide spectrum of disease severity (ie, New York Heart Association class 2–4). The benefit is additive to that of ACE inhibitors and other standard therapies for CHF but can be seen in patients not receiving ACE inhibitors as well [72].

The benefit of beta blockers has not been directly demonstrated in patients with kidney transplants. Biologically, there is no compelling reason to believe RTRs will respond differently from the general population. A recent cohort study' of nontransplant patients with chronic kidney disease presenting with acute myocardial infarction showed beta-blocker use was associated with improved survival [52]. Another cohort study has indicated beta-blocker use is independently associated with improved survival on dialysis [91]. It is highly probable that beta blockers will confer benefit in transplant recipients with myocardial infarction or CHF.

Anemia management

There has been little investigation of the role of anemia management in the prevention of cardiomyopathy and CHF in RTRs. Rigatto et al data suggest that a hemoglobin level below 120 g/L may be a causal risk factor for CHF in RTRs. Clinical trials in dialysis patients, however, have not shown survival benefit with higher hemoglobin targets [92]. Achievement of higher hemoglobin targets did not lead to regression of LVH in CKD [93]. It seems reasonable to treat anemia in the setting of a failing allograft in the same way it is treated in native kidney failure (target hemoglobin, 110–120 g/L). Whether higher targets are desirable is at present unknown.

Nontraditional risk factors

Several novel and nontraditional risk factors for cardiac disease in patients with renal disease, such as homocysteine, lipoprotein (a), C-reactive protein, hyperparathyroidism, and oxidative stress, are the subject of much active research. The strength of the epidemiologic evidence available so far is weaker for these factors than for those discussed previously, and recommendations cannot be made.

Revascularization

Coronary artery disease before transplantation is associated with adverse events after transplantation [94]. One small trial in patients with diabetes showed benefit from identifying and revascularizing significant coronary artery disease before transplantation [95]. This trial is limited by its small numbers and by the poor quality, by modern standards, of the perioperative medical management in the control arm. Nevertheless, this study has had great impact on practice, and most transplantation centers investigate all but the lowest-risk patients and aggressively revascularize any significant coronary lesions (Fig. 3) [96]. A more detailed review of cardiac risk assessment before renal transplantation is beyond the scope of this article.

The issue of when and how to revascularize after transplantation is less clear, and the evidence base is sparse. Patients with kidney disease in general are at a higher risk of cardiovascular events. In the author and colleagues' experience, however, they tend to be less aggressively investigated and revascularized, in part because of a widely held belief that revascularization is either impossible (because of diffuse coronary involvement) or futile (because of high rates of restenosis and bypass graft occlusion). The data in renal transplant patients do not support the futility of revascularization, however. Herzog et al [97] showed that an aggressive revascularization modality (coronary artery bypass grafting [CABG] with and without inferior mammary grafting [IMG]) was associated with lower risk of cardiac death or myocardial infarction than less aggressive modalities (percutaneous transluminal coronary angioplasty [PTCA]/stent) after adjustment

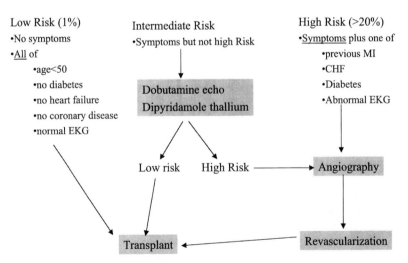

Fig. 3. Pretransplantation assessment of cardiac disease. CHF, congestive heard failure; EKG, electrocardiogram; MI, myocardial infarction.

for comorbid conditions. The data suggest that techniques known to be associated with better patency (CABG with IMG > CABG without IMG > stent > PTCA) are associated with improved outcome. Because these data are observational, selection bias cannot be completely excluded as an explanation for the results. Moreover, the study did not compare revascularization with medical management alone. Despite these major limitations, the author believes that coronary revascularization, including CABG, should be considered for the same indications in RTRs as in nonrenal patients. A randomized, controlled trial of medical management versus coronary revascularization in RTRs would be necessary to prove benefit, but an adequately powered study is probably unfeasible.

Summary

RTRs are at high risk for ischemic heart disease and heart failure. Although some differences pertain, most of the major risk factors are similar to those in the general population. It is highly probable that interventions of proven benefit in the general population will also be of benefit in RTRs. A combination of lifestyle modifications (smoking cessation, maintenance of ideal body weight, healthy diet), aggressive blood pressure control (<130/80 mm Hg), use of ACE inhibitors or ARBs, lipid lowering with statins, antiplatelet therapy for diabetics and those with established coronary disease, and beta blockers for CHF or after myocardial infarction is likely to have a major benefit on patient survival and cardiac morbidity among transplant recipients. Coronary revascularization should be considered for the same indications as in the general population.

References

[1] Kasiske BL. Risk factors for accelerated atherosclerosis in renal transplant patients. Am J Med 1988;84: 985–92.

[2] Lindholm A, Albrechtsen D, Frodin L, et al. Ischemic heart disease—major cause of death and graft loss after transplantation in Scandinavia. Transplantation 1995;60:451–7.

[3] Huting J, Kramer W, Schutterle G, et al. Analysis of left ventricular changes associated with chronic hemodialysis: a non-invasive follow-up study. Nephron 1988;49:284–90.

[4] Parfrey PS, Foley RN, Harnett JD, et al. The outcome and risk factors for left ventricular disorders in chronic uremia. Nephrol Dial Transplant 1996; 11:1277–85.

[5] Foley RN, Parfrey PS, Harnett JD, et al. The impact of anemia on cardiomyopathy, morbidity and mortality in end stage renal disease. Am J Kidney Dis 1996;28:53–61.

[6] Levin A, Thompson CR, Ethier J, et al. Left ventricular mass index increase in early renal disease: impact of decline in hemoglobin. Am J Kidney Dis 1999;34:125–34.

[7] Rigatto C, Parfrey P, Foley R, et al. Congestive heart failure in renal transplant recipients: risk factors, outcomes, and relationship to ischemic heart disease. J Am Soc Nephrol 2002;13:1084–90.

[8] Rigatto C, Foley R, Jeffrey J, et al. Electrocardiographic left ventricular hypertrophy in renal transplant recipients: prognostic value and impact of blood pressure and anemia. J Am Soc Nephrol 2003;14:462–8.

[9] Parfrey PS, Harnett JD, Foley RN, et al. Impact of renal transplantation on uremic cardiomyopathy. Transplantation 1995;60:908–14.

[10] Rigatto C, Foley RN, Kent GM, et al. Long-term changes in left ventricular hypertrophy after renal transplantation. Transplantation 2000;70:570–5.

[11] Kasiske BL, Guijarro C, Massy ZA, et al. Cardiovascular disease after renal transplantation. J Am Soc Nephrol 1996;7:158–65.

[12] Culleton BF, Larson MG, Wilson PWF, et al. Cardiovascular disease and mortality in a community based cohort with mild renal insufficiency. Kidney Int 1999;56:2214–9.

[13] Senni M, Tribouilly C, Rodeheffer R, et al. Congestive heart failure in the community: trends in incidence and survival in a 10 year period. Arch Intern Med 1999;159:29–34.

[14] Ho K, Pinsky J, Kannel W, et al. The epidemiology of heart failure: the Framingham Study. J Am Coll Cardiol 1993;22:6A–13A.

[15] Himelman RB, Landzberg JS, Simonson JS, et al. Cardiac consequences of renal transplantation: changes in left ventricular morphology and function. J Am Coll Cardiol 1988;12:915–23.

[16] Larsson O, Attman PO, Beckman-Suurkula M, et al. Left ventricular function before and after kidney transplantation. A prospective study in patients with juvenile-onset diabetes mellitus. Eur Heart J 1986;7:779–91.

[17] Deligiannis A, Paschalidou E, Sakellariou G, et al. Changes in left ventricular anatomy during haemodialysis, continuous ambulatory peritoneal dialysis and after renal transplantation. Proc Eur Dial Transplant Assoc Eur Ren Assoc 1985;21:185–9.

[18] Lai KN, Barnden L, Mathew TH. Effect of renal transplantation on left ventricular function in hemodialysis patients. Clin Nephrol 1982;18:74–8.

[19] Ikaheimo M, Linnaluoto M, Huttunen K, et al. Effects of renal transplantation on left ventricular size and function. Br Heart J 1982;47:155–60.

[20] Huting J. Course of left ventricular hypertrophy and function in end-stage renal disease after renal transplantation. Am J Cardiol 1992;70:1481–4.

[21] Torres S, Maximino J, Pereira S, et al. Evolucao morfologica do ventriculo esquerdo apos transplante renal. Estudo ecocardiografico. Rev Port Cardiol 1991;10:497–501.

[22] Peteiro J, Alvarez N, Calvino R, et al. Changes in left ventricular mass and filling after renal transplantation are related to changes in blood pressure: an echocardiographic and pulsed Doppler study. Cardiology 1994;85:273–83.

[23] Levin A, Thompson CR, Ethier J, et al. Left ventricular mass index increase in early renal disease: impact of decline in hemoglobin. Am J Kidney Dis 1999;34:125–34.

[24] Foley RN, Parfrey PS, Harnett JD, et al. Hypoalbuminemia, cardiac morbidity and mortality in end stage renal disease. J Am Soc Nephrol 1996;7: 728–36.

[25] Rigatto C, Parfrey P, London G. Cardiac hypertrophy in end-stage renal failure. In: Loscalzo J, London G, editors. Cardiovascular disease in end-stage renal failure. Oxford (UK): Oxford University Press; 2000. p. 157–75.

[26] Kasiske B, Harini C, Roel J. Explained and unexplained ischemic heart disease risk after renal transplantation. J Am Soc Nephrol 2000;11:1735–43.

[27] Aker S, Ivens K, Grabensee B, et al. Cardiovascular complications after renal transplantation. Transplant Proc 1998;30:2039–42.

[28] Ducloux D, Motte G, Challier B, et al. Serum total homocysteine and cardiovascular disease occurrence in chronic stable transplant recipients: a prospective study. J Am Soc Nephrol 2000;11: 134–7.

[29] Mange K, Cizman B, Joffe M, et al. Arterial hypertension and renal allograft survival. JAMA 2000; 283:633–8.

[30] Kasiske BL, Anjum S, Shah R, et al. Hypertension after kidney transplantation. Am J Kidney Dis 2004;43:1071–81.

[31] Ridker P, Nader R, Clearfield M, et al. Measurement of C-reactive protein for the targeting of statin therapy in the primary prevention of acute coronary events. N Engl J Med 2001;344:1959–65.

[32] Kasiske BL, Snyder JJ, Gilbertson D, et al. Diabetes mellitus after kidney transplantation in the United States. Am J Transplant 2003;3:178–85.

[33] Eikelboom J, Lonn E, Genest J, et al. Homocysteine and cardiovascular disease: a critical review of the epidemiological evidence. Ann Intern Med 1999; 131:363–75.

[34] Kark J, Selhub J, Adler B, et al. Nonfasting plasma homocysteine level and mortality in middle aged and elderly men and women in Jerusalem. Ann Intern Med 1999;131:321–30.

[35] Bostom A, Rosenberg I, Silbershatz H, et al. Nonfasting plasma total homocysteine levels and stroke

incidence in elderly persons: the Framingham Study. Ann Intern Med 1999;131:352–5.

[36] Kasiske B. Hyperlipidemia with chronic renal disease. Am J Kidney Dis 1998;32:S142–56.

[37] Holdaas H, Fellstrom B, Jardine AG, et al, for the Assessment of LEscol in Renal Transplantation (ALERT) Study Investigators. Effect of fluvastatin on cardiac outcomes in renal transplant recipients: a multicentre, randomised, placebo-controlled trial. Lancet 2003;361:2024–31.

[38] Jardine AG, Holdaas H, Fellstrom B, et al, for the ALERT Study Investigators. Fluvastatin prevents cardiac death and myocardial infarction in renal transplant recipients: post-hoc subgroup analyses of the ALERT study. Am J Transplant 2004;4: 988–95.

[39] The sixth report of the Joint National Committee on Prevention, Detection, Evaluation and Treatment of High Blood Pressure. Arch Intern Med 1997;157: 2413–46.

[40] Wilson P, D'Agostino R, Levy D, et al. Prediction of coronary heart disease using risk factor categories. Circulation 1998;97:1837–47.

[41] Levy D, Savage DD, Garrison RJ, et al. Echocardiographic criteria for left ventricular hypertrophy: the Framingham Study. Am J Cardiol 1987;59:956–60.

[42] National High Blood Pressure Education Program Working Group. 1995 Update of the working group reports on chronic renal failure and renovascular hypertension. Arch Intern Med 1996;156:1938–47.

[43] Levin A, Thompson CR, Ethier J, et al. Left ventricular mass index increase in early renal disease: impact of decline in hemoglobin. Am J Kidney Dis 1999;34:125–34.

[44] Rigatto C, Parfrey P, Foley R, et al. Congestive heart failure in renal transplant recipients: risk factors, outcomes, and relationship to ischemic heart disease. J Am Soc Nephrol 2002;13:1084–90.

[45] Rigatto C, Foley R, Kent G, et al. Long-term changes in left ventricular hypertrophy after renal transplantation. Transplantation 2000;70:570–5.

[46] Mailloux L, Levey A. Hypertension in patients with chronic renal disease. Am J Kidney Dis 1998;32: S120–41.

[47] Klahr S, Levey A, Beck G, et al. The effects of dietary protein restriction and blood pressure control on the progression of chronic renal disease. N Engl J Med 1994;330:877–84.

[48] Peterson J, Adler S, Burkart J, et al. Blood pressure control, proteinuria, and the progression of renal disease. Ann Intern Med 1995;123:754–62.

[49] Hansson L, Zanchetti A, Carruthers S, et al. Effects of blood pressure lowering and low-dose aspirin in patients with hypertension: principal results of the Hypertension Optimal Treatment (HOT) randomised trial. Lancet 1998;351:1755–62.

[50] Chobanian AV, Bakris GL, Black HR, et al, for the Joint National Committee on Prevention, Detection, Evaluation, and Treatment of High Blood

Pressure, National Heart, Lung, and Blood Institute, National High Blood Pressure Education Program Coordinating Committee. Seventh report of the Joint National Committee on Prevention, Detection, Evaluation, and Treatment of High Blood Pressure. Hypertension 2003;42:1206–52.

[51] Lewis EJ, Hunsicker LG, Bain RP, et al. The effect of angiotensin-converting-enzyme inhibition on diabetic nephropathy. N Engl J Med 1993;329:1456–61.

[52] Maschio G, Alberti D, Janin J, et al. Effect of the angiotensin converting enzyme inhibitor benazepril on the progression of CRI. The Angiotensin Converting Enzyme Inhibition in Progressive Renal Insufficiency Study Group. N Engl J Med 1996;334:939–45.

[53] The GISEN Group. Randomized placebo controlled trial of effect of ramipril on decline in glomerular filtration and risk of terminal renal failure in proteinuric non-diabetic nephropathy (REIN). Lancet 1997;349:1857–63.

[54] Cohn J, Johnson G, Ziesche S, et al. A comparison of enalapril with hydralazine-isosorbide dinitrate in the treatment of chronic congestive heart failure (V-HeFT II). J Am Coll Cardiol 1996;27:642–9.

[55] The CONSENSUS Trial Study Group. Effects of enalapril on mortality in severe congestive heart failure. Results of the Cooperative North Scandinavian Enalapril Survival Study (CONSENSUS). N Engl J Med 1987;316:1429–35.

[56] Pfeffer M, Braunwald E, Moye L, et al. Effect of captopril on mortality and morbidity in patients with left ventricular dysfunction after myocardial infarction. Results of the Survival and Ventricular Enlargement trial (SAVE). N Engl J Med 1992;327:669–77.

[57] Rutherford J, Pfeffer M, Moye L, et al. Effects of captopril on ischemic events after myocardial infarction. Results of the SAVE Trial. Circulation 1994;90:1731–8.

[58] The HOPE Study Investigators. Effects of an angiotensin-converting-enzyme inhibitor, ramipril, on cardiovascular events in high risk patients. N Engl J Med 2000;342:145–53.

[59] Yusuf S, Pepine C, Garces C, et al. Effect of enalapril on myocardial infarction and unstable angina in patients with low ejection fractions. Lancet 1992;340:1173–8.

[60] Lewis E, Hunsicker L, Clarke W, et al. Renoprotective effect of the angiotensin-receptor antagonist irbesartan in patients with nephropathy due to type 2 diabetes. N Engl J Med 2001;345:851–60.

[61] Brenner B, Cooper M, Zeeuw D, et al. Effects of losartan on renal and cardiovascular outcomes in patients with type 2 diabetes and nephropathy. N Engl J Med 2001;345:861–9.

[62] Parving H-H, Lehnert H, Brochner-Mortensen J, et al. The effect of irbesartan on the development of diabetic nephropathy in patients with type 2 diabetes. N Engl J Med 2001;345:870–8.

[63] McMurray JJ, Ostergren J, Swedberg K, et al, for the CHARM Investigators and Committees. Effects of candesartan in patients with chronic heart failure and reduced left-ventricular systolic function taking angiotensin-converting-enzyme inhibitors: the CHARM-Added trial. Lancet 2003;362(9386):767–71.

[64] Granger CB, McMurray JJ, Yusuf S, et al, for the CHARM Investigators and Committees. Effects of candesartan in patients with chronic heart failure and reduced left-ventricular systolic function intolerant to angiotensin-converting-enzyme inhibitors: the CHARM-Alternative trial. Lancet 2003;362(9386):772–6.

[65] Yusuf S, Pfeffer MA, Swedberg K, et al, for the CHARM Investigators and Committees. Effects of candesartan in patients with chronic heart failure and preserved left-ventricular ejection fraction: the CHARM-Preserved Trial. Lancet 2003;362(9386):777–81.

[66] Pfeffer MA, McMurray JJ, Velazquez EJ, et al, for the Valsartan in Acute Myocardial Infarction Trial Investigators. Valsartan, captopril, or both in myocardial infarction complicated by heart failure, left ventricular dysfunction, or both. N Engl J Med 2003;349:1893–906.

[67] Lindholm L, Ibsen H, Dahlof B, et al. Cardiovascular morbidity and mortality in patients with diabetes in the Losartan Intervention For Endpoint reduction in hypertension study (LIFE): a randomised trial against atenolol. Lancet 2002;359:1004–10.

[68] Pitt B, Poole-Wilson P, Segal R, et al. Effects of losartan compared with captopril on mortality in patients with symptomatic heart failure: randomised trial: the Losartan Heart Failure Survival Study. Lancet 2000;355:1582–7.

[69] Dickstein K, Kjekshus J. Effects of losartan and captopril on mortality and morbidity in high risk patients after acute myocardial infarction: the OPTIMAAL randomised trial. Lancet 2002;360:752–60.

[70] Nakao N, Yoshimura A, Morita H, et al. Combination therapy of angiotensin-II receptor blocker and angiotensin-converting-enzyme inhibitor in non-diabetic renal disease (COOPERATE): a randomised controlled trial. Lancet 2003;361:117–24.

[71] Cohn J, Tognoni G. A randomized trial of the angiotensin receptor blocker valsartan in chronic heart failure. N Engl J Med 2001;345:1667–75.

[72] Mann J, Gerstein H, Pogue J, et al. Renal insufficiency as a predictor of cardiovascular outcomes and the impact of ramipril: the HOPE randomized trial. Ann Intern Med 2001;134:707–9.

[73] Sizeland PC, Bailey RR, Lynn KL, et al. Anemia and angiotensin-converting enzyme inhibition in renal transplant recipients. J Cardiovasc Pharmacol 1990;16(Suppl 7):S117–9.

[74] Pratt MC, Lewis-Barned NJ, Walker RJ, et al. Effect of angiotensin converting enzyme inhibitors on

erythropoietin concentrations in healthy volunteers. Br J Clin Pharmacol 1992;34:363–5.

[75] Antiplatelet Trialists Collaboration. Collaborative overview of randomised trials of antiplatelet therapy—I: prevention of death, myocardial infarction, and stroke by prolonged antiplatelet therapy in various categories of patients. BMJ 1994;308: 81–106.

[76] Antiplatelet Trialists' Collaboration. Secondary prevention of vascular disease by prolonged antiplatelet treatment. Br Med J (Clin Res Ed) 1988;296: 320–31.

[77] Wright R, Reeder G, Herzog C, et al. Acute myocardial infarction and renal dysfunction: a high risk combination. Ann Intern Med 2002;137:563–70.

[78] Zusman R, Chesebro J, Comerota A, et al. Antiplatelet therapy in the prevention of ischemic vascular events: literature review and evidence-based guidelines for drug selection. Clin Cardiol 1999;22:559–73.

[79] Hayden M, Pignone M, Phillips C, et al. Aspirin for the primary prevention of cardiovascular events: a summary of the evidence for the US Preventive Services Task Force. Ann Intern Med 2002;136: 161–72.

[80] Matsumoto C, Swanson SJ, Agodoa LY, et al. Hospitalized gastrointestinal bleeding and procedures after renal transplantation in the United States. J Nephrol 2003;16(1):49–56.

[81] ISIS Collaborative Group. Randomised trial of intravenous atenolol among 16027 cases of suspected acute myocardial infarction: ISIS-1. Lancet 1986;2: 57–66.

[82] The MIAMI Trial Research Group. Metoprolol in acute myocardial infarction (MIAMI). Eur Heart J 1985;6:199–226.

[83] Timolol-induced reduction in mortality and reinfarction in patients surviving acute myocardial infarction. N Engl J Med 1981;304:801–7.

[84] Hennekens C, Albert C, Godfried S, et al. Adjunctive drug therapy of acute myocardial infarction-evidence from clinical trials. N Engl J Med 1996; 335:1660–7.

[85] Teo KK, Yusuf S, Furberg C. Effects of prophylactic antiarrhythmic drug therapy in acute myocardial infarction. An overview of results from randomized controlled trials. JAMA 1993;270:1589–95.

[86] Packer M, Coats A, Fowler M, et al. Effect of carvedilol on survival in severe chronic heart failure. N Engl J Med 2001;344:1651–8.

[87] Shibata M, Flather M, Wang D. Systematic review of the impact of beta blockers on mortality and hospital admissions in heart failure. Eur J Heart Fail 2001;3:351–7.

[88] Hjalmarson A, Goldstein S, Fagerberg B, et al. Effects of controlled release metoprolol on total mortality, hospitalizations, and well being in patients with heart failure: the metoprolol CR/XL randomised intervention trial in congestive heart failure (MERIT-HF). The MERIT-HF study group. JAMA 2000;283:1295–302.

[89] The MERIT-HF Study Group. Effect of metoprolol CR/XL in chronic heart failure: Metoprolol CR/XL Randomosed Intervention Trial in Heart Failure (MERIT-HF). Lancet 1999;353:2001–7.

[90] The CIBIS-II Study group. The Cardiac Insufficiency Bisoprolol Study II (CIBIS-II): a randomised trial. Lancet 1999;353:9–13.

[91] Foley R, Herzog C, Collins A. Blood pressure and long term mortality in US hemodialysis patients: USRDS Waves 3 and 4 Study. Kidney Int 2002;62: 1784–90.

[92] Besarab A, Bolton W, Browne J, et al. The effects of normal as compared with low hematocrit values in patients with cardiac disease who are receiving hemodialysis and epoietin. N Engl J Med 1998;339: 584–90.

[93] Roger SD, McMahon LP, Clarkson A, et al. Effects of early and late intervention with epoetin alpha on left ventricular mass among patients with chronic kidney disease (stage 3 or 4): results of a randomized clinical trial. J Am Soc Nephrol 2004;15(1): 148–156.

[94] Manske CL, Thomas W, Wang Y, et al. Screening diabetic transplant candidates for coronary artery disease: identification of a low risk subgroup. Kidney Int 1993;44(3):617–21.

[95] Manske CL, Wang Y, Rector T, et al. Coronary revascularisation in insulin-dependent diabetic patients with chronic renal failure. Lancet 1992; 340(8826):998–1002.

[96] de Lemos JA, Hillis LD. Diagnosis and management of coronary artery disease in patients with end-stage renal disease on hemodialysis. J Am Soc Nephrol 1996;7(10):2044–54.

[97] Herzog CA, Ma JZ, Collins AJ. Long-term outcome of renal transplant recipients in the United States after coronary revascularization procedures. Circulation 2004;109:2866–71.

ELSEVIER
SAUNDERS

Cardiol Clin 23 (2005) 343–362

CARDIOLOGY
CLINICS

Chronic Kidney Disease: A Risk Factor for Cardiovascular Disease

Ravinder K. Wali, MD[a],*, William L. Henrich, MD[b]

[a]Division of Nephrology, Department of Medicine, University of Maryland School of Medicine,
22 South Greene Street, Baltimore, MD 21201, USA
[b]Department of Medicine, University of Maryland School of Medicine,
22 South Greene Street, Baltimore, MD 21201, USA

Chronic kidney disease (CKD) is a poorly recognized but important risk factor for cardiovascular disease (CVD). Evidence has demonstrated that persons with CKD are more likely to die of events related to CVD than from consequences of progression in renal failure per se [1,2] and CVD is the main cause of death in patients with CKD. Almost half of all deaths in patients with CKD are caused by cardiovascular events, particularly congestive cardiac failure, acute myocardial infarction (AMI) and sudden cardiac death.

During the past 10 years, the burden of CVD-related morbidity and mortality in the general population has improved remarkably, thanks to well-designed randomized, controlled trials that have unequivocally shown that treatment of targeted risk factors decreases cardiovascular and all-cause mortality. CVD-related morbidity and mortality in patients with CKD has remained almost unchanged, however, perhaps because of poor recognition of the impact of CKD on the biology of CVD and, to some extent, the lack of well-designed prospective studies to define the role of treatment of targeted risk factors in patients with CKD.

A recent analysis of a managed care database showed that, in persons with advanced CKD, death before the initiation of renal replacement therapy is twice as likely to occur than initiation of dialysis therapy [3]. In 1998, the National Kidney Foundation established a task force on CKD and CVD, which recommended that patients with CKD be considered in the highest risk group for the onset and progression of subsequent events related to CVD. The task force recommends that patients with CKD should be evaluated thoroughly for the risk factors for CVD and that treatment recommendations for CVD risk stratification should consider the highest-risk status of patients with CKD [1].

Stages of chronic kidney disease

The National Kidney Foundation published clinical practice guidelines (K/DOIQ) on evaluation, classification, and risk stratification of CKD [4]. These guidelines, define CKD in five different stages as (Table 1)

1. Kidney damage for more than 3 months determined either by kidney biopsy or the presence of markers of kidney damage, with or without a decrease in estimated glomerular filtration rate (eGFR). The markers of kidney damage include proteinuria (albumin/creatinine ratio or total protein/creatinine ratio, in an untimed spot urine sample), abnormal urinary sediment, abnormalities on kidney imaging studies, or a combination of these markers.
2. eGFR of more than 60 but less than 89 mL/min/1.73m^2 is considered mild CKD.
3. eGFR of more than 30 but less than 59/mL/min/1.73m^2 for 3 months or longer with or without markers of kidney damage is considered moderate CKD.

* Corresponding author.
E-mail address: rwali@medicine.umaryland.edu
(R.K. Wali).

Table 1
Stages of chronic kidney disease and prevalence in the general population

Stage	Description	GFR mL/min/1.73m^2	Prevalence N (1000)	%
1[a,b]	Kidney damage with normal or increased GFR	≥90	5900	3.3
2[a,b]	Kidney damage with mildly decreased GFR	60–89	5300	3.0
3[a]	Moderately decreased GFR	30–59	7600	4.3
4[a]	Severely decreased GFR	15–29	400	0.2
5[c]	Kidney failure	<15 or dialysis	300	0.1

Abbreviation: GFR, glomerular filtration rate.

[a] Data for stages 1–4 from National Health and Nutrition Examination Survey III (1988–1994). Population of 177 million aged 20 years or more.

[b] For stages 1 and 2, kidney damage was assessed by spot albumin/creatinine ratio greater than 17 mg/g (men) or 15 mg/g (women) on two measurements.

[c] Data for stage 5 include approximately 230,000 patients treated by dialysis and assumes 70,000 additional patients not receiving dialysis. Percentages total more than 100% because the National Health and Nutrition Examination Survey III may not have included patients receiving dialysis. GFR estimated from serum creatinine using MDRD study equation based on age, gender, race, and calibration for serum creatinine (*Data from* US Renal Data System. USRDS 1998 annual data report. Bethesda, National Institutes of Health National Institute of Diabetes; 1998.)

From National Kidney Foundation. K/DOQI clinical practice guidelines for chronic kidney disease: evaluation, classification, and stratification. Am J Kidney Dis 2002;39(2 Suppl 1):S1–266; with permission from the National Kidney Foundation.

4. eGFR of more than 15 but less than 29 mL/min/1.73m^2 for 3 months or longer with or without markers of kidney damage is considered severe CKD.
5. eGFR of less than 15 mL/min/1.73m^2 is considered indication for renal replacement therapy (dialysis or renal transplantation).

This categorization is arbitrary and to some extent is based on the results of small observational studies that have demonstrated inevitable progression in the decline of eGFR in persons with eGFRs of less than 60 mL/min/1.73m^2. The GFR estimation is based on the Modification for Diet and Renal Disease (MDRD) formula, taking into consideration serum creatinine level, age, race, and body size to avoid inadvertent mistakes in quantifying GFR based on the serum creatinine level alone [5–7]. The National Kidney Foundation GFR calculator (MDRD equation) is

available at http://www.kidney.org/professional/doqi/index.cfm) (Table 2).

The stages of CKD are based on the severity of impairment in the levels of GFR. As of 2000, 20 million adults in the United States adult population (10.8% of the population) had various stages of CKD. Although there are several different etiologic factors for the development of CKD, these can be broadly classified as diabetic and nondiabetic in nature, because these two categories have different rates of progression of CVD and different associated comorbidities [7,8].

Early stages of chronic kidney disease and its impact on cardiovascular biology

Onset of CKD is associated with an increased predilection for the development of CVD-related events [9,10]. Persons with CKD are predisposed

Table 2
Equations to predict glomerular filtration rate based on serum creatinine

Cockcroft-Gault equation[24]	$C_{Cr}(\text{mL/min}) = \frac{(140-\text{age}) \times \text{weight}^a}{72 \times S_{Cr}} \times (0.85 \text{ if female})$
Abbreviated MDRD Study equation[22,23]	$GFR(\text{mL/min}^{-1}/1.73m^2) = 186 \times (S_{Cr})^{-1.154} \times (\text{age}^a)^{-0.203}$ $\times (0.742 \text{ if female}) \times (1.210 \text{ if black})$

Abbreviations: C_{cr}, creatinine clearance; GFR, glomerular filtration rate; MDRD, Modification of Diet in Renal Disease; S_{cr}, serum creatinine in mg/dL.

[a] Age is given in years and weight in kilograms.

From Sarnak MJ, Levey AS, Schoolwerth AC, et al. Kidney disease as a risk factor for development of CVD. Hypertension 2003;42:1050–65; with permission.

to three types of CVD—atherosclerosis, arteriosclerosis, and cardiomyopathy—when compared with age- and gender-matched persons with normal kidney function.

Atherosclerotic disease in CKD patients is somewhat different from that in the general population with atherosclerosis. In both groups, atherosclerosis is an intimal disease characterized by the presence of atheromatous plaques. In patients with CKD and in dialysis-dependent patients, however, this atherosclerotic burden is further complicated by an increased frequency of calcific lesions, an increase in medial thickness and calcification involving medium- to large-sized blood vessels.

In addition, CKD patients have an increased prevalence of arteriosclerosis and remodeling of large arteries [11]. Remodeling of large arteries is caused by a combination of factors such as pressure overload leading to wall hypertrophy and an increased wall/lumen ratio resulting from flow overload. There is also a proportional increase in arterial diameter and wall thickness with a reduction in arterial compliance as determined by aortic pulse wave velocity and impedance measurements.

These vascular processes work in concert to result in a significant loss of vessel wall compliance, decreased aortic compliance, and increased pulse pressure, and these factors are independent risk factors for CVD [12]. The loss of compliance is often associated with an increase in systolic blood pressure and pulse pressure, resulting in accelerated left ventricular hypertrophy (LVH), decreased coronary artery functional reserve, and coronary perfusion and hence could jeopardize myocardial microcirculatory reserves.

Chronic kidney disease is a risk factor for cardiovascular disease

The burden of CVD in early CKD before the need for renal replacement therapy has been demonstrated by prospective and retrospective population-based epidemiologic studies. Although small studies have refuted an association between CKD and CVD, several different studies indicate that onset of CKD is associated with an increased risk for events caused by CVD. Even if the association is now strongly established, the biologic reasons for this association remain poorly understood.

The Hoorn study

The Hoorn study was a population-based cohort study of glucose tolerance and other cardiovascular risk factors in a white population aged 50 to 75 years. Baseline measurements were obtained from 1989 to 1992 and were followed until January 1, 2000 (N = 631). The eGFR by the MDRD formula ranged from 16.8 to 116.9 mL/min/1.73m^2. During the follow-up of 10.2 years, 117 subjects died, 50 (43%) from cardiovascular causes. Renal function was inversely associated with all-cause and cardiovascular mortality across a range of serum creatinine levels. Within this range of eGFR, a decrease in eGFR by 5 mL/min/1.73m^2 was associated with a 26% increase in risk of cardiovascular death. These associations persisted even after adjustments for baseline hypertension, diabetes mellitus, age, sex, and other traditional risk factors for cardiovascular disease [13]. Based on eGFR tertiles, the lowest survival rate was noted in the cohort with worst renal function, although it is not clear from the study description whether survival was confounded by the initiation of renal replacement therapy (Fig. 1).

The Cardiovascular Health Study

The Cardiovascular Health Study was a prospective, population-based study of persons older than 65 years with a median follow-up of 7.3 years. Renal insufficiency was defined as serum

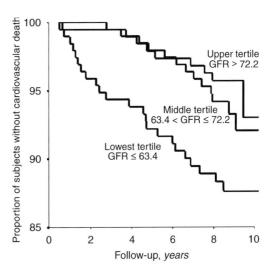

Fig. 1. Cardiovascular survival (Kaplan-Meier) according to tertiles of glomerular filtration rate (GFR), estimated by the Modification of Diet in Renal Disease equation and expressed in mL/min/1.73m^2. (*From* Henry RMA, Kostense PJ, Bos G, et al. Mild renal insufficiency is associated with increased cardiovascular mortality: the Hoorn Study. Kidney Int 2002;62:1406; with permission.)

creatinine level of 1.5 mg/dL or higher in men and 1.3 mg/dL or higher in women. In patients with renal insufficiency, the rates of all-cause mortality and CVD mortality were almost twice those in persons with lower creatinine levels. In addition, there was a linear increase in the risk of CVD, peripheral vascular disease, and congestive heart failure with an increasing serum creatinine level [14]. In the same cohort of patients, Shlipak et al [15] reported that the prevalence of clinical and subclinical cardiovascular disease was 64% in patients with renal insufficiency, as compared with 43% in those with normal renal function.

Subgroup analyses of Heart Outcome and Prevention Evaluation (HOPE Study)

Mann et al [16] studied the subset of subjects with renal insufficiency (serum creatinine $\geq$ 1.4 mg/dL; N = 980) from the enrollees of Heart Outcome and Prevention Evaluation and compared the outcome with 8307 persons with serum creatinine levels below 1.4 mg/dL. Cumulative incidence of each primary outcome measure (cardiovascular death, myocardial infarction, or stroke) was higher in patients with renal insufficiency than in persons with normal creatinine levels (22.2% versus 15.1%; $P < 0.001$; 11.4% versus 6.6%; $P < 0.001$; and 17.8% versus 10.6%, $P < 0.001$, respectively). The use of an angiotensin-converting enzyme (ACE) inhibitor (ramipril) was associated with similar reductions in the incidence of these primary outcomes in patients with and without renal insufficiency.

British population-based study

The relationships between serum creatinine concentration and the risk of major events related to ischemic heart disease and stroke and all-cause mortality were examined in a prospective study in a general population of middle-aged men (aged 40 to 59 years) drawn from 24 British towns who have been followed for an average of 14.75 years (N = 7690). There were 287 major stroke events, 967 major ischemic heart disease events, and 1259 deaths from all causes during the follow-up. Stroke risk was significantly increased at serum creatinine levels above 116 μmol/L (1.3 mg/dL, 90th percentile) even after adjustment for a wide range of cardiovascular risk factors (relative risk [RR], 1.6). Risk of a major ischemic heart disease event was significantly increased at serum creatinine levels at or above 130 μmol/L (1.5 mg/dL, 97.5 percentile), but this risk was attenuated after

adjustments for age and diabetes mellitus (RR, 1.2). An increased creatinine concentration (≥116 μmol/L, 1.3 mg/dL) was associated with a significant increase in stroke in both normotensive and hypertensive men. Both all-cause mortality and overall cardiovascular mortality were significantly increased in those with serum creatinine levels above 1.5 mg/dL (97.5 percentile), and no significant association was seen with cancer or other noncardiovascular mortality. It was concluded that even a borderline increase in the serum creatinine concentration is a marker for increased risk of cerebrovascular disease in both normotensive and hypertensive persons [17].

Framingham Offspring community study

The Framingham Offspring community-based study followed a cohort of 6233 subjects for 15 years. CVD was almost twice as prevalent in persons with mild-to-moderate CKD (based on serum creatinine levels) as in those without underlying renal disease [18].

Second National Health and Nutrition Examination Survey mortality study

The association between renal insufficiency and increased CVD-related and all-cause mortality rates during 16 years of follow-up was examined among participants in the second National Health and Nutrition Examination Survey Mortality Study (NHANES II). Study subjects were 30 to 74 years of age at the baseline examinations from 1976 to 1980, with proteinuria (n = 8786) or serum creatinine levels of 3.0 mg/dL or lower (n = 6354); GFR was estimated by using the MDRD formula. CVD-related mortality rates were 6.2, 17.9, and 37.2 deaths/1000 person-years among subjects with urinary protein levels of less than 30, 30 to 299, and 300 mg/dL or higher, respectively. There were 4.1, 8.6, and 20.5 deaths/ 1000 person-year among participants with eGFRs of 90 or higher, 70 to 89, and 70 mL/min or lower, respectively. After adjustment for potential confounders, in this representative sample of the United States general population, renal insufficiency was independently associated with increased CVD-related and all-cause mortality [19].

Managed care group database analysis

A recent retrospective study from 1996 to June 30, 2001, of a managed care database with 27,998 enrollees with eGFR of less than 90 mL/min/ 1.73m^2 until renal replacement therapy, death, disenrollment from the health plan, or the last date of follow-up. Only 3.1% of persons with stage 2 to stage 4 CKD progressed and required dialysis; whereas 24.9% of this cohort died before the need for dialysis therapy. Another important finding was that patients with CKD had a significantly increased frequency of comorbidities during the follow-up period as compared with those without CKD. During the follow-up period, persons with CKD were at greater risk of developing other comorbid conditions than those with an eGFR of 90 mL/min/1.73m^2 or higher. Comorbidities included coronary artery disease (11.5% versus 7.4%), congestive heart failure (10.4% versus 5.2%), and anemia (24.5% versus 0.1%). These results indicate that CKD is a strong risk factor for the development of different spectrums of cardiovascular disease and anemia (Table 3) [3].

Antihypertensive and Lipid-Lowering Treatment to Prevent Heart Attack Trial

Rahman et al [20] analyzed the data from the Antihypertensive and Lipid-Lowering Treatment to Prevent Heart Attack Trial (ALLHAT), which enrolled 42,418 high-risk hypertensive participants aged 55 years and older with more than one risk factor for CVD at the time of enrollment. A total of 40,514 subjects had a baseline serum creatinine measured at the time of randomization in the study. Based on the MDRD equation and the practice guidelines promulgated by the Dialysis Outcome Quality Initiative (K/DOQI), 15.1% had normal or increased eGFR (≥ 90 mL/min/1.73m^2), 56.7% had a mild reduction in eGFR (60–89 mL/min/1.73m^2), 17.2% had a moderate decrease in eGFR (30–59 mL/min/1.73m^2),

and 0.6% had severe of CKD (≤ 29 mL/min/1.73m^2). A history of previous AMI and stroke was present in 19.2%, 23.4%, 28.7%, and 26.9% of persons with stage 2, 3, 4, and 5 CKD, respectively. A history of coronary bypass surgery or angioplasty or other revascularization procedure was noted in 9.2%, 13.6%, 17.2%, and 14.4% of patients with stage 2 to 5 CKD, respectively. A history of CHD was present in 21.2%, 26.4%, 31.3%, and 28.7% of patients with stage 2 to 5 CKD strata, respectively. At the time of enrollment, EKG criteria for LVH were noted in 3.9%, 4.2%, 6.0%, and 11.2% of patients with stages 2 to 5 CKD, respectively (Fig. 2).

Although patients with a serum creatinine level of 2.0 mg or higher were excluded from enrollment in the ALLHAT study, the prevalence of moderate CKD (following the definition of K/DOQI practice guidelines: eGFR < 60 mL/min/1.73m^2) was present in 18% of the cohort at the time of randomization, as compared with 4.6% in NHANES III cohort of the general adult population. This inconsistency is explained mostly by the overall greater age and the presence of more than one risk factor for CVD in the ALLHAT participants at the time of enrollment in the study.

Conclusions from the prospective and retrospective studies of chronic kidney disease

These observational data suggest a strong association between even a modest decrease in eGFR and an increased prevalence of clinical and subclinical CVD and different degrees of LVH. The association between renal function and CVD may reflect an unmeasured risk factor associated with impaired renal function. These putative factors

Table 3

Changes in the prevalence of comorbidities in patients with chronic kidney disease and controls matched for age and sex*

Comorbidity	Patients with chronic kidney disease (n = 27998)		Control patients (n = 27998)	
	Baseline	Change	Baseline	Change
None	44.4	−24.1	73.7	−26.6
Coronary artery disease	13.1	11.5	6.2	7.4
Congestive heart failure	6.0	10.4	1.8	5.2
Hypertipidemia	13.6	14.1	7.4	10.5
Hypertension	37.4	21.2	16.8	19.3
Diabetes	15.8	9.2	5.3	5.7
Anemia	8.6	24.5	2.1	0.1

* Values are given as percentage.

Modified from Keith DS, Nichols GA, Gullion CM, et al. Longitudinal follow-up and outcomes among a population with CKD in a large managed care organization. Arch Intern Med 2004;164(6):659–63; with permission.

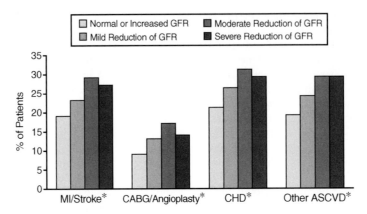

Fig. 2. History of cardiovascular disease at baseline in the Antihypertensive and Lipid-Lowering Treatment to Prevent Heart Attack Trial. Participants stratified by glomerular filtration rate (GFR). ASCVD, arteriosclerotic cardiovascular disease; CABG, coronary artery bypass grafting; CHD, coronary artery disease; MI, myocardial infarction. (*From* Rahman M, Brown CD, Coresh J, et al. The prevalence of reduced glomerular filtration rate in older hypertensive patients and its association with cardiovascular disease: a report from the Antihypertensive and Lipid-Lowering Treatment to Prevent Heart Attack Trial. Arch Intern Med 2004;164:972; with permission.)

may cause CVD or be an outcome of an underlying pathologic process that affects both GFR and the risk factors for CVD [1]. Whether an association between moderate renal insufficiency and CVD demonstrated in these retrospective and observational studies is caused by the co-occurrence of renal insufficiency with traditional cardiovascular risk factors or whether renal insufficiency per se is an independent risk factor for CVD events and cardiovascular mortality remains an interesting question.

Lack of association between CVD and CKD: Culleton et al [18] reported results from 6233 adult participants of the Framingham Heart Study with mild CKD based on serum creatinine levels of 1.5 to 3.0 mg/dL in men and 1.4 to 3.0 mg/dL in women. At baseline, 8.7% of men (n = 246) and 8.0% women (n = 270) had chronic renal impairment. During 15 years of follow-up, there were 1000 CVD events and 1406 deaths. After adjusting for covariates other than coexisting CVD (eg, diabetes, hypertension), mild renal impairment was not associated with either an increased risk of CVD events or all-cause mortality in either men or women. Garg et al [21] studied the cohort of participants in NHANES I (1974–1975) and NHANES I Epidemiologic Follow-up Study (18-year follow-up, 1992). The primary analysis was limited to 2352 adults with complete data, without baseline CVD and an approximate GFR of 30 to 60 mL/min/1.73m^2 (defined as moderate renal insufficiency). Supplementary analyses included participants with marked renal impairment and

baseline CVD. Moderate renal insufficiency was not identified as an independent risk factor for CVD after adjusting for traditional cardiovascular risk factors.

These variable results from different retrospective studies could be caused by multiple factors, particularly because Culleton et al [18] and Garg et al [21] used narrower definitions of renal impairment and used serum creatinine alone as the measurement of renal function. In addition, CVD-event data were captured after the actual event and could have been a major confounder in the final analysis. Most of the prospective cohort studies, on the other hand, consistently demonstrated an inverse association between the degree of renal function and cardiovascular morbidity and mortality.

The pathologic basis for the increased risk of CVD in patients with CKD can result from several factors, these can be summarized as follows [22]:

1. Associated comorbidities such as hypertension and diabetes mellitus that are almost always present in patients with CKD.
2. An abnormal milieu that could result in accelerated atherosclerotic burden presence of traditional and nontraditional risk factors and the presence of microinflammatory state in patients with CKD.
3. Poor use of primary preventive measures in patients with CKD because of the lack of prior randomized studies (Multicenter studies

usually have excluded patients with a serum creatinine level of 2 mg/dL or higher from the randomized studies.)

4. Unexpected or underreported toxic effects following therapeutic and diagnostic studies in patients with CKD.

5. The concept of reverse epidemiology, a paradoxical association of the triad of increased blood pressure, cholesterol, and body mass index with improved survival in dialysis patients, in contrast to the poor outcomes in the presence of any of these three factors in the general population.

Cardiovascular disease in patients with end-stage renal disease and renal replacement therapy

Despite advances in the understanding of the dynamics of dialysis therapy, including use of the biocompatible membranes and nonacetate dialysate, and of the physiologic principles governing the adequacy of dialysis, CVD remains the most important cause of death in patients receiving maintenance dialysis therapy. CVD accounts for almost 44% of overall mortality in long-term dialysis patients [23].

Acute coronary syndrome leading to AMI in patients receiving dialysis has a malignant course. An analysis of the United States Renal Data System (USRDS) revealed that almost 60% of all patients receiving dialysis between 1990 and 1995 had an AMI. The in-hospital mortality for this group was 26%. These data also revealed an early risk of acute coronary syndrome soon after initiation of dialysis, with 29% of AMIs occurring during the first year and 52% of AMIs developing within first 2 years after initiation of dialysis therapy. During the period from 1977 to 1995, 34,189 patients receiving maintenance dialysis experienced an AMI. The 1-year and 2-year survival rates were 41% and 27%, respectively (Fig. 3).

In addition, even during the era of reperfusion therapy from 1990 to 1995, overall mortality rates at 1 year and 2 years were 61% and 74%, respectively. Two-year mortality from cardiac causes was 50% in patients with an AMI between 1977 and 1984 and 52% for patients experiencing an AMI between 1990 and 1995 (the era of reperfusion therapy). This increased mortality (all-cause mortality and mortality from cardiac causes) was noted in patients with or without diabetes mellitus, but the overall risk of death (18%) and risk of death from cardiac causes (19%) was lower in African American than in white patients [24].

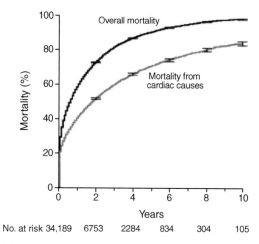

Fig. 3. Estimated cumulative mortality after acute myocardial infarction among patients receiving dialysis. (*From* Herzog CA, Ma JZ, Collins AJ. Poor long-term survival after acute myocardial infarction among patients on long-term dialysis. N Engl J Med 1998;339(12): 801; with permission.)

In view of these catastrophic outcomes after AMI in maintenance dialysis patients, every effort should be made to evaluate the presence of atherosclerotic coronary artery disease (CAD) during the early stages of the evolution of CKD.

Cardiac disease also remains an important cause of death in recipients of kidney transplantation. Among recipients of kidney transplants from 1977 to 1996, there were approximately 79,000 patients with a functioning graft, and 4250 of these had a first AMI, with an estimated in-hospital mortality of 11.5%. The overall mortality at 2 years was 30.4%, and mortality from cardiac causes was 11.5%. African American transplant recipients had no survival advantage after AMI as was described in African American dialysis patients following AMI. On the other hand, Native American renal transplant recipients had a twofold-increased risk for cardiac death. In contrast to the dialysis population, there was a significant (almost 50%) reduction of all-cause and cardiac mortality after AMI in recipients of kidney transplants in the era from 1990 to 1996 as compared with the years from 1977 to 1984. This reduction in mortality suggests a benefit of reperfusion therapy in the recipients of a functioning renal transplant.

The American Society of Transplant Physicians recommends that all potential candidates for transplantation (except those at the lowest possible cardiac risk) should have pretransplant screening for CAD [25]. There are no such established guidelines in the United States or in Europe concerning the evaluation of CAD in patients receiving maintenance dialysis. In view of the catastrophic outcome after the onset of AMI, it is prudent to recommend that all high-risk CKD patients be screened for the presence of CAD before the initiation of dialysis therapy.

Cardiac valvular abnormalities and valve replacement in patients with chronic kidney disease

Different published series have demonstrated that dialysis-dependent patients are at an increased risk for valvular sclerosis and valvular calcification. Premature aortic valve calcification and mitral valve calcification are common in dialysis patients. The precise mechanisms for ectopic calcification in patients with CKD are not well known. The accumulation of calcium phosphate (hydroxyapatite, $Ca_3[-PO_4]_2- \times Ca[OH]_2$, containing 40% of elemental calcium in weight) precipitates in ectopic places including coronary arteries and cardiac valves. Several factors, such as an abnormal calcium–phosphate product, hyperparathyroidism, intake of calcium-based phosphate binders, increased mechanical stress, and as yet unknown factors, have been implicated in the pathogenesis of ectopic calcification including valvular calcification [26]. Several studies suggest that the presence of vascular calcification is associated with an increased risk of cardiac events in uremic patients [27].

In a small but important group of patients receiving long-term dialysis, premature valve calcification can progress to hemodynamically significant aortic stenosis or, less frequently, mitral stenosis. Cardiac valvular disease is a common complication in hemodialysis patients, with a prevalence of up to 9%. The estimated annual incidence of valvular heart disease that leads to significant hemodynamic effects and requires valve replacement was reported to be 1.5 to 1.9 cases per 1000 dialyzed patients between 1988 and 1992 [28].

In dialysis patients, cardiac surgery, including valve replacement and coronary artery bypass grafting, is fraught with increased mortality. The reported perioperative mortality was 17.0% for aortic valve replacement only, 22.4% for mitral valve replacement only, 24.5% for combined coronary artery bypass grafting and aortic valve replacement, and 36.8% for combined coronary artery bypass grafting with mitral valve

replacement. Similar observations were reported on the retrospective analysis of USRDS database in dialysis patients requiring valve surgery.

In addition, an analysis of the USRDS database revealed, contrary to the previous belief, that bioprosthetic valves in dialysis-dependent patients function as well as the nonprosthetic (metallic) valves (Fig. 4). Undoubtedly, long-term survival in dialysis patients after cardiac valve replacement is poor, but this poor outcome does not seem to be related to the type of the prosthetic valve. There is currently a debate as to whether the American Heart Association Task force should upgrade the use of bioprosthetic valves in dialysis-dependent patients to class II status from the current class III status [29].

Pathophysiology of accelerated cardiovascular disease in patients with chronic kidney disease

Traditional modifiable risk factors in patients with chronic kidney disease

Hypertension

Early CKD is associated with an increase in diastolic and, to a lesser extent, systolic blood pressure. With the onset of CKD, already existing hypertension may worsen, or new-onset hypertension could develop because of an increase in plasma volume (salt and water retention), increased activity of the renin-angiotensin-aldosterone system and sympathetic activity, and accumulation of circulating endogenous vasoactive substances.

Without effective control of hypertension and salt-water retention, blood pressure gradually worsens and causes further progression in renal damage, thereby triggering a vicious cycle. Although the impact of different degrees of hypertension in patients with CKD has not been studied, observational studies from the general population have demonstrated a linear relationship between diastolic, systolic, and pulse pressure and the development of CAD, congestive heart failure, and stroke. Such an association could be substantially higher among young individuals who develop CKD at an early age.

Proteinuria or microalbuminuria

Microalbuminuria is associated with an increased risk of CAD, LVH, and myocardial infarction in patients with hypertension and without diabetes mellitus [30,31]. The presence of proteinuria during the 6 years of follow-up was consistently associated with an increased all-cause, CVD, and coronary heart disease mortality, even after

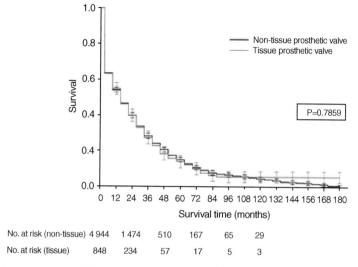

Fig. 4. Estimated all-cause survival of dialysis patients after heart valve replacement surgery with tissue and nontissue prosthetic valves. (*From* Herzog CA, Ma JZ, Collins AJ. Long-term survival of dialysis patients in the United States with prosthetic heart valves: should ACC/AHA practice guidelines on valve selection be modified? Circulation 2002,105:1338; with permission.)

adjusting for other risk factors. Proteinuria was an independent risk factor for CVD mortality [32]. Similar observations were noted in the analysis of the fifteenth biennial examination of the Framingham Heart Study [33].

Proteinuria could be the result of different types of glomerular injury, but the downstream effect is uniformly similar, whatever the nature of the glomerular injury. Proteinuria of any magnitude and of any cause results in tubular injury, which, in turn, is almost invariably associated with progression of renal failure [34,35].

Microalbuminuria of any cause results in increased vascular permeability, endothelial dysfunction, and increased levels of the markers of oxidative stress [36–38]. Different types of interventions in different stages of microalbuminuria, in particular the use of angiotensin-receptor blockers [40] and blockage of the aldosterone axis [41], are associated with improved outcome of renal function and cardiovascular morbidity and mortality [39].

Diabetes mellitus

Diabetes mellitus (particularly type 2 diabetes) is a common cause of CKD; between 40% and 45% of the current dialysis patients in the United States have diabetes mellitus. The presence of diabetes is an independent risk factor for CVD. The combination of diabetes and CKD is perhaps additive with regard to the onset and progression

of CVD in patients receiving renal replacement therapy and recipients of organ transplantation. Recipients of solid-organ transplantation and bone marrow transplantation can develop new-onset diabetes (posttransplant diabetes mellitus [PTDM]) and complications caused by the development of insulin-resistant syndrome in such patients with PTDM. The effects of PTDM on CVD remain to be elucidated.

The microvascular complications of type 1 and type 2 diabetes can be modified or prevented modified by intensive glycemic control [42,43]. It is well established that tight glycemic control prevents end-organ damage and prevents progression in CVD and CKD. The use of angiotensin-receptor blockers in patients with diabetes mellitus can delay the progression of CKD and the need for renal replacement therapy [44].

The optimal glycemic control meeting the American Diabetes Association's defined goal of glycosylated hemoglobin levels is essential to prevent new-onset atherosclerotic disease and to ameliorate the progression of atherosclerosis in patients with diabetes mellitus and CKD.

Dyslipidemia in chronic kidney disease

During the progression of CKD, dyslipidemia is characterized by an accumulation of partially metabolized triglyceride-rich particles resulting in the production of predominantly very-low-density lipoprotein and intermediate-density lipoprotein remnants, either because of abnormal lipoprotein lipase levels or its function, resulting in hypertriglyceridemia and significantly reduced high-density lipoprotein (HDL) cholesterol levels [45]. Several prospective studies in the general population have demonstrated that the relationship between the risk of CAD and blood cholesterol is almost log-linear. The minimum threshold below which a lower total cholesterol is not associated with a risk of atherosclerosis is not known. On the contrary, recent evidence has demonstrated that a low-density lipoprotein (LDL) cholesterol goal should be approximately 70 mg/dL in patients with established CAD [46,47].

Microalbuminuria and macroalbuminuria are associated with increased cholesterol, and the combination of microalbuminuria and early renal impairment is usually associated with an increase in LDL [48]. Most often, nephrotic-range proteinuria (ie, proteinuria of > 3 g/24 hours) further accentuates the increase in LDL cholesterol [49]. In addition, accurate estimation of LDL cholesterol in patients with CKD with or without a microinflammatory state may be hampered by the presence of other unmeasured and unknown lipid abnormalities (eg, the presence of a high proportion of small, dense LDL particles, an increase in the levels of oxidized-LDL [50], and increased fragments of lipoprotein (a) as a part of total LDL cholesterol) [51].

There are no known randomized, controlled, interventional studies to test the hypothesis that dyslipidemia is directly related to atherosclerosis in patients with CKD or receiving renal replacement therapy. Seliger et al [52,53] in a retrospective, observational study, however, analyzed the USRDS database and identified a cohort of 3716 patients who were placed on dialysis in 1996. Patients receiving statin therapy had better CVD outcomes and a reduced rate of all-cause mortality during the follow-up. The major caveat of this retrospective study was that patients receiving statins might have had other favorable factors that prevented them from developing accelerated atherosclerosis and that could not be recognized in the final analyses.

An inverse association between blood cholesterol and all-cause mortality or cardiovascular mortality has been termed reverse causality [54]. The paradoxical association of lower cholesterol and increased mortality (the so-called "U-shaped curve") in dialysis patients is partly explained by the presence of markers of malnutrition, systemic inflammation, and concurrent illness [55,56]. In a cohort of 1167 hemodialysis patients, Iseki et al [55] demonstrated low serum cholesterol levels and decreased serum albumin levels were associated with increased all-cause mortality. In patients with normal serum albumin levels, the opposite was true: high serum cholesterol was associated with increased mortality. Increased levels of C-reactive protein and other markers of inflammation, such as serum ferritin, interleukin-6, and tumor necrosis factor alpha, are associated with low serum cholesterol levels [56]. Hence, low total cholesterol is often associated with microinflammation, malnutrition, or the combination of these factors.

Nevertheless, these observations support the notion that there is a paradoxical association (reverse epidemiology) between low serum cholesterol and increased mortality in hemodialysis patients. These observations do not refute the hypothesis that dyslipidemia is important in the pathogenesis of atherosclerosis. Rather, it is more likely that high cholesterol levels impart the same degree of risk for atherosclerosis in patients with CKD as in the general population and that other conditions, such as systemic inflammation, infection, and poor nutritional intake, account for the increased mortality in patients with low cholesterol levels.

Because of the lack of prospective studies, the K/DOQI work group for dyslipidemia in CKD evaluated the prevalence of dyslipidemia in a large cross-section of 1047 hemodialysis patients enrolled in the Dialysis Morbidity and Mortality study. Based on National Cholesterol Educational Program, Adult Treatment Panel III definitions, 20% of patients had a normal lipid profile, 62% had dyslipidemia that would warrant therapy, 56% had LDL levels of 100 mg/dL or higher, and another 6% had triglyceride levels of 200 mg/dL or higher, and non-HDL cholesterol (total cholesterol–HDL cholesterol) levels of 130 mg/dL or higher in the presence of LDL cholesterol levels of less than 100 mg/dL. Also, based on these definitions, the prevalence of dyslipidemia that would need treatment was slightly higher in peritoneal dialysis patients (73%); another 6% had triglyceride levels of 200 mg/dL or higher and non-HDL cholesterol levels of 130 mg/dL, respectively, in the presence of LDL levels of less than 100 mg/dL [57].

Several studies have demonstrated the impact of dyslipidemia on cardiovascular morbidity and mortality after kidney transplantation [58,59]. The effects are almost similar to the observations in the general population. Only one prospective, randomized study has evaluated the role of statin therapy on CVD-related events in the recipients of kidney transplantation [60].

High-density lipoprotein cholesterol

Low levels of HDL cholesterol are associated with an increased risk of arteriosclerotic cardiovascular disease (ASCVD), independent of LDL cholesterol levels. Based on the results of a meta-analysis of observational studies in the general population [61], patients with early renal disease (progressive CKD) demonstrate a significant decrease in HDL cholesterol in the early stages of the disease [62]. These low levels of HDL cholesterol persist in more than 50% of patients receiving dialysis [63–65] and in more than 20% of patients in the posttransplant period [58,59,66].

The crucial questions, however, are:

1. The optimal dose and the type of statin that is safe and effective as a lipid-lowering agent in patients with CKD (in early-stage disease, after initiation of dialysis therapy, and after transplantation);
2. The dose and type of statin that could decrease the levels of different fractions of cholesterol, including LDL cholesterol and triglyceride levels have not been studied so far;
3. Whether such therapy could prevent the progression and ameliorate the burden of atherosclerosis in patients with CKD and in patients receiving renal replacement therapy yet to be proven [67].

Nontraditional modifiable factors in patients with chronic kidney disease

A study by Fathi et al [67] showed the lack of improvement in the burden of CVD with the use of statin therapy, despite an appropriate response to lipid-lowering agents with reduction in lipid levels. This finding suggests that other factors (so-called "nontraditional factors") may be involved in the development and progression of ASCVD in patients with CKD [68].

Several nontraditional risk factors, such as increased levels of C-reactive protein, lipoprotein (a), homocysteine, and fibrinogen, have been associated with an increased risk for CVD in the general population [69–71].

Muntner et al [68] analyzed the NHANES III database and demonstrated that the lowest level of kidney function was associated with increased levels of apolipoprotein B, lipoprotein (a), homocysteine, fibrinogen, and C-reactive protein in

patients with CKD and associated CVD. The prevalence of these risk factors was directly proportional to the decrease in kidney function. Similarly, observational studies have demonstrated an increase in the levels of C-reactive protein, lipoprotein (a), fibrinogen, and homocysteine, and increased mortality in dialysis patients [72].

As in the general population, the biologic and clinical significance of these nontraditional risk factors in patients with CKD is uncertain. These risk factors may be merely an epiphenomenon or may be etiologically related to the onset and progression of ASCVD. Other studies have also demonstrated similar association of CKD with increased levels of markers of inflammation and oxidative stress. Thus, an important triad (inflammation, oxidative stress, and the presence of other traditional risk factors) could play a significant role in the pathogenesis of the complex syndrome of ASCVD in patients with different degrees of CKD [73].

Cardiovascular Health Study and markers of inflammation

Shlipak et al [74] studied the association of renal insufficiency with inflammatory and procoagulant markers as potential mediators both for CVD and kidney disease. Several inflammatory and procoagulant factors were evaluated using baseline data from the Cardiovascular Health Study, a population-based cohort study of 5888 persons aged 65 years or older. C-reactive protein, fibrinogen, factor VIIc, and factor VIIIc levels were measured in nearly all participants; interleukin-6, intercellular adhesion molecule-1, plasmin–antiplasmin complex, and D-dimer levels were measured in nearly half of the participants. Renal insufficiency was defined as a serum creatinine level of 1.3 mg/dL of higher in women and 1.5 mg/dL or higher in men. Based on these criteria, renal insufficiency was present in 647 participants in the study (11%). After adjustment for baseline differences, levels of C-reactive protein, fibrinogen, interleukin-6, factor VIIc, factor VIIIc, plasmin–antiplasmin complex, and D-dimer were significantly higher among persons with renal insufficiency ($P < 0.001$ for each risk factor). The positive associations of renal insufficiency with these inflammatory and procoagulant markers were similar regardless of CVD status (clinical, subclinical, or no CVD disease) at baseline. Therefore, renal insufficiency is independently associated with increased levels of these biomarkers (putative risk factors) and may be an important link between CVD and CKD.

Uremia-related risk factors for arteriosclerotic cardiovascular disease

The effects of uremia may be independent of established traditional and nontraditional risk factors. CKD is generally considered to be a vasculopathic state [75]. The factors that may contribute to this increased risk for CVD because of progressive decline in renal function could be: such as anemia, left ventricular hypertrophy and increased left ventricular mass index, chronic microinflammation, increase oxidative stress, vascular calcification, and increased levels of biomarkers of myocardial damage or stress.

Anemia

Anemia is a frequent complication of CKD. Anemia resulting from a deficiency of erythropoietin (EPO) is present in the majority of patients when the eGFR is less than 60 mL/min. Levin et al [76] reported that even in early stages of kidney disease (creatinine clearance rate > 50 mL/min), approximately 25% of patients have anemia. The decrease in hemoglobin begins as early as the onset of stage 2 or 3 CKD and continues to progress with progression in CKD. Anemia is an important risk factor for CVD, because its presence is associated with LVH in the general population [77]. Anemia is an important and the most common manifestation of end-stage renal disease (ESRD) and continues to remain an important and the most common feature (in >40% of patients) following kidney transplantation. In one cross-sectional study, an estimated creatinine clearance rate below 50 mL/min was associated with a threefold increased risk of anemia in women and a fivefold increased risk in men [78].

The effect of milder decreases in kidney function on hemoglobin levels was analyzed in a population-based sample of 15,419 participants aged 20 years and older in the NHANES III conducted from 1988 to 1994. There was a strong correlation between decreased kidney function and hemoglobin level. The prevalence of anemia (hemoglobin level < 12 g/dL in men and < 11 g/dL in women) increased from 1% at an eGFR of 60 mL/min/1.73m^2 to 9% at an eGFR of 30 mL/min/1.73m^2 and to 33% in men and 67% in women at an eGFR of 15 mL/min/1.73m^2 [79]. The burden of anemia in these patients was independent of the iron stores and the markers of chronic inflammatory state.

A prospective study of 446 subjects (86% white) with a mean duration of renal disease of 6.6 years and a mean creatinine clearance rate of 36.3 mL/min without an arteriovenous fistula and without previous exposure to EPO therapy. Follow-up at 12 months showed that LVH increased from the baseline with a decrease in hemoglobin (odds ratio [OR], 1.32) for every 0.5 g/dL decrease in hemoglobin. Systolic blood pressure increased (OR, 1.11) for every 5 mm increase in hemoglobin. The use of ACE inhibitors had no impact on either the baseline or follow-up LVH. The progression in LVH was associated with worsening of cardiac symptoms (15%) and increased rate of hospitalization (22%), and both of these were related to cardiac causes in such a short period of follow-up [80]. It is possible that in the presence of less-than-optimal hemoglobin values, ACE inhibitors and angiotensin-receptor blockers are unable to exert left ventricular remodeling effect.

Similarly, in patients receiving dialysis, a decrease in hemoglobin concentration by 1 g/dL was associated with about 1.3-fold greater incidence of congestive heart failure [81]. Correction of anemia in dialysis patients has been shown to reduce left ventricular mass and the incidence of congestive heart failure [82].

LVH is present in 80% of incident dialysis patients. Because hemoglobin decreases in the early stages of the evolution of CKD, and because anemia is a leading cause of progression in LVH, treatment with EPO in the early stages of the CKD might be more effective in preventing the development and progression of LVH and growth.

A recently published study in patients with CKD reported a significant improvement in hemoglobin levels and in quality of life with the use of EPO therapy administered every week. This study did not evaluate the effects of an increase in hemoglobin level on the progression of LVH [83,84].

Other advantages of the use of erythropoietin therapy

Several studies have demonstrated that anemia is common in patients with congestive heart failure and is associated with worsening of symptoms and decreased survival. When anemia in these patients is treated with EPO, a significant improvement in cardiac function, skeletal muscle function, and symptoms has been observed [85,86]. Although it was originally believed that EPO acted specifically on hematopoietic cells, recent evidence has demonstrated several nonhematopoietic effects of erythropoietin therapy. Ischemia/reperfusion experiments on the heart [87] and brain [88,89] in rat models showed a significant reduction in infarct size when treated with EPO therapy. Other effects of EPO are related to its proangiogenic effects on endothelial cells, which could be of potential value in patients with ischemic heart disease [89,90]. These preclinical findings suggest that EPO may have potential effects in cardiovascular disease well beyond the correction of hemoglobin levels [82,89].

Left ventricular hypertrophy or Increase in left ventricular mass index

LVH is present in more than 80% of incident dialysis patients. It is assumed that the LVH develops early and gradually worsens with the progression of CKD.

A prospective study evaluated 146 hemodialysis patients who achieved the target hemoglobin level of 10 g/dL (versus 13 g/dL). Follow-up EKGs in 48 weeks showed that achieving the target hemoglobin of 13 g/dL did not lead to regression of established concentric LVH or left ventricular dilation. EPO therapy, however, prevented new-onset left ventricular dilation and was associated with improved quality of life [91]. The follow-up of this study, however, was very short, only 48 weeks.

Left ventricular hypertrophy and cardiac events

The impact of LVH on mortality was studied in ESRD patients enrolled in the Dialysis Morbidity and Mortality Study Wave 2. EKG data about the presence and absence of LVH were analyzed in 64% (n = 2584) of the entire cohort. The prevalence of LVH was 16.4%. Multivariate analysis showed that progression in LVH was dependent on age, presence of hypertension, diabetes mellitus, hyperparathyroidism, and hypoalbuminemia. The effect of LVH on subsequent mortality was highest in the first 6 months of follow-up, and the event rate became less pronounced thereafter [92].

In ESRD patients, hypertension is also a leading cause of LVH, but structural left ventricular changes and myocardial fibrosis could be caused by nonhemodynamic factors, such as increased levels of angiotensin II, parathyroid hormone, endothelins, and aldosterone and increased sympathetic nerve activity with increased plasma catecholamine levels [93].

Anemia management, volume control, and the use of ACE inhibitors and angiotensin-receptor blockers are the cornerstones of preventing the progression of LVH and making possible the regression of LVH in patients with CKD either before or after the initiation of dialysis [94]. A Brazilian study demonstrated that renal transplantation resulted in resolution of systolic dysfunction, regression of LVH, and improvement of left ventricular dilatation. The reduction of LVH was dependent on optimal renal function and, to a greater extent, dependent on the degree of blood pressure control as assessed by ambulatory blood pressure monitoring [95].

Left ventricular hypertrophy and sudden cardiac death

The mortality of dialysis patients is almost 3.5 times higher than the age matched healthy controls. Analysis of USRDS data base revealed that nearly 60% of all cardiac deaths in dialysis population is due to cardiac arrest [96].

The relative contribution of prevalent cardiovascular risk factors for sudden cardiac death is not known, and the relative importance of these risk factors for increased risk for death have not been studied or are poorly understood. In a small study of 123 hemodialysis patients followed for 10 years with annual echocardiographic examination, Paoletti et al [97] demonstrated that progressive LVH (defined by delta-left ventricular mass index [LVMI]) was associated with increased risk of sudden cardiac death.

Another study followed the LVMI in 161 hemodialysis patients with repeated EKG examinations. An increase in LVMI was associated with an increased risk of cardiovascular events. The cardiovascular event–free survival in patients with changes in LVMI below the 25th percentile was significantly higher ($P = 0.004$) than in those with changes above the 75th percentile. An increase in LVMI by 1 $g/m^{2.7}$ per month was associated with a 62% increase in the incident risk of fatal and nonfatal cardiovascular events (hazard ratio, 1.62; 95% CI, 1.13–2.3; $P = 0.009$) [98].

Chronic microinflammation and increased oxidant stress

Acute or chronic microinflammation results in the production of acute-phase proteins. C-reactive protein, fibrinogen, and interleukin-6 are positive acute-phase proteins; albumin and cholesterol are negative acute-phase proteins. Increased levels of C-reactive protein, fibrinogen, and interleukin-6 are associated with an increased risk for cardiovascular events in both the general population and in dialysis-dependent persons. The precise mechanism by which hypoalbuminemia and increased levels of C-reactive protein are associated with increased risk for CVD remains unclear. An acute-phase response could lead to hypoalbuminemia caused by decreased synthesis of albumin or to an increase in the level of C-reactive protein. Increased levels of C-reactive protein have been shown to predict all-cause mortality and increased morbidity in hemodialysis patients (Fig. 5) [99].

Fibrinogen is another acute-phase protein, and hyperfibrinoginemia is a nontraditional risk factor for CVD. Fibrinogen has an important modulating effect on coagulation and increases blood viscosity. Several prospective studies in the general population have shown increased mortality with increased levels of fibrinogen [71]. The fibrinogen levels tend to increase in the early stages of CKD, and even higher levels are seen in patients with CKD, without or with associated proteinuria [100]. Although there are genetic variations in the synthesis of fibrinogen [101], Prinsen et al [102] demonstrated by using isoptic methods that in vivo absolute fibrinogen synthesis rate is increased in the early stages of CKD and in patients receiving peritoneal dialysis.

A meta-analysis of prospective studies in the general population has demonstrated that an increase in the fibrinogen level of about 0.1 mg/dL results in almost 1.8-fold increased the risk of cardiovascular events [71]. If there is a cause-and-

effect relationship between increased levels of fibrinogen and cardiovascular events (because early renal insufficiency is often associated with similar degrees of increase in fibrinogen levels), an increase in fibrinogen level could portend a similar degree of risk for CVD-related events in patients with CKD.

Increased levels of fibrinogen are independently associated with concentric LVH and systolic dysfunction in ESRD patients [103]. The exact mechanisms of how increased fibrinogen levels result in an increased left ventricular mass remain unclear. The increased left ventricular mass could be secondary to the microinflammatory state. These relationships may contribute to the negative prognostic effect of elevated fibrinogen levels in ESRD. Chronic inflammation could be the mechanism of cardiovascular damage in dialysis patients, because interleukin-6 polymorphism has been shown to be different in patients with and without LVH [104].

Biomarkers of increased oxidative stress accumulate in patients with CKD and in dialysis-dependent patients. These markers include advanced glyoxidation products, lipid peroxidation products and oxidized LDL, and advanced protein oxidation products. In addition, increased oxidative stress is associated with nitric oxide (NO) dysregulation and increased diathesis for vascular injury [105].

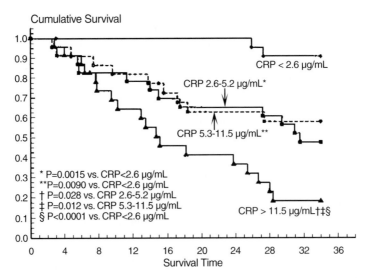

Fig. 5. Kaplan-Meier estimate of survival in hemodialysis patients with serum C-reactive protein (CRP) levels in the highest quartile, middle two quartiles, and lowest quartile. (*From* Yeun JY, Levine RA, Mantadilok V, et al. C-reactive protein predicts all-cause and cardiovascular mortality in hemodialysis patients. Am J Kidney Dis 2000;35:472; with permission.)

The endogenous inhibitor of NO, asymmetric dimethylarginine (ADMA), is a strong predictor of adverse cardiovascular outcomes in patients with ESRD. Interaction of ADMA with the NO system results in the decreased availability of NO, thus resulting in the altered vascular relaxation, and may be an important factor in the pathogenesis of LVH and vascular calcification in CKD patients. The relationship between plasma ADMA and left ventricular geometry and function was studied in a cohort of 198 hemodialysis patients. Plasma ADMA levels were significantly higher in patients with significant LVH and increased LVMI. In addition, ADMA levels were inversely related to left ventricular ejection fraction. How increased levels of ADMA affect left ventricular remodeling and left ventricular dysfunction remains poorly understood. It could be another marker of a microinflammatory state [106] or an epiphenomenon.

Vascular calcification

Ectopic calcification is common in patients receiving dialysis therapy. The exact mechanism for the process of calcification within the arterial wall in patients with CKD and in dialysis-dependent patients is not known. Coronary artery calcification in the general population represents the burden of atherosclerotic disease and has been shown to predict cardiovascular outcomes [107]. Soft tissue, coronary, and valvular calcifications are relatively common in patients receiving maintenance dialysis. Calcification in the vessel wall can be either intimal calcification (a hallmark of atherosclerosis, this process starts as early as in childhood and adolescence) or medial calcification. Medial calcification (Mönckeberg's medial calcinosis) is relatively more common in patients with diabetes mellitus and CKD. The progression in coronary artery calcification in the general population has been associated with both traditional and nontraditional risk factors for CAD. The progression of coronary artery calcification in patients with CKD is further confounded by the duration of dialysis (dialysis vintage), duration and degree of hyperphosphatemia and its associated complications such as hyperparathyroidism, and the use of calcium-containing phosphate binders. The picture is complicated further by the presence of other atherogenic factors such as increased oxidative stress and the degree of associated microinflammation. The major caveat is the unpredictability of the severity of coronary

artery calcification as measured on electron beam CT and the degree of occlusive CAD [108]. Some studies have demonstrated that mere presence of coronary artery calcification is associated with increased all-cause mortality [109,110]. The most optimistic observations, however, suggest that the degree of coronary artery calcification in dialysis patients can be ameliorated with the use of non–calcium-containing phosphate binders (sevelamer) [111] Also, lipid-lowering therapy has resulted in a significant decrease in the degree of coronary artery calcification in the general population [112] and in the dialysis population [113].

Increased levels of cardiac troponin I and T as biomarkers of myocardial stress or damage

Troponin I and T, identified as cardiac troponins (cTnT and cTnI), have emerged as new markers of cardiac ischemia and infarction and follow similar kinetics of release from the myocardium after AMI. After an AMI, levels of both troponins are elevated within 3 to 6 hours. Troponin T tends to peak at 12 hours, and troponin I peaks closer to 24 hours; both remain elevated for up to 5 days. These biomarkers may remain detectable up to 2 weeks after the ischemic event.

cTnT levels are useful in risk stratification of patients with suspected acute coronary syndrome. Its role in patients with CKD remains questionable, because cTnT is excreted by the kidneys.

Aviles et al [114] studied the impact of positive cTnT (third-generation recombinant human cTnT assay) in the patients enrolled in the Global Use of Strategies to Open Occluded Coronary Arteries IV trial. They included patients with decreased creatinine clearance rates (measured by Cockcroft and Gault formula, with adjustment for gender) in four different groups: abnormal creatinine clearance and detectable or increased cTnT levels (n = 950), abnormal creatinine clearance only (n = 783), abnormal cTnT levels only (n = 2695), and normal creatinine clearance and cTnT levels (n = 2605). Based on the quartiles of creatinine clearance (first to fourth: <58.4 mL/min, 58.4–76.9 mL/min, 77.0–98.6 mL/min, and >98.6mL/min, respectively), cTnT levels were independently associated with the risk of death or myocardial infarction within 30 days (primary outcome) across a wide range of creatinine clearance rates. The odds ratio for short-term outcome (30 days) actually rose with declining creatinine clearance rates (Fig. 6). There were, however, only 11 patients with a creatinine

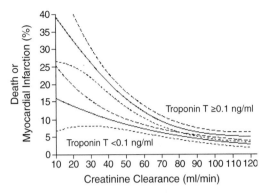

Fig. 6. Incidence of the primary end point of death or myocardial infarction, according to the baseline troponin T level and creatinine clearance rate. (*From* Aviles RJ, Askari AT, Lindahl B, et al. Troponin T levels in patients with acute coronary syndromes, with or without renal dysfunction. N Engl J Med 2002;346:2050; with permission.)

clearance rate of less than 10 mL/min; therefore the value of positive cTnT in establishing the diagnosis and prognosis in dialysis patients was not clarified by this study. The value of increased cTnT level in asymptomatic patients with CKD using the third-generation troponin assay is not known at present [115].

DeFilipi et al [116] measured cTnT and C-reactive protein in patients with ESRD and assessed the combined value of these markers to predict outcomes and associated cardiac pathology. A prospective cohort of patients receiving maintenance hemodialysis (n = 224) was enrolled in this study with a mean follow-up of more than 2 years. Increased quartiles of both C-reactive protein and cTnT predicted increased risk of death compared with the lowest quartiles, and this risk was independent of other potential confounders for cardiovascular disease. In addition, increased levels of cTnT, but not C-reactive protein, were a predictor of diffuse CAD, and the prevalence of multivessel CAD was significantly higher in the group with highest quartiles of cTnT levels. It also became evident from this study that neither troponin nor C-reactive protein could predict the presence of LVH and reduced left ventricular ejection fraction (<40%) [116].

A similar observation was reported in a cross-sectional study by Iliou et al [117,118]. They measured cTnT and performed EKGs in asymptomatic maintenance hemodialysis patients. Almost 19% of patients had increased levels of cTnT at the time of enrollment into the study. Increased

levels of predialysis cTnT levels were associated with LVH, all-cause mortality, and major cardiovascular events (cardiac death, myocardial infarction, or unstable angina).

Although the spectrum of increased cTnT in patients with CKD is still evolving, it is unclear from the observational studies whether increased levels of these biomarkers are perhaps an expression of underlying myocardial hypoxia-ischemia or microinfarction. Whether troponin assays will offer a new tool for risk stratification of underlying CVD in patients with CKD remains to be proven.

Summary

The goal of risk stratification of CVD in patients with CKD is to lead to effective and early intervention and to prevent the adverse outcomes associated with this complex multisystem disease that is characteristic of growing number of patients with CKD in the general population [119] and of patients receiving dialysis therapy or kidney transplantation [120]. By 2030, there will be 2.24 million patients with ESRD in the United States, and approximately 1.3 million of these cases of ESRD will be caused by diabetes mellitus. Thus, CVD in this high-risk population presents a challenge for the nephrology and the cardiology community.

References

[1] Levey AS, Beto JA, Coronado BE, et al. Controlling the epidemic of cardiovascular disease in chronic renal disease: what do we know? what do we need to learn? where do we go from here? National Kidney Foundation Task Force on Cardiovascular Disease. Am J Kidney Dis 1998;32: 853–906.

[2] Shulman NB, Ford CE, Hall WD, et al. Prognostic value of serum creatinine and effect of treatment of hypertension on renal function. Results from the Hypertension Detection and Follow-Up Program. The Hypertension Detection and Follow-Up Program Cooperative Group. Hypertension 1989;13: 180–93.

[3] Keith DS, Nichols GA, Gullion CM, et al. Longitudinal follow-up and outcomes among a population with chronic kidney disease in a large managed care organization. Arch Intern Med 2004;164:659–63.

[4] K/DOQI clinical practice guidelines for chronic kidney disease. Evaluation, classification, and stratification. Am J Kidney Dis 2002;39:S49–52.

[5] Cockcroft DW, Gault MH. Prediction of creatinine clearance from serum creatinine. Nephron 1976;16: 31–41.

[6] Levey AS, Bosch JP, Lewis JB, et al. A more accurate method to estimate glomerular filtration rate from serum creatinine: a new prediction equation. Modification of Diet in Renal Disease Study Group. Ann Intern Med 1999;130: 461–70.

[7] Levey AS. Clinical practice. Nondiabetic kidney disease. N Engl J Med 2002;347:1505–11.

[8] Remuzzi G, Schieppati A, Ruggenenti P. Clinical practice. Nephropathy in patients with type 2 diabetes. N Engl J Med 2002;346:1145–51.

[9] Jungers P, Massy ZA, Khoa TN, et al. Incidence and risk factors of atherosclerotic cardiovascular accidents in predialysis chronic renal failure patients: a prospective study. Nephrol Dial Transplant 1997;12:2597–602.

[10] Tonelli M, Bohm C, Pandeya S, et al. Cardiac risk factors and the use of cardioprotective medications in patients with chronic renal insufficiency. Am J Kidney Dis 2001;37:484–9.

[11] London GM, Marchais SJ, Guerin AP, et al. Impairment of arterial function in chronic renal disease: prognostic impact and therapeutic approach. Nephrol Dial Transplant 2002;17(Suppl 11):13–5.

[12] Klassen PS, Lowrie EG, Reddan DN, et al. Association between pulse pressure and mortality in patients undergoing maintenance hemodialysis. JAMA 2002;287:1548–55.

[13] Henry RM, Kostense PJ, Bos G, et al. Mild renal insufficiency is associated with increased cardiovascular mortality: the Hoorn study. Kidney Int 2002; 62:1402–7.

[14] Fried LF, Shlipak MG, Crump C, et al. Renal insufficiency as a predictor of cardiovascular outcomes and mortality in elderly individuals. J Am Coll Cardiol 2003;41:1364–72.

[15] Shlipak MG, Fried LF, Crump C, et al. Cardiovascular disease risk status in elderly persons with renal insufficiency. Kidney Int 2002;62:997–1004.

[16] Mann JF, Gerstein HC, Pogue J, et al. Renal insufficiency as a predictor of cardiovascular outcomes and the impact of ramipril: the HOPE randomized trial. Ann Intern Med 2001;134:629–36.

[17] Wannamethee SG, Shaper AG, Perry IJ. Serum creatinine concentration and risk of cardiovascular disease: a possible marker for increased risk of stroke. Stroke 1997;28:557–63.

[18] Culleton BF, Larson MG, Wilson PW, et al. Cardiovascular disease and mortality in a community-based cohort with mild renal insufficiency. Kidney Int 1999;56:2214–9.

[19] Muntner P, He J, Hamm L, et al. Renal insufficiency and subsequent death resulting from cardiovascular disease in the united States. J Am Soc Nephrol 2002; 13:745–53.

[20] Rahman M, Brown CD, Coresh J, et al. The prevalence of reduced glomerular filtration rate in older hypertensive patients and its association with cardiovascular disease: a report from the Antihypertensive and Lipid-Lowering Treatment to Prevent Heart Attack Trial. Arch Intern Med 2004;164: 969–76.

[21] Garg AX, Clark WF, Haynes RB, et al. Moderate renal insufficiency and the risk of cardiovascular mortality: results from the NHANES I. Kidney Int 2002;61:1486–94.

[22] McCullough PA. Cardiorenal risk: an important clinical intersection. Rev Cardiovasc Med 2002;3: 71–6.

[23] USRDS. The United States renal data system. Am J Kidney Dis 2003;42:202–14.

[24] Herzog CA, Ma JZ, Collins AJ. Poor long-term survival after acute myocardial infarction among patients on long-term dialysis. N Engl J Med 1998;339:799–805.

[25] Kasiske BL, Ramos EL, Gaston RS, et al. The evaluation of renal transplant candidates: clinical practice guidelines. Patient Care and Education Committee of the American Society of Transplant Physicians. J Am Soc Nephrol 1995;6:1–34.

[26] Rubel JR, Milford EL. The relationship between serum calcium and phosphate levels and cardiac valvular procedures in the hemodialysis population. Am J Kidney Dis 2003;41:411–21.

[27] Salgueira M, del Toro N, Moreno-Alba R, et al. Vascular calcification in the uremic patient: a cardiovascular risk? Kidney Int Suppl 2003;S119–21.

[28] Baglin A, Hanslik T, Vaillant JN, et al. Severe valvular heart disease in patients on chronic dialysis. A five-year multicenter French survey. Ann Med Interne (Paris) 1997;148:521–6.

[29] Herzog CA, Ma JZ, Collins AJ. Long-term survival of dialysis patients in the United States with prosthetic heart valves: should ACC/AHA practice guidelines on valve selection be modified? Circulation 2002;105:1336–41.

[30] Gerstein HC, Mann JF, Yi Q, et al. Albuminuria and risk of cardiovascular events, death, and heart failure in diabetic and nondiabetic individuals. JAMA 2001;286:421–6.

[31] Bakris GL. Microalbuminuria: what is it? why is it important? what should be done about it? J Clin Hypertens (Greenwich) 2001;3:99–102.

[32] Grimm RH Jr, Svendsen KH, Kasiske B, et al. Proteinuria is a risk factor for mortality over 10 years of follow-up. MRFIT Research Group. Multiple Risk Factor Intervention Trial. Kidney Int Suppl 1997;63:S10–4.

[33] Culleton BF, Larson MG, Parfrey PS, et al. Proteinuria as a risk factor for cardiovascular disease and mortality in older people: a prospective study. Am J Med 2000;109:1–8.

[34] Ruggenenti P, Gambara V, Perna A, et al. The nephropathy of non-insulin-dependent diabetes: predictors of outcome relative to diverse patterns of renal injury. J Am Soc Nephrol 1998;9: 2336–43.

[35] Remuzzi G, Bertani T. Pathophysiology of progressive nephropathies. N Engl J Med 1998;339: 1448–56.

[36] Yudkin JS, Forrest RD, Jackson CA. Microalbuminuria as predictor of vascular disease in non-diabetic subjects. Islington Diabetes Survey. Lancet 1988;2:530–3.

[37] Stehouwer CD, Gall MA, Twisk JW, et al. increased urinary albumin excretion, endothelial dysfunction, and chronic low-grade inflammation in type 2 diabetes: progressive, interrelated, and independently associated with risk of death. Diabetes 2002;51:1157–65.

[38] Murtaugh MA, Jacobs DR Jr, Yu X, et al. Correlates of urinary albumin excretion in young adult blacks and whites: the Coronary Artery Risk Development in Young Adults Study. Am J Epidemiol 2003;158:676–86.

[39] De Zeeuw D, Remuzzi G, Parving HH, et al. Albuminuria, a therapeutic target for cardiovascular protection in type 2 diabetic patients with nephropathy. Circulation 2004;110:921–7.

[40] Keane WF. Metabolic pathogenesis of cardiorenal disease. Am J Kidney Dis 2001;38:1372–5.

[41] Hollenberg NK. Aldosterone in the development and progression of renal injury. Kidney Int 2004; 66:1–9.

[42] Intensive blood-glucose control with sulphonylureas or insulin compared with conventional treatment and risk of complications in patients with type 2 diabetes (UKPDS 33). UK Prospective Diabetes Study (UKPDS) Group. Lancet 1998;352: 837–53.

[43] Retinopathy and nephropathy in patients with type 1 diabetes four years after a trial of intensive therapy. The Diabetes Control and Complications Trial/Epidemiology of Diabetes Interventions and Complications Research Group. N Engl J Med 2000;342:381–9.

[44] Hostetter TH. Prevention of end-stage renal disease due to type 2 diabetes. N Engl J Med 2001;345: 910–2.

[45] Oda H, Keane WF. Lipid abnormalities in end stage renal disease. Nephrol Dial Transplant 1998;13(Suppl 1):45–9.

[46] Nissen SE, Tuzcu EM, Schoenhagen P, et al. Effect of intensive compared with moderate lipid-lowering therapy on progression of coronary atherosclerosis: a randomized controlled trial. JAMA 2004; 291:1071–80.

[47] Cannon CP, Braunwald E, McCabe CH, et al. Intensive versus moderate lipid lowering with statins after acute coronary syndromes. N Engl J Med 2004;350:1495–504.

[48] Bianchi S, Bigazzi R, Campese VM. Microalbuminuria in essential hypertension: significance, pathophysiology, and therapeutic implications. Am J Kidney Dis 1999;34:973–95.

[49] Demant T, Mathes C, Gutlich K, et al. A simultaneous study of the metabolism of apolipoprotein b and albumin in nephrotic patients. Kidney Int 1998;54:2064–80.

[50] Warwick GL, Waller H, Ferns GA. Antioxidant vitamin concentrations and LDL oxidation in nephrotic syndrome. Ann Clin Biochem 2000;37(Pt 4):488–91.

[51] Kronenberg F, Lingenhel A, Lhotta K, et al. Lipoprotein(a)- and low-density lipoprotein-derived cholesterol in nephrotic syndrome: impact on lipid-lowering therapy? Kidney Int 2004;66: 348–54.

[52] Seliger SL, Stehman-Breen CO. Are HMG-CoA reductase inhibitors underutilized in dialysis patients? Semin Dial 2003;16:179–85.

[53] Seliger SL, Weiss NS, Gillen DL, et al. HMG-CoA reductase inhibitors are associated with reduced mortality in ESRD patients. Kidney Int 2002;61: 297–304.

[54] Kalantar-Zadeh K, Block G, Humphreys MH, et al. Reverse epidemiology of cardiovascular risk factors in maintenance dialysis patients. Kidney Int 2003;63:793–808.

[55] Iseki K, Yamazato M, Tozawa M, et al. Hypocholesterolemia is a significant predictor of death in a cohort of chronic hemodialysis patients. Kidney Int 2002;61:1887–93.

[56] Bologa RM, Levine DM, Parker TS, et al. Interleukin-6 predicts hypoalbuminemia, hypocholesterolemia, and mortality in hemodialysis patients. Am J Kidney Dis 1998;32:107–14.

[57] National Kidney Foundation, DOQI Work Group. K/DOQI clinical practice guidelines for management of dyslipidemias in patients with kidney disease. Am J Kidney Dis 2003;41:I–91.

[58] Brown JH, Murphy BG, Douglas AF, et al. Influence of immunosuppressive therapy on lipoprotein(a) and other lipoproteins following renal transplantation. Nephron 1997;75:277–82.

[59] Aakhus S, Dahl K, Wideroe TE. Hyperlipidaemia in renal transplant patients. J Intern Med 1996; 239:407–15.

[60] Holdaas H, Fellstrom B, Jardine AG, et al. Effect of fluvastatin on cardiac outcomes in renal transplant recipients: a multicentre, randomised, placebo-controlled trial. Lancet 2003;361:2024–31.

[61] Gordon DJ, Probstfield JL, Garrison RJ, et al. High-density lipoprotein cholesterol and cardiovascular disease. Four prospective American studies. Circulation 1989;79:8–15.

[62] Grutzmacher P, Marz W, Peschke B, et al. Lipoproteins and apolipoproteins during the progression of chronic renal disease. Nephron 1988;50:103–11.

[63] Senti M, Romero R, Pedro-Botet J, et al. Lipoprotein abnormalities in hyperlipidemic and normolipidemic men on hemodialysis with chronic renal failure. Kidney Int 1992;41:1394–9.

[64] Hernandez E, Praga M, Alamo C, et al. Lipoprotein(a) and vascular access survival in patients on chronic hemodialysis. Nephron 1996;72:145–9.

[65] Avram MM, Antignani A, Goldwasser P, et al. Lipids in diabetic and nondiabetic hemodialysis and CAPD patients. ASAIO Trans 1988;34:314–6.

[66] Gonyea JE, Anderson CF. Weight change and serum lipoproteins in recipients of renal allografts. Mayo Clin Proc 1992;67:653–7.

[67] Fathi R, Isbel N, Short L, et al. The effect of long-term aggressive lipid lowering on ischemic and atherosclerotic burden in patients with chronic kidney disease. Am J Kidney Dis 2004;43:45–52.

[68] Muntner P, Hamm LL, Kusek JW, et al. The prevalence of nontraditional risk factors for coronary heart disease in patients with chronic kidney disease. Ann Intern Med 2004;140:9–17.

[69] Stampfer MJ, Malinow MR, Willett WC, et al. A prospective study of plasma homocyst(e)ine and risk of myocardial infarction in US physicians. JAMA 1992;268:877–81.

[70] Ridker PM, Cushman M, Stampfer MJ, et al. Inflammation, aspirin, and the risk of cardiovascular disease in apparently healthy men. N Engl J Med 1997;336:973–9.

[71] Danesh J, Collins R, Appleby P, et al. Association of fibrinogen, C-reactive protein, albumin, or leukocyte count with coronary heart disease: meta-analyses of prospective studies. JAMA 1998;279:1477–82.

[72] Wanner C, Zimmermann J, Schwedler S, et al. Inflammation and cardiovascular risk in dialysis patients. Kidney Int Suppl 2002;99–102.

[73] Oberg BP, McMenamin E, Lucas FL, et al. Increased prevalence of oxidant stress and inflammation in patients with moderate to severe chronic kidney disease. Kidney Int 2004;65:1009–16.

[74] Shlipak MG, Fried LF, Crump C, et al. Elevations of inflammatory and procoagulant biomarkers in elderly persons with renal insufficiency. Circulation 2003;107:87–92.

[75] Luke RG. Chronic renal failure—a vasculopathic state 2. N Engl J Med 1998;339:841–3.

[76] Levin A. Cardiac disease in chronic kidney disease: current understanding and opportunities for change. Blood Purif 2004;22:21–7.

[77] Astor BC, Arnett DK, Brown A, et al. Association of kidney function and hemoglobin with left ventricular morphology among African Americans: the Atherosclerosis Risk in Communities (ARIC) Study. Am J Kidney Dis 2004;43:836–45.

[78] Cumming RG, Mitchell P, Craig JC, et al. Renal impairment and anaemia in a population-based study of older people. Intern Med J 2004;34:20–3.

[79] Astor BC, Muntner P, Levin A, et al. Association of kidney function with anemia: the Third National Health and Nutrition Examination Survey (1988–1994). Arch Intern Med 2002;162:1401–8.

[80] Levin A. Prevalence of cardiovascular damage in early renal disease. Nephrol Dial Transplant 2001;16(Suppl 2):7–11.

[81] Foley RN, Parfrey PS, Harnett JD, et al. The impact of anemia on cardiomyopathy, morbidity, and mortality in end-stage renal disease. Am J Kidney Dis 1996;28:53–61.

[82] Pascual J, Teruel JL, Moya JL, et al. Regression of left ventricular hypertrophy after partial correction of anemia with erythropoietin in patients on hemodialysis: a prospective study. Clin Nephrol 1991;35:280–7.

[83] Provenzano R, Garcia-Mayol L, Suchinda P, et al. Once-weekly epoetin alfa for treating the anemia of chronic kidney disease 1. Clin Nephrol 2004;61:392–405.

[84] Henry DH, Bowers P, Romano MT, et al. Epoetin alfa. Clinical evolution of a pleiotropic cytokine 2. Arch Intern Med 2004;164:262–76.

[85] Marrades RM, Alonso J, Roca J, et al. Cellular bioenergetics after erythropoietin therapy in chronic renal failure. J Clin Invest 1996;97:2101–10.

[86] Marrades RM, Roca J, Campistol JM, et al. Effects of erythropoietin on muscle O2 transport during exercise in patients with chronic renal failure. J Clin Invest 1996;97:2092–100.

[87] Parsa CJ, Matsumoto A, Kim J, et al. A novel protective effect of erythropoietin in the infarcted heart. J Clin Invest 2003;112:999–1007.

[88] Celik M, Gokmen N, Erbayraktar S, et al. Erythropoietin prevents motor neuron apoptosis and neurologic disability in experimental spinal cord ischemic injury. Proc Natl Acad Sci U S A 2002;99:2258–63.

[89] Wang L, Zhang Z, Wang Y, et al. Treatment of stroke with erythropoietin enhances neurogenesis and angiogenesis and improves neurological function in rats. Stroke 2004;35:1732–7.

[90] Ribatti D, Vacca A, Roccaro AM, et al. Erythropoietin as an angiogenic factor. Eur J Clin Invest 2003;33:891–6.

[91] Foley RN, Parfrey PS, Morgan J, et al. Effect of hemoglobin levels in hemodialysis patients with asymptomatic cardiomyopathy. Kidney Int 2000;58:1325–35.

[92] Stack AG, Saran R. Clinical correlates and mortality impact of left ventricular hypertrophy among new ESRD patients in the United States. Am J Kidney Dis 2002;40:1202–10.

[93] London GM. Left ventricular alterations and end-stage renal disease. Nephrol Dial Transplant 2002;17(Suppl 1):29–36.

[94] Bech-Hanssen O, Wallentin I, Larsson O, et al. Reduced left ventricular hypertrophy in type 1 diabetic patients with end-stage renal failure. A comparison between groups investigated 1977–80 and 1991–93. Nephrol Dial Transplant 1996;11:1547–52.

[95] Ferreira SR, Moises VA, Tavares A, et al. Cardio-vascular effects of successful renal transplantation: a 1-year sequential study of left ventricular morphology and function, and 24-hour blood pressure profile. Transplantation 2002;74:1580–7.

[96] Herzog CA. Cardiac arrest in dialysis patients: approaches to alter an abysmal outcome. Kidney Int Suppl 2003;S197–200.

[97] Paoletti E, Specchia C, Di Maio G, et al. The worsening of left ventricular hypertrophy is the strongest predictor of sudden cardiac death in haemodialysis patients: a 10 year survey. Nephrol Dial Transplant 2004;19:1829–34.

[98] Zoccali C, Benedetto FA, Mallamaci F, et al. Left ventricular mass monitoring in the follow-up of dialysis patients: prognostic value of left ventricular hypertrophy progression. Kidney Int 2004;65: 1492–8.

[99] Yeun JY, Levine RA, Mantadilok V, et al. C-reactive protein predicts all-cause and cardiovascular mortality in hemodialysis patients. Am J Kidney Dis 2000;35:469–76.

[100] Irish A. Cardiovascular disease, fibrinogen and the acute phase response: associations with lipids and blood pressure in patients with chronic renal disease 2. Atherosclerosis 1998;137:133–9.

[101] Scarabin PY, Bara L, Ricard S, et al. Genetic variation at the beta-fibrinogen locus in relation to plasma fibrinogen concentrations and risk of myocardial infarction. The ECTIM Study. Arterioscler Thromb 1993;13:886–91.

[102] Prinsen BH, Rabelink TJ, Beutler JJ, et al. Increased albumin and fibrinogen synthesis rate in patients with chronic renal failure. Kidney Int 2003;64:1495–504.

[103] Zoccali C, Benedetto FA, Mallamaci F, et al. Fibrinogen, inflammation and concentric left ventricular hypertrophy in chronic renal failure. Eur J Clin Invest 2003;33:561–6.

[104] Losito A, Kalidas K, Santoni S, et al. Association of interleukin-6 -174G/C promoter polymorphism with hypertension and left ventricular hypertrophy in dialysis patients. Kidney Int 2003;64:616–22.

[105] Himmelfarb J, Stenvinkel P, Ikizler TA, et al. The elephant in uremia: oxidant stress as a unifying concept of cardiovascular disease in uremia. Kidney Int 2002;62:1524–38.

[106] Zoccali C, Mallamaci F, Maas R, et al. Left ventricular hypertrophy, cardiac remodeling and asymmetric dimethylarginine (ADMA) in hemodialysis patients. Kidney Int 2002;62:339–45.

[107] Wong ND, Hsu JC, Detrano RC, et al. Coronary artery calcium evaluation by electron beam computed tomography and its relation to new cardiovascular events. Am J Cardiol 2000; 86:495–8.

[108] Sharples EJ, Pereira D, Summers S, et al. Coronary artery calcification measured with electron-beam

computerized tomography correlates poorly with coronary artery angiography in dialysis patients. Am J Kidney Dis 2004;43:313–9.

[109] London GM, Guerin AP, Marchais SJ, et al. Arterial media calcification in end-stage renal disease: impact on all-cause and cardiovascular mortality 2. Nephrol Dial Transplant 2003;18:1731–40.

[110] Matsuoka M, Iseki K, Tamashiro M, et al. Impact of high Coronary Artery Calcification Score (CACS) on survival in patients on chronic hemodialysis. Clin Exp Nephrol 2004;8:54–8.

[111] Chertow GM, Burke SK, Raggi P. Sevelamer attenuates the progression of coronary and aortic calcification in hemodialysis patients. Kidney Int 2002;62:245–52.

[112] Achenbach S, Ropers D, Pohle K, et al. Influence of lipid-lowering therapy on the progression of coronary artery calcification: a prospective evaluation. Circulation 2002;106:1077–82.

[113] Chertow GM, Burke SK, Dillon MA, et al. Long-term effects of sevelamer hydrochloride on the calcium x phosphate product and lipid profile of haemodialysis patients. Nephrol Dial Transplant 1999;14:2907–14.

[114] Aviles RJ, Askari AT, Lindahl B, et al. Troponin T levels in patients with acute coronary syndromes, with or without renal dysfunction. N Engl J Med 2002;346:2047–52.

[115] Mockel M, Schindler R, Knorr L, et al. Prognostic value of cardiac troponin T and I elevations in renal disease patients without acute coronary syndromes: a 9-month outcome analysis. Nephrol Dial Transplant 1999;14:1489–95.

[116] deFilippi C, Wasserman S, Rosanio S, et al. Cardiac troponin T and C-reactive protein for predicting prognosis, coronary atherosclerosis, and cardiomyopathy in patients undergoing long-term hemodialysis. JAMA 2003;290:353–9.

[117] Iliou MC, Fumeron C, Benoit MO, et al. Factors associated with increased serum levels of cardiac troponins T and I in chronic haemodialysis patients: Chronic Haemodialysis and New Cardiac Markers Evaluation (CHANCE) Study. Nephrol Dial Transplant 2001;16:1452–8.

[118] Iliou MC, Fumeron C, Benoit MO, et al. Prognostic value of cardiac markers in ESRD: Chronic Hemodialysis and New Cardiac Markers Evaluation (CHANCE) Study. Am J Kidney Dis 2003;42: 513–23.

[119] Coresh J, Astor BC, Greene T, et al. Prevalence of chronic kidney disease and decreased kidney function in the adult us population: third National Health and Nutrition Examination Survey. Am J Kidney Dis 2003;41:1–12.

[120] Eknoyan G. On the epidemic of cardiovascular disease in patients with chronic renal disease and progressive renal failure: a first step to improve the outcomes. Am J Kidney Dis 1998;32:S1–4.

ELSEVIER
SAUNDERS

Cardiol Clin 23 (2005) 363–372

CARDIOLOGY
CLINICS

Kidney Disease and Cardiovascular Disease: Implications of Dyslipidemia

William F. Keane, MD[a],*, Paulette A. Lyle, BS[b]

[a]US Human Health, Merck & Co., Inc., 351 N. Sumneytown Pike, UG4A-025, North Wales, PA 19454, USA
[b]Merck Research Laboratories, 1 Walnut Grove, Horsham, PA 19044, USA

Chronic kidney disease causes significant burdens to patients and health care systems worldwide. The incidence and prevalence of chronic kidney disease and end-stage renal disease (ESRD) are high and are increasing at impressive rates. The National Health and Nutrition Examination Survey III (1989–1994) reported that 7.6 million persons (or 4.3% of the population) in the United States had moderately decreased glomerular filtration rate (30–59 mL/min/1.73 m^2) (Table 1). Furthermore, between 1998 and 2010, the incidence of kidney failure in the United States is expected to double, from 320,000 to 650,000 cases [1].

Chronic kidney disease and ESRD are often associated with diabetes, hypertension, and dyslipidemia. The leading cause of ESRD in the United States is diabetes, which was associated with 40% of new cases of ESRD between 1994 and 1999 [2]. Diabetes is associated with increased risks for renal disease and cardiovascular disease and is often associated with dyslipidemia. The worldwide prevalence of type 2 diabetes has been increasing in recent years; the increase is thought to be related to obesity from increasing caloric intake and reduced physical activity. The number of patients requiring dialysis or transplantation is expected to increase as the number of patients with type 2 diabetes continues to grow and as patients with hypertension live longer.

Cardiovascular disease (coronary heart disease, cerebrovascular disease, peripheral vascular disease, and disorders of cardiovascular perfusion [heart failure and left ventricular hypertrophy]) is common in patients with kidney disease, with and without concurrent diabetes, and carries high risks for morbidity and mortality in these patients. The risks of coronary heart disease and death from myocardial infarction are increased in patients with microalbuminuria or proteinuria evidence of kidney disease [3]. Atherosclerosis is common in patients with kidney disease [4], and these patients also have a high prevalence of cardiomyopathy [5]. Mortality resulting from cardiovascular disease is 10 to 30 times more common in patients undergoing dialysis than in the general population [6]. More than half of the deaths of patients with ESRD are from cardiovascular causes [7]. Because of their high mortality from cardiovascular disease, many patients with chronic renal disease may not survive long enough to develop ESRD.

The risk factors for cardiovascular disease in patients with chronic kidney disease parallel those in the general population (eg, age, diabetes, hypertension [especially systolic], left ventricular hypertrophy, and dyslipidemia) but may be different in their level of impact and duration in patients with kidney disease [8]. Given that they occur early in the progression of kidney disease (as was shown, for example, by Culleton [9], the Hypertension Detection and Follow-up Program [10], and the Hypertension Optimal Treatment Study [11]), it is important to treat them as early and effectively as possible to slow the development of irreversible cardiac and renal changes [12].

Urinary protein excretion is an important additional risk factor for cardiovascular disease in kidney disease and is also an important method for measuring the severity and progression of

---

* Corresponding author. Merck & Co., Inc. P.O. Box 1000, UG4A-025, North Wales, PA 19454.
  E-mail address: williamf_keane@merck.com (W.F. Keane).

Table 1
Stages of chronic kidney disease

Stage	Description	GFR mL/min/1.73 m^2	Prevalence[d]	
			N (1000)	%
1[a,b]	Kidney damage with normal or increased GFR	≥90	5900	3.3
2[a,b]	Kidney damage with mildly decreased GFR	60–89	5300	3.0
3[a]	Moderately decreased GFR	30–59	7600	4.3
4[a]	Severely decreased GFR	15–29	400	0.2
5[c]	Kidney failure	<15 or dialysis	300	0.1

Abbreviation: GFR, glomerular filtration rate.

[a] Data for stages 1–4 from National Health and Nutrition Examination Survey III (1988–1994). Population of 177 million aged 20 years or more.

[b] For stages 1 and 2, kidney damage was assessed by spot albumin/creatinine ratio greater than 17 mg/g (men) or 15 mg/g (women) on two measurements.

[c] Data for stage 5 include approximately 230,000 patients treated by dialysis and assumes 70,000 additional patients not receiving dialysis. Percentages total more than 100% because the National Health and Nutrition Examination Survey III may not have included patients receiving dialysis. GFR estimated from serum creatinine using MDRD study equation based on age, gender, race, and calibration for serum creatinine.

[d] For stages 1–4 (*Data from* US Renal Data System. USRDS 1998 annual data report. Bethesda, National Institutes of Health National Institute of Diabetes; 1998.)

From National Kidney Foundation. K/DOQI clinical practice guidelines for chronic kidney disease: evaluation, classification, and stratification. Am J Kidney Dis 2002;39(2 Suppl 1):S1–266; with permission from the National Kidney Foundation.

kidney disease. Proteinuria is often assessed with untimed spot urine sample collection [2]. Micro-albuminuria is diagnosed when urinary albumin excretion is 30 to 300 mg/24 hours or more than 3 mg/dL (dipstick). Microalbuminuria and overt proteinuria are considered to be markers of glomerular and endothelial damage and are risk predictors for cardiovascular morbidity and mortality in patients with essential hypertension, type 1 and type 2 diabetes, diabetic or nondiabetic renal disease, and in the general population [13–30].

Dyslipidemia is present in up to 60% of patients with chronic kidney disease or undergoing dialysis [31] and in 60% of patients who have had kidney transplantation [32]. This article reviews the nature of dyslipidemia in the context of chronic kidney disease; diabetes, lipids, and kidney disease; renal failure and lipids; possible mechanisms for the interaction between kidney disease and dyslipidemia; and treatment interventions for patients with kidney disease and dyslipidemia.

The nature of dyslipidemia in the context of chronic kidney disease

Dyslipidemia has been shown to be associated with cardiovascular disease in patients with and without diabetes and frequently accompanies diabetic nephropathy. Abnormal lipid levels are thought to play a role in acceleration of atherosclerotic micro- and macrovascular disease.

Patients with normal renal function and common types of hyperlipidemia generally do not develop renal insufficiency, indicating that the normal glomerulus has mechanisms to prevent accumulation of lipoproteins. A pre-existing renal disorder with mesangial dysfunction seems to be a prerequisite for lipoprotein accumulation in the glomeruli [33].

The roles that lipids may play in development and progression of renal disease have been studied since 1860 [34] and have been investigated in several animal models [35]. Kamanna et al [34] have summarized the study of the cell biology and histopathology of kidney disease and hyperlipidemia. Hyperlipidemia is common in patients with renal disease. The abnormalities in lipids and lipoproteins in renal disease have varied in experimental reports, however, and have often included hypertriglyceridemia, hypercholesterolemia, and increased low-density lipoprotein cholesterol (LDL) with low, normal, or high levels of high-density lipoprotein (HDL) cholesterol [36]. Increased triglyceride-rich very-low-density lipoprotein (VLDL) and intermediate-density lipoprotein (IDL) have been reported in chronic kidney disease [34]. Some [37–39], but not all [40], studies in patients with proteinuria have shown an association between total cholesterol and deterioration of renal function after controlling for proteinuria in multivariate models. Observational [37,41–47] and prospective studies [48] have shown that low HDL was one of the determinants of rate of decline of renal function. The community-based Atherosclerosis Risk in Communities study showed a relationship between glomerular filtration rate (GFR) and atherosclerotic cardiovascular disease [49]. The relative risk for an increase of 0.3 mg/dL in serum creatinine over 3 years in patients with serum creatinine levels higher than 1.6 mg/dL (men) or 1.4 mg/dL (women) was 1.40 for triglycerides, 1.18 for total cholesterol, 1.16 for lipoprotein (a), 1.13 for LDL, and 0.78 for HDL [49]. In patients with microalbuminuria and essential hypertension, which commonly accompany chronic renal disease, high levels of LDL, triglycerides, apolipoprotein B (apoB), lipoprotein (a), and low HDL may be present [50].

Lipoproteins are characterized by density properties or apolipoprotein composition. Studies that include measurements of apolipoprotein levels have shown that early- and later-stage kidney disease may not be associated with a classic atherogenic hyperlipidemia profile but may involve characteristic changes in lipoprotein metabolism, plasma apolipoprotein profile, and individual apoB-containing proteins [51–53]. apoB-containing lipoproteins are found in VLDL, IDL, and LDL. There are several types of apoB-containing lipoproteins, which are characterized by specific composition of minor apolipoproteins (apoC, apoE, and others) and lipid constituents (triglycerides and cholesterol), metabolic properties, and relative atherogenicity [54]. Whereas nephrotic syndrome and heavy proteinuria are associated with increased formation of cholesterol-rich apoB-containing lipoprotein in LDL and VLDL, the characteristic feature in renal failure is the accumulation of intact or partially metabolized triglyceride-rich lipoprotein in IDL and VLDL [54]. A significantly decreased plasma apoA-I/apoC-III ratio is the hallmark lipid abnormality in renal disease [52,55]. This ratio reflects the reduced apoA-I and apoA-II levels, moderately elevated apoB and apoE, and significantly increased apoC-III levels [56]. This hyperlipidemic profile seems to be caused by faulty catabolism and removal of cholesterol-rich apoB-containing lipoproteins because of reduced activity of lipolytic enzymes, compositional changes in the lipoproteins that

render them poor substrates for lipolysis, and decreased receptor-mediated uptake of lipoproteins [51]. Clinical studies have reported on the possible relationship between apoB-containing lipoproteins and kidney disease: a reduced plasma apoA-1/apoB ratio was associated with a slightly steeper decline of creatinine clearance in patients with moderate renal insufficiency [41]; plasma apoB and LDL significantly correlated with the rate of progression of renal insufficiency [42]; and total cholesterol, LDL, and apoB were significantly associated with rate of decline in renal function [57]. In another study, baseline total cholesterol, LDL, and apoB (but not triglycerides) were associated with decline of renal function in patients with chronic renal insufficiency [57].

Diabetes, lipids, and kidney disease

In diabetic patients, even small amounts of urinary albumin may be associated with substantial changes in lipid profile [58]. Studies in patients with type 1 or type 2 diabetes have shown an association between total cholesterol or LDL level and the rate of progression of renal disease [54]. For example, in a study of patients with type 1 diabetes and nephropathy, higher total cholesterol, triglycerides, and apoB levels were correlated with more rapid renal function decline [37]. Total triglyceride and VLDL triglyceride concentrations were markedly increased in a type 2 diabetes population [59], whereas total cholesterol was not increased in another type 2 diabetes population after correction for gender, age, and duration of diabetes [60]. A review of dyslipidemia in type 2 diabetes was recently published [61].

Renal failure and lipids

The particularly high risk of cardiovascular complications in patients with ESRD is associated with traditional risk factors (including dyslipidemia); factors associated with chronic renal failure; and emerging risk factors, such as inflammation and hyperhomocysteinemia [62]. Total cholesterol levels may be similar or even lower in nondiabetic patients with ESRD versus the general population; this finding is attributed to the pervasive malnutrition in ESRD. In fact, a low cholesterol level has been associated with worse outcome in some patients [63], but in other studies higher total cholesterol and LDL levels predicted cardiac death in diabetic patients receiving dialysis [64]. As in chronic kidney disease, renal failure is accompanied by an abnormal apolipoprotein profile. The current recommendation is that dyslipidemia in patients with renal failure should be treated [62,65].

High triglycerides, decreased HDL, and high lipoprotein (a) levels may be seen in patients receivng hemodialysis and peritoneal dialysis [66]. Hemodialysis can moderately attenuate dyslipidemia, sometimes resulting in normal levels of total cholesterol and LDL with or without increased levels of atherogenic lipoproteins [67]. Peritoneal dialysis may aggravate lipid abnormalities, in particular by increasing LDL levels through increased cholesterol-rich apoB-containing lipoproteins [68]. The associations between lipid abnormalities and ESRD outcome have been inconsistent [66].

Dyslipidemias are common in transplantation patients. Total cholesterol and LDL levels are typically elevated, and triglycerides are often increased. The HDL level is usually normal [36].

Possible mechanisms for the interactions between kidney disease and dyslipidemia

There are several hypotheses regarding the relationship between urinary albumin excretion, kidney disease, and lipid abnormalities [50,69]. Kidney disease may increase lipid levels, and some of the lipid abnormalities associated with kidney disease may cause cardiovascular complications. In patients with kidney disease, increased total cholesterol, LDL, and lipoprotein (a) levels could be secondary to urinary protein loss [70–73]. Even early renal disease may cause changes in lipoprotein profile that can be atherogenic [52]. The IDLs that are elevated in kidney disease are atherogenic because of their size and ability to penetrate the arterial intima [53].

On the other hand, lipid abnormalities could contribute to kidney damage. In the presence of renal disease, lipoproteins may play a role in renal injury in a way that is analogous to their involvement in atherosclerosis [74–76]. This possibility is supported by studies showing that kidney function may be improved by pharmacologic agents that lower lipid levels [77,78]. Experimental data support the hypothesis that dyslipidemia contributes to glomerular and interstitial injury of the renal parenchyma [74]. Glomerular mesangial cells and vascular smooth muscle cells have similarities that suggest that accumulation of lipids in mesangial cells, analogous to an atherosclerotic

process in smooth muscle cells, may cause or accelerate glomerulosclerosis [79,80]. LDL causes monocytes to adhere to endothelial cells, and this adhesion may be an important factor in inflammatory glomerular disease [81,82].

Treatment interventions for patients with kidney disease and dyslipidemia

Nonpharmacologic interventions are important for the control of lipids in all patient populations. The Steno-2 study showed a significant benefit of intensive, multifactorial treatment (diet, exercise, smoking cessation, therapy with angiotensin-converting enzyme inhibitors or angiotensin-receptor blockers, vitamin and mineral supplementation, oral hypoglycemic agent [if needed], and treatment of hypertension or dyslipidemia) on risk factors for cardiovascular disease in patients with type 2 diabetes and microalbuminuria [83].

Clinical trials have shown that statin therapy reduces the risk of adverse cardiovascular outcomes in patients at risk of cardiovascular disease, even in those with normal lipid levels. For example, in the Heart Protection Study [84] simvastatin therapy significantly reduced the incidence of major coronary events and ischemic stroke in patients with normal lipid levels who had cerebrovascular disease, other occlusive arterial disease, or diabetes. Patients with type 2 diabetes and at least one other risk factor for cardiovascular disease (hypertension, retinopathy, high cholesterol level, or smoking) who were treated with atorvastatin experienced significant decreases in serious cardiovascular outcomes and stroke in the Collaborative AtoRvastatin Diabetes Study [85,86].

Treatments that lower proteinuria (eg, angiotensin-converting enzyme inhibitors or angiotensin-receptor blockers) may lower lipid levels. Lipid-lowering therapy is often desirable in patients with kidney disease and hyperlipidemia, however. At present, it seems that lipid regulation decreases the incidence of coronary vascular events and other vascular complications in patients with kidney disease, but there are not yet enough data to determine definitively whether lipid regulation slows progression of kidney disease. A meta-analysis of controlled clinical trials showed that lipid-lowering therapy slowed the rate of decline in GFR and showed a tendency toward decreased proteinuria in patients with renal disease. The reduction in GFR was 0.16 (0.03–0.27) mL/min per month, which compares favorably to the effect of angiotensin-converting enzyme inhibitor therapy on rate of change in renal function [87]. Statin therapy has been shown to be effective for improving lipid levels and kidney function [78,88] and for secondary prevention of cardiovascular events in patients with chronic renal insufficiency [89]. In the Heart Protection Study, simvastatin significantly decreased the aging-related rise in serum creatinine levels in diabetic and nondiabetic patients [90]. Similarly, patients in the simvastatin group had a significantly smaller decrease in estimated GFR during the trial.

Currently, there are no prospective, randomized trial results reporting the effects of the management of dyslipidemia on cardiovascular outcomes in patients with chronic kidney disease. The statin (simvastatin)-selective intestinal cholesterol absorption inhibitor (ezetimibe) combination is being tested in the Study of Heart and Renal Protection study, which includes patients with chronic kidney disease or receiving dialysis without dyslipidemia and no history of myocardial infarction or coronary revascularization [91]. The primary outcome being investigated is a composite of serious cardiovascular events.

In more advanced kidney disease, lipid-lowering treatment with statin therapy reduced cholesterol-rich apoB-containing lipoproteins in patients with nephrotic syndrome [92]; reduced total cholesterol, LDL and triglycerides levels and increased HDL levels in patients undergoing continuous peritoneal dialysis [93]; and has been associated with reduced cardiovascular and total mortality in patients in patients with ESRD [94]. The extent of lipid lowering with statin therapy in patients with peritoneal dialysis or hemodialysis is similar to that in patients without renal disease [95–98].

The Assessment of Lescol in Renal Transplantation study was the first prospective, randomized trial of the effects of dyslipidemia management on cardiovascular outcomes in transplantation patients [99]. It assessed the effect of fluvastatin in renal transplant recipients with mild-to-moderate hypercholesterolemia (total cholesterol of 4.0–9.0 mmol/L; 155–348 mg/dL), except for those with a history of myocardial infarction, for whom the upper limit of total cholesterol was 7.0 mmol/L (270 mg/dL). The primary objective was to investigate the effects of fluvastatin on major adverse cardiac events. Fluvastatin lowered LDL levels by 32%. Although there was not a significant effect on the combined cardiovascular end point (cardiac death, nonfatal myocardial infarction, or coronary revascularization), there were significant reductions in cardiovascular deaths and nonfatal myocardial infarction. The observed cardiac event rate was lower than predicted in this trial, and it had insufficient power to detect a significant reduction in the chosen primary end point. The beneficial proportional reduction in cardiovascular events was similar to those of statins in other populations.

Additional lipid-related studies are underway in the ESRD population. One example is the Die Deutsche Diabetes Dialyse Studie [100], which will test the hypothesis that atorvastatin decreases the rate of cardiovascular mortality and of non-fatal myocardial infarction in patients with type 2 diabetes receiving hemodialysis. A secondary end point is mean percentage change in lipid profile from baseline in patients for whom the baseline LDL level is 80 to 190 mg/dL (2.1–4.9 mmol/L) and triglyceride level is less than 1000 mg/dL (11.4 mmol/L). The results of this study should be published in 2005.

Lipid-lowering measures are indicated in patients with all stages of renal disease because of their increased risk of cardiovascular complications. The number of patients who reach lipid goals has been disappointing; reasons given have included failure of physicians to test for and treat dyslipidemia (before and concurrently with cardiovascular disease) and failure of patients to follow treatment recommendations, including taking medication as directed. Although little information is currently available about the impact of lipid treatment in patients with chronic kidney disease (no available data) or transplantation (one study), the National Kidney Foundation cites the benefit of lipid therapy in the general population as additional support for lipid management in patients with kidney disease. Currently, the National Kidney Foundation recommends strict control of lipoprotein levels for patients with kidney disease (Fig. 1) [36,65].

Summary

Cardiovascular complications are common in patients with kidney disease. Regulating the lipid levels in these patients is important so that the risks of kidney and cardiovascular complications can be minimized. Lipid regulation decreases the incidence of coronary vascular events and other vascular complications in patients with kidney disease; however, whether lipid regulation slows

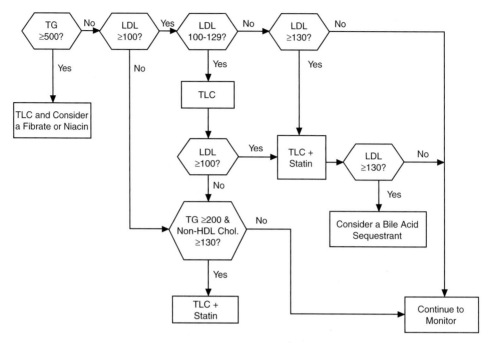

Fig. 1. Treatment of dyslipidemia in adults with kidney disease as recommended by the National Kidney Foundation. Units are mg/dL. HDL, high-density lipoprotein; LDL, low-density lipoprotein; TG, triglycerides, TLC, therapeutic lifestyle changes. (*From* National Kidney Foundation. K/DOQI clinical practice guidelines for managing dyslipidemias in chronic kidney disease. Am J Kidney Disease 2003;41(Suppl 3):S40; with permission and Kasiske B, Cosio FG, Beto J, et al. Clinical practice guidelines for managing dyslipidemias in kidney transplant patients: a report from the Managing Dyslipidemias in Chronic Kidney Disease Work Group of the National Kidney Foundation Kidney Disease Outcomes Quality Initiative. Am J Transplant 2004;4(Suppl 7):28; with permission from the National Kidney Foundation.)

progression of kidney disease is not yet known. Additional studies of the implications of dyslipidemia in patients with kidney disease are needed.

References

[1] US Renal Data System. USRDS 1998 annual data report. Bethesda: National Institutes of Health National Institute of Diabetes; 1998.

[2] National Kidney Foundation. K/DOQI clinical practice guidelines for chronic kidney disease: evaluation, classification, and stratification. Am J Kidney Dis 2002;39(2 Suppl 1):S1–266.

[3] Watkins PJ. Cardiovascular disease, hypertension, and lipids. BMJ 2003;326(7394):874–6.

[4] Jungers P, Massy ZA, Khoa TN, et al. Incidence and risks of atherosclerotic cardiovascular accidents in predialysis chronic renal failure patients: a prospective study. Nephrol Dial Transplant 1997;12(12):2597–602.

[5] Foley RN, Parfrey PS, Harnett JD, et al. Clinical and echocardiographic disease in patients starting end-stage renal disease therapy. Kidney Int 1995; 47(1):186–92.

[6] Levey AS, Beto JA, Coronado BE, et al. Controlling the epidemic of cardiovascular disease in chronic renal disease: what do we know? What do we need to learn? Where do we go from here? National Kidney Foundation Task Force on Cardiovascular Disease. Am J Kidney Dis 1998; 32(5):853–906.

[7] Foley RN, Parfrey PS, Hefferton D, et al. Advance prediction of early death in patients starting maintenance dialysis. Am J Kidney Dis 1994;23(6): 836–45.

[8] Sarnak MJ, Levey AS, Schoolwerth AC, et al. Kidney disease as a risk factor for development of cardiovascular disease: a statement from the American Heart Association Councils on Kidney in Cardiovascular Disease, High Blood Pressure Research, Clinical Cardiology, and Epidemiology and Prevention. Circulation 2003;108(17):2154–69.

[9] Culleton BF, Larson MG, Wilson PW, et al. Cardiovascular disease and mortality in a community-based cohort with mild renal insufficiency. Kidney Int 1999;56(6):2214–9.

[10] Shulman NB, Ford CE, Hall WD, et al. Prognostic value of serum creatinine and effect of treatment of hypertension on renal function. Results from the

Hypertension Detection and Follow-up Program. The Hypertension Detection and Follow-up Program Cooperative Group. Hypertension 1989; 13(Suppl 5):I80–93.

[11] Ruilope LM, Salvetti A, Jamerson K, et al. Renal function and intensive lowering of blood pressure in hypertensive participants of the Hypertension Optimal Treatment (HOT) Study. J Am Soc Nephrol 2001;12(2):218–25.

[12] Locatelli F, Del Vecchio L, Pozzoni P. The importance of early detection of chronic kidney disease. Nephrol Dial Transplant 2002;17(Suppl 11):2–7.

[13] Hillege HL, Janssen WM, Bak AA, et al. Microalbuminuria is common, also in a nondiabetic, nonhypertensive population, and an independent indicator of cardiovascular risk factors and cardiovascular morbidity. J Intern Med 2001;249(6): 519–26.

[14] Romundstad S, Holmen J, Hallan H, et al. Microalbuminuria, cardiovascular disease and risk factors in a nondiabetic/nonhypertensive population. The Nord-Trondelag Health Study (HUNT, 1995–97), Norway. J Intern Med 2002;252(2): 164–72.

[15] Yudkin JS, Forrest RD, Jackson CA. Microalbuminuria as predictor of vascular disease in non-diabetic subjects. Islington Diabetes Survey. Lancet 1988;2(8610):530–3.

[16] Dinneen SF, Gerstein HC. The association of microalbuminuria and mortality in non-insulin-dependent diabetes mellitus. A systematic overview of the literature. Arch Intern Med 1997;157(13): 1413–8.

[17] Gerstein HC, Mann JF, Yi Q, Zinman B, et al. Albuminuria and risk of cardiovascular events, death, and heart failure in diabetic and nondiabetic individuals. JAMA 2001;286(4):421–6.

[18] Hillege HL, Fidler V, Diercks GF, et al. Urinary albumin excretion predicts cardiovascular and noncardiovascular mortality in general population. Circulation 2002;106(14):1777–82.

[19] Rossing P, Hougaard P, Borch-Johnsen K, et al. Predictors of mortality in insulin dependent diabetes: 10 year observational follow up study. BMJ 1996;313(7060):779–84.

[20] Jager A, Kostense PJ, Ruhe HG, et al. Microalbuminuria and peripheral arterial disease are independent predictors of cardiovascular and all-cause mortality, especially among hypertensive subjects: five-year follow-up of the Hoorn Study. Arterioscler Thromb Vasc Biol 1999;19(3):617–24.

[21] Damsgaard EM, Froland A, Jorgensen OD, et al. Microalbuminuria as predictor of increased mortality in elderly people. BMJ 1990;300(6720): 297–300.

[22] Roest M, Banga JD, Janssen WM, et al. Excessive urinary albumin levels are associated with future cardiovascular mortality in postmenopausal women. Circulation 2001;103(25):3057–61.

[23] Borch-Johnsen K, Feldt-Rasmussen B, Strandgaard S, et al. Urinary albumin excretion. An independent predictor of ischemic heart disease. Arterioscler Thromb Vasc Biol 1999;19(8):1992–7.

[24] Gerstein HC, Mann JF, Pogue J, et al. Prevalence and determinants of microalbuminuria in high-risk diabetic and nondiabetic patients in the Heart Outcomes Prevention Evaluation Study. The HOPE Study Investigators. Diabetes Care 2000; 23(Suppl 2):B35–9.

[25] Winocour PH, Harland JO, Millar JP, et al. Microalbuminuria and associated cardiovascular risk factors in the community. Atherosclerosis 1992; 93(1–2):71–81.

[26] Goligorsky MS, Chen J, Brodsky S. Workshop: endothelial cell dysfunction leading to diabetic nephropathy: focus on nitric oxide. Hypertension 2001;37(2 Part 2):744–8.

[27] Grimm RH Jr, Svendsen KH, Kasiske B, et al. Proteinuria is a risk factor for mortality over 10 years of follow-up. MRFIT Research Group. Multiple Risk Factor Intervention Trial. Kidney Int 1997; 52(Suppl 63):S10–4.

[28] Nelson RG, Pettitt DJ, Carraher MJ, et al. Effect of proteinuria on mortality in NIDDM. Diabetes 1988;37(11):1499–504.

[29] Ballard DJ, Humphrey LL, Melton LJ III, et al. Epidemiology of persistent proteinuria in type II diabetes mellitus. Population-based study in Rochester, Minnesota. Diabetes 1988;37(4): 405–12.

[30] Stephenson JM, Kenny S, Stevens LK, et al. Proteinuria and mortality in diabetes: the WHO Multinational Study of Vascular Disease in Diabetes. Diabet Med 1995;12(2):149–55.

[31] Harris K, Thomas M, Short C, et al. Assessment of the efficacy of treatment of dyslipidaemia in renal outpatients. J Nephrol 2002;15(3):263–9.

[32] Kasiske BL. Hyperlipidemia in patients with chronic renal disease. Am J Kidney Dis 1998;32(5 Suppl 3):S142–56.

[33] Attman PO. Progression of renal failure and lipids: is there evidence for a link in humans? Nephrol Dial Transplant 1998;13(3):545–7.

[34] Kamanna VS, Roh DD, Kirschenbaum MA. Hyperlipidemia and kidney disease: concepts derived from histopathology and cell biology of the glomerulus. Histol Histopathol 1998;13(1):169–79.

[35] Crook ED, Thallapureddy A, Migdal S, et al. Lipid abnormalities and renal disease: is dyslipidemia a predictor of progression of renal disease? Am J Med Sci 2003;325(6):340–8.

[36] Kasiske B, Cosio FG, Beto J, et al. Clinical practice guidelines for managing dyslipidemias in kidney transplant patients: a report from the Managing Dyslipidemias in Chronic Kidney Disease Work Group of the National Kidney Foundation Kidney Disease Outcomes Quality Initiative. Am J Transplant 2004;4(Suppl 7):13–53.

[37] Mulec H, Johnsen SA, Wiklund O, et al. Cholesterol: a renal risk factor in diabetic nephropathy? Am J Kidney Dis 1993;22(1):196–201.

[38] Washio M, Okuda S, Ikeda M, et al. Hypercholesterolemia and the progression of the renal dysfunction in chronic renal failure patients. J Epidemiol 1996;6(4):172–7.

[39] Hsu CY, Bates DW, Kuperman GJ, et al. Diabetes, hemoglobin A_{1c}, cholesterol, and the risk of moderate chronic renal insufficiency in an ambulatory population. Am J Kidney Dis 2000;36(2):272–81.

[40] Yokoyama H, Tomonaga O, Hirayama M, et al. Predictors of the progression of diabetic nephropathy and the beneficial effect of angiotensin-converting enzyme inhibitors in NIDDM patients. Diabetologia 1997;40(4):405–11.

[41] Cappelli P, Evangelista M, Bonomini M, et al. Lipids in the progression of chronic renal failure. Nephron 1992;62(1):31–5.

[42] Samuelsson O, Aurell M, Knight-Gibson C, et al. Apolipoprotein-B-containing lipoproteins and the progression of renal insufficiency. Nephron 1993; 63(3):279–85.

[43] Krolewski AS, Warram JH, Christlieb AR. Hypercholesterolemia—a determinant of renal function loss and deaths in IDDM patients with nephropathy. Kidney Int 1994;45(Suppl 45):S125–31.

[44] Ravid M, Neumann L, Lishner M. Plasma lipids and the progression of nephropathy in diabetes mellitus type II: effect of ACE inhibitors. Kidney Int 1995;47(3):907–10.

[45] Mänttäri M, Tiula E, Alikoski T, et al. Effects of hypertension and dyslipidemia on the decline in renal function. Hypertension 1995;26(4):670–5.

[46] Wirta O, Pasternack A, Laippala P, et al. Glomerular filtration rate and kidney size after six years disease duration in non-insulin-dependent diabetic subjects. Clin Nephrol 1996;45(1):10–7.

[47] Klag MJ, Whelton PK, Randall B, et al. Serum cholesterol and ESRD incidence in men screened for the MRFIT [abstract]. J Am Soc Nephrol 1996;6:393.

[48] Hunsicker LG, Adler S, Caggiula A, et al. Predictors of the progression of renal disease in the Modification of Diet in Renal Disease Study. Kidney Int 1997;51(6):1908–19.

[49] Manjunath G, Tighiouart H, Ibrahim H, et al. Level of kidney function as a risk factor for atherosclerotic cardiovascular outcomes in the community. J Am Coll Cardiol 2003;41(1):47–55.

[50] Campese VM, Bianchi S, Bigazzi R. Is microalbuminuria a predictor of cardiovascular and renal disease in patients with essential hypertension? Curr Opin Nephrol Hypertens 2000;9(2):143–7.

[51] Attman PO, Samuelsson O, Alaupovic P. Lipoprotein metabolism and renal failure. Am J Kidney Dis 1993;21(6):573–92.

[52] Samuelsson O, Attman PO, Knight-Gibson C, et al. Lipoprotein abnormalities without hyperlipidaemia in moderate renal insufficiency. Nephrol Dial Transplant 1994;9(11):1580–5.

[53] Alaupovic P. Apolipoprotein composition as the basis for classifying plasma lipoproteins. Characterization of ApoA- and ApoB-containing lipoprotein families. Prog Lipid Res 1991;30(2–3):105–38.

[54] Attman PO, Samuelsson O, Alaupovic P. Progression of renal failure: role of apolipoprotein B-containing lipoproteins. Kidney Int 1997;52(Suppl 63):98–101.

[55] Moberly JB, Attman PO, Samuelsson O, et al. Apolipoprotein C–III, hypertriglyceridemia and triglyceride-rich lipoproteins in uremia. Miner Electrolyte Metab 1999;25(4–6):258–62.

[56] Attman PO, Samuelsson OG, Moberly J, et al. Apolipoprotein B-containing lipoproteins in renal failure: the relation to mode of dialysis. Kidney Int 1999;55(4):1536–42.

[57] Samuelsson O, Mulec H, Knight-Gibson C, et al. Lipoprotein abnormalities are associated with increased rate of progression of human chronic renal insufficiency. Nephrol Dial Transplant 1997;12(9): 1908–15.

[58] Kapelrud H, Bangstad HJ, Dahl-Jorgensen K, et al. Serum Lp(a) lipoprotein concentrations in insulin dependent diabetic patients with microalbuminuria. BMJ 1991;303(6804):675–8.

[59] Nielsen FS, Voldsgaard AI, Gall MA, et al. Apolipoprotein (a) and cardiovascular disease in type 2 (non-insulin-dependent) diabetic patients with and without diabetic nephropathy. Diabetologia 1993;36(5):438–44.

[60] Bruno G, Cavallo-Perin P, Bargero G, et al. Prevalence and risk factors for micro- and macroalbuminuria in an Italian population-based cohort of NIDDM subjects. Diabetes Care 1996;19(1):43–7.

[61] Battisti WP, Palmisano J, Keane WF. Dyslipidemia in patients with type 2 diabetes. Relationships between lipids, kidney disease and cardiovascular disease. Clin Chem Lab Med 2003;41(9): 1174–81.

[62] Zoccali C, Mallamaci F, Tripepi G. Traditional and emerging cardiovascular risk factors in end-stage renal disease. Kidney Int 2003;63(Suppl 85): S105–10.

[63] Lowrie EG, Lew NL. Death risk in hemodialysis patients: the predictive value of commonly measured variables and an evaluation of death rate differences between facilities. Am J Kidney Dis 1990; 15(5):458–82.

[64] Tschöpe W, Koch M, Thomas B, et al. Serum lipids predict cardiac death in diabetic patients on maintenance hemodialysis. Results of a prospective study. The German Study Group Diabetes and Uremia. Nephron 1993;64(3):354–8.

[65] National Kidney Foundation. K/DOQI clinical practice guidelines for managing dyslipidemias in chronic kidney disease. Am J Kidney Dis 2003; 41(Suppl 3):S1–91.

[66] Foley RN, Parfrey PS. Cardiovascular disease and mortality in ESRD. J Nephrol 1998;11(5):239–45.

[67] Wanner C, Krane V. Non-high density lipoprotein cholesterol: a target of lipid-lowering in dialysis patients. Am J Kidney Dis 2003;41(3 Suppl 1): S72–5.

[68] Attman PO, Samuelsson O, Johansson AC, et al. Dialysis modalities and dyslipidemia. Kidney Int 2003;63(Suppl 84):S110–2.

[69] Campese VM, Bianchi S, Bigazzi R. Hypertension, hyperlipidemia and microalbuminuria. Contrib Nephrol 1997;120:11–21.

[70] Kaysen GA. Hyperlipidemia of the nephrotic syndrome. Kidney Int 1991;39(Suppl 31):S8–15.

[71] Keane WF, St. Peter JV, Kasiske BL. Is the aggressive management of hyperlipidemia in nephrotic syndrome mandatory? Kidney Int 1992;42(Suppl 38):S134–41.

[72] Newmark SR, Anderson CF, Donadio JV, et al. Lipoprotein profiles in adult nephrotics. Mayo Clin Proc 1975;50(7):359–64.

[73] Karådi I, Romics L, Pålos G, et al. Lp(a) lipoprotein concentration in serum of patients with heavy proteinuria of different origin. Clin Chem 1989; 35(10):2121–3.

[74] Keane WF. Proteinuria: its clinical importance and role in progressive renal disease. Am J Kidney Dis 2000;35(4 Suppl 1):S97–105.

[75] Tolins JP, Stone BG, Raij L. Interactions of hypercholesterolemia and hypertension in initiation of glomerular injury. Kidney Int 1992;41(5): 1254–61.

[76] Moorhead JF, Chan MK, El Nahas M, et al. Lipid nephrotoxicity in chronic progressive glomerular and tubulo-interstitial disease. Lancet 1982; 2(8311):1309–11.

[77] Keane WF, Mulcahy WS, Kasiske BL, et al. Hyperlipidemia and progressive renal disease. Kidney Int 1991;39(Suppl 31):S41–8.

[78] Tonelli M, Moyé L, Sacks FM, et al, for the Cholesterol and Recurrent Events (CARE) Trial Investigators. Effect of pravastatin on loss of renal function in people with moderate chronic renal insufficiency and cardiovascular disease. J Am Soc Nephrol 2003;14(6):1605–13.

[79] Rovin BH, Tan LC. LDL stimulates mesangial fibronectin production and chemoattractant expression. Kidney Int 1993;43(1):218–25.

[80] Klahr S, Schreiner G, Ichikawa I. The progression of renal disease. N Engl J Med 1988;318(25): 1657–66.

[81] Alderson LM, Endemann G, Lindsey S, et al. LDL enhances monocyte adhesion to endothelial cells in vitro. Am J Pathol 1986;123(2):334–42.

[82] Pai R, Kirschenbaum MA, Kamanna VS. Low-density lipoprotein stimulates the expression of macrophage colony-stimulating factor in glomerular mesangial cells. Kidney Int 1995;48(4): 1254–62.

[83] Gaede P, Vedel P, Larsen N, et al. Multifactorial intervention and cardiovascular disease in patients with type 2 diabetes. N Engl J Med 2003;348(5): 383–93.

[84] Collins R, Armitage J, Parish S, et al. Effects of cholesterol-lowering with simvastatin on stroke and other major vascular events in 20536 people with cerebrovascular disease or other high-risk conditions. Lancet 2004;363(9411):757–67.

[85] Colhoun HM, Thomason MJ, Mackness MI, et al. Design of the Collaborative AtoRvastatin Diabetes Study (CARDS) in patients with type 2 diabetes. Diabet Med 2002;19(3):201–11.

[86] Colhoun HM, Betteridge DJ, Durrington PN, et al. Primary prevention of cardiovascular disease with atorvastatin in type 2 diabetes in the Collaborative Atorvastatin Diabetes Study (CARDS): multicentre randomised placebo-controlled trial. Lancet 2004;364:685–96.

[87] Fried LF, Orchard TJ, Kasiske BL. Effect of lipid reduction on the progression of renal disease: a meta-analysis. Kidney Int 2001;59(1):260–9.

[88] Imai Y, Suzuki H, Saito T, et al. The effect of pravastatin on renal function and lipid metabolism in patients with renal dysfunction with hypertension and hyperlipidemia. Pravastatin and Renal Function Research Group. Clin Exp Hypertens 1999; 21(8):1345–55.

[89] Tonelli M, Moye L, Sacks FM, et al. Pravastatin for secondary prevention of cardiovascular events in persons with mild chronic renal insufficiency. Ann Intern Med 2003;138(2):98–104.

[90] Heart Protection Study Collaborative Group. MRC/BHF heart protection study of cholesterol-lowering with simvastatin in 5693 people with diabetes: a randomised placebo-controlled trial. Lancet 2003;361:2005–16.

[91] Baigent C, Landry M. Study of Heart and Renal Protection (SHARP). Kidney Int 2003;63(Suppl 84):S207–10.

[92] Massy ZA, Ma JZ, Louis TA, et al. Lipid-lowering therapy in patients with renal disease. Kidney Int 1995;48(1):188–98.

[93] Harris KP, Wheeler DC, Chong CC. A placebo-controlled trial examining atorvastatin in dyslipidemic patients undergoing CAPD. Kidney Int 2002;61(4):1469–74.

[94] Seliger SL, Weiss NS, Gillen DL, et al. HMG-CoA reductase inhibitors are associated with reduced mortality in ESRD patients. Kidney Int 2002; 61(1):297–304.

[95] Hufnagel G, Michel C, Vrtovsnik F, et al. Effects of atorvastatin on dyslipidaemia in uraemic patients on peritoneal dialysis. Nephrol Dial Transplant 2000;15(5):684–8.

[96] Saltissi D, Morgan C, Rigby RJ, et al. Safety and efficacy of simvastatin in hypercholesterolemic patients undergoing chronic renal dialysis. Am J Kidney Dis 2002;39(2):283–90.

[97] Nishikawa O, Mune M, Miyano M, et al. Effect of simvastatin on the lipid profile of hemodialysis patients. Kidney Int 1999;56(Suppl 71):S219–21.

[98] Matthys E, Schurgers M, Lamberigts G, et al. Effect of simvastatin on the dyslipoproteinemia in CAPD patients. Atherosclerosis 1991;86(2–3):183–92.

[99] Holdaas H, Fellstrom B, Jardine AG, et al. Effect of fluvastatin on cardiac outcomes in renal transplant recipients: a multicentre, randomised, placebo-controlled trial. Lancet 2003;361(9374): 2024–31.

[100] Wanner C, Krane V, Ruf G, et al. Rationale and design of a trial improving outcome of type 2 diabetics on hemodialysis. Die Deutsche Diabetes Dialyse Studie Investigators. Kidney Int 1999;71: S222–6.

ELSEVIER
SAUNDERS

Cardiol Clin 23 (2005) 373–384

CARDIOLOGY
CLINICS

Vascular Calcification in Patients With Renal Failure: Culprit or Innocent Bystander?

Santo Dellegrottaglie, MD[a], Rajiv Saran, MD[b], Sanjay Rajagopalan, MD[a],*

[a]*Zena and Michael A. Wiener Cardiovascular Institute and Marie-Josée and Henry R. Kravis Center
for Cardiovascular Health, Mount Sinai Medical Center,
One Gustave L. Levy Place, New York, NY 10029, USA*
[b]*Division of Nephrology, University of Michigan, 315 W. Huron, Ann Arbor, MI 48103, USA*

There is an emerging epidemic of chronic kidney disease (CKD) in developed countries, driven primarily by the aging of the global population and the escalating numbers of patients who have type 2 diabetes mellitus [1]. Recent reports suggest that as many as 6% to 11% of the adult population could have some degree of CKD, and this estimate is supported by the dramatic rise in the number of people with end-stage renal disease (ESRD) [2]. What is not readily appreciated is that the preponderance of patients who have CKD are more likely to die from cardiovascular disease than to go on to ESRD requiring renal replacement therapy [3]. This likelihood is reflected in the increased referrals to cardiologists of patients who have cardiovascular disease and coexisting CKD.

CKD has clearly emerged as an independent risk factor for cardiovascular events, particularly in higher-risk populations [4–6]. Recently, an independent and graded association between reduced renal function and risk of cardiovascular events has been demonstrated in a single large cohort of patients (approximately 1 million individuals) [7]. The concomitance of a higher incidence of traditional cardiovascular risk factors, such as older age, hypertension, dyslipidemia, and diabetes, and risk factors specific to CKD (ie, albuminuria, anemia, abnormal calcium and phosphate metabolism, extracellular fluid volume overload, electrolyte imbalance) may partly explain the high prevalence of cardiovascular disease in these patients [8]. A number of other pathophysiologic variables that are driven by the uremic milieu, such as oxidative stress, inflammation, and endothelial dysfunction, may promote the atherosclerotic process.

The interaction among this multiplicity of factors has been hypothesized to promote the myocardial and vascular complications commonly encountered in CKD patients. In particular, atherosclerosis is common in patients who have CKD; the lesions typically are associated with marked vascular calcification (VC) [9,10].

The traditional variables of risk are poorly predictive of cardiovascular events in this population. With the availability of feasible and reproducible imaging modalities, however, there has been a great interest in surrogate markers of cardiovascular risk in patients who have renal failure. Specifically, in view of the higher predilection for VC in patients who have CKD, it has been hypothesized that determining vessel calcium scores by CT may be a helpful marker of the extension of atherosclerosis and in predicting events in this population.

This article briefly summarizes the current knowledge regarding (1) the mechanisms responsible for VC and its relationship to the atherosclerotic process (with a focus on uremic patients) and (2) the detection of VC and its prevalence in patients who have CKD and ESRD.

* Corresponding author: Sanjay Rajagopalan, MD Cardiovascular Institute, Mount Sinai Medical Center Box 1030, One Gustave L. Levy Place, New York, NY 10029.
E-mail address: sanjay.rajagopalan@mssm.edu (S. Rajagopalan).

cardiology.theclinics.com

Mechanisms of vascular calcification in renal failure

In patients who have renal failure, VC frequently may be observed in two distinct pathologic sites: in the intima, where it is invariably associated with atherosclerosis, and in the tunica media, where it is relevant to the loss of vascular elasticity and compliance. Medial calcification (Mönckeberg's sclerosis) is particularly common in patients who have ESRD and may occur independently of atherosclerosis, thus suggesting etiologic mechanisms different from those involved with intimal calcification [11]. The hemodynamic consequences of medial wall calcification are quite different from those caused by atherosclerotic calcification, and they are less widely understood [12]. Medial wall calcification increases vascular stiffness and reduces vascular compliance. As a result, systolic blood pressure rises, pulse pressure widens, and pulse wave velocity increases. The amount of coronary calcium correlates with arterial stiffness and the extent of calcification in abdominal aorta in dialysis patients [13].

In atherosclerosis, VC probably occurs throughout the course of plaque development, but it is most pronounced in larger, presumably more mature lesions [14]. Heavily calcified plaques are traditionally considered to be associated with a stable phenotype. Whether the presence of small areas of VC contributes to plaque rupture and subsequent arterial thrombosis is still unclear [15,16].

Based on biomechanical considerations, the lipid-rich areas, rather than areas with VC, have heightened stress [16]. Another possibility is that the risk of plaque rupture caused by calcification is biphasic and dose dependent. Model calculations support an increased mural tension in the transition area between the calcified plaque and the circumferential nonatherosclerotic wall [17]. As the degree of calcification increases, the initial transition area between rigid and distensible plaque increases until the calcified plaques coalesce (Fig. 1). In theory, calcification beyond this point may reduce transition zones, resulting in lower mural tension, and may be associated with a lowered risk of plaque rupture. Thus, the most relevant prognostic parameter may not be the extent of VC but rather the extent of the total transition area [18]. Although this concept is appealing, arriving at such a metric in the clinical realm remains unrealistic.

General mechanisms of vascular calcification

Numerous mechanisms have been proposed to explain VC. Traditionally, VC was considered a passive process associated with atherosclerosis or normal aging, but recent evidence indicates that intimal and medial VC may be determined by an active process [19–21].

Bone and mineral metabolism

Experimental works indicate that the plethora of genes and proteins that normally function as key modulators of bone and mineral metabolism are also involved, either directly or indirectly, in the process of VC [19,22]. Bone-related proteins, such as osteonectin, parathyroid hormone, parathyroid hormone–related peptide, and bone morphogenic protein 7, are expressed in the atherosclerotic plaques as well as in sites of medial arterial calcification [21–25].

The recent discovery of osteoprotegerin, a member of the tumor necrosis factor-α receptor family with inhibitory effects on osteoclastogenesis, introduces another link between bone and vascular metabolism [26]. Osteoprotegerin is a soluble molecule that binds and inhibits the ligand for receptor activator of NF-κB, a member of the tumor necrosis factor-α superfamily member demonstrated in the vasculature and essential for the maturation of osteoclast progenitors [27]. In keeping with the possible role of osteoprotegerin in promoting VC, serum levels of osteoprotegerin are elevated in patients who have ESRD (Fig. 2) [28].

The expression of various mineral-regulating proteins in vascular tissue may reflect predominantly phenotypic alterations in vascular smooth muscle cell (VSMC) and possibly vascular endothelial cells [29]. VSMCs can be induced to transform into an osteoblast-like phenotype in vitro. VSMCs and osteoblasts derive from a common mesenchymal precursor cell, and core-binding factor (Cbfa)-1 is a transcription factor thought to be responsible for the switch that converts this precursor to the osteoblast phenotype [30].

Conventionally, phosphate levels were thought to influence mineralization only through physicochemical means. New evidence, however, indicates that phosphate regulates and coordinates cell signaling and gene expression by dynamic transport processes. Primary cultures of human VSMCs express bone proteins and mineralize when treated with β-glycerophosphate, which serves as an inorganic phosphate donor in the

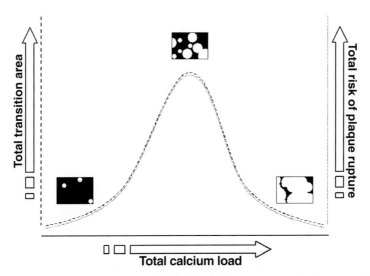

Fig. 1. Hypothetical relationships of total calcium load with transition area (between rigid and nonrigid vessel wall) and risk of plaque rupture. As the degree of vascular calcification increases, the total area of transition initially increases and then decreases (*dashed line*), with the coalescence of the foci of calcification (*insets*). The risk of plaque rupture in relation to the amount of calcium in the vessel wall should follow the same trend (*dotted line*). (*Modified from* Abedin M, Tintut Y, Demer LL. Vascular calcification: mechanisms and clinical ramifications. Arterioscler Thromb Vasc Biol 2004;24(7):1165; with permission.)

presence of alkaline phosphatase [29]. Moreover, high intracellular phosphate levels reduce the expression of typical VSMC genes and induce various osteoblastic-like phenotypic changes in VSMCs (see Fig. 2). In particular, phosphate stimulates the expression of alkaline phosphatase on the surface of VSMCs and the production of Cbfa-1 and of calcium-binding proteins, such as osteocalcin and osteopontin (OPN) [31,32]. Recent studies demonstrate that Cbfa-1, alkaline phosphatase, and OPN are present in calcified arteries but are absent from the vessel wall of noncalcified arteries [20,21].

Molecular inhibitors of calcification

Elevated serum phosphorus levels and high values for the calcium–phosphorus ion product in serum have often been associated with VC, supporting their obligatory involvement in the calcification process [21]. Plasma calcium and phosphate levels, however, are already at or above their theoretic solubility limits in healthy persons, who normally do not develop VC. Why then do normal persons not develop VC?

Plasma components (such as citrate and magnesium) play a key physiologic role by maintaining mineral in solution. Furthermore, specific proteins at sites other than bone may serve an inhibitory function and prevent ectopic calcification. For instance, fetuin-A, matrix Gla protein (MGP), and OPN are important inhibitors of calcification in vivo (see Fig. 2). Serum levels of fetuin-A are significantly reduced in patients who have renal failure [33,34]. Furthermore, circulating levels of fetuin-A decline with increasing inflammation in patients receiving dialysis [33]. MGP is a small protein found in normal arterial wall, and its expression seems to be increased in atherosclerotic plaques [22]. The MGP knockout mouse has extensive aortic calcification, and recent evidence indicates that MGP inhibits mesenchymal cell differentiation to the osteogenic lineage [35,36]. OPN is another important negative regulator of calcification. It operates mostly by inducing mineral resorption [37,38]. Giachelli and colleagues [39] showed that OPN colocalizes with calcified atherosclerotic plaques; within the plaque, OPN is expressed by macrophages, smooth muscle cells, and endothelial cells. Mice deficient in both OPN and MGP have accelerated aortic calcification compared with mice deficient only in MGP, a finding consistent with the concept that OPN inhibits mineralization [40].

Mechanisms of vascular calcification in renal failure

The high prevalence of traditional risk factors for atherosclerosis combined with specific factors

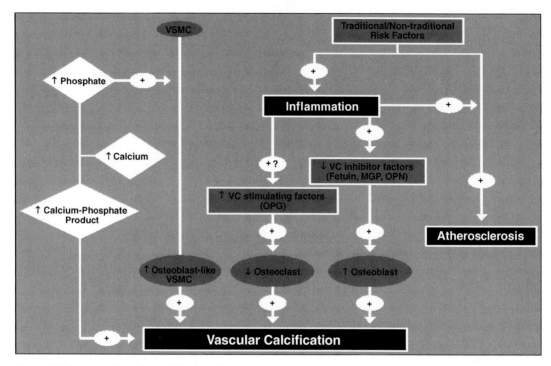

Fig. 2. Mechanisms of vascular calcification. The common coexistence of atherosclerosis and vascular calcification may in part relate to the crucial role of inflammation in inducing both the processes. VC, vascular calcification; VSMC, vascular smooth muscle cells; MGP, matrix Gla protein; OPN, osteopontin; OPG, osteoprotegerin.

related to renal failure may be responsible for the increased VC observed in patients who have renal failure. In particular, some of the major risk factors for atherosclerosis (ie, age, cigarette smoking, and diabetes mellitus) may contribute to intimal or medial wall calcification (Table 1) [41].

Inflammation may play a central role in the predisposition of patients who have renal failure to VC. Inflammation is a common link between the development of atherosclerosis and VC [23]. Inflammation is a fundamental component of the atherosclerotic process, and high serum levels of inflammatory markers (ie, C-reactive protein) have been reported in patients who have ESRD [42]. The role of inflammation in VC is strengthened further by recent observations linking levels of circulating inhibitors of VC, such as fetuin-A and OPN, with increasing inflammatory markers [33]. Thus, multiple factors that are proinflammatory at the vessel wall level may promote VC (see Fig. 2).

Recent evidence suggests that abnormalities in calcium and phosphorus metabolism, including therapeutic interventions affecting total body calcium balance, may also influence the development and progression of VC (primarily medial) in

patients who have renal failure. Thus it has been postulated that accelerated VC at the medial level may be promoted in patients who have ESRD by the putative systemic calcium load arising from the use of calcium-containing phosphate binders and the use of high concentrations of calcium salts in the dialysate [43]. This accelerated medial VC may be distinct from the concomitant intimal VC that may occur in the same patients through different (perhaps proinflammatory) mediators. Supporting these hypotheses is the correlation between VC and calcium–phosphate product observed in studies involving young patients who have ESRD, who have predominantly medial VC. Studies including older patients with ESRD, who may have concomitant intimal VC, do not show this association [13,44–46].

Detection and significance of vascular calcification in patients who have renal failure

Assessment of vascular calcification in clinical practice

Various noninvasive methods (ie, ultrasound, optical coherence tomography, fluoroscopy, and

Table 1
Risk factors for intimal and medial vascular calcification

Risk factor	Intimal vascular calcification	Medial vascular calcification
Advanced age	+	+
Male sex	+	–
Diabetes mellitus	+	+
Dyslipidemia	+	–
Hypertension	+	–
Smoking	+	–
Renal failure		
Reduced glomerular filtration rate	–	+
Hypercalcemia	–	+
Hyperphosphatemia	+	+
Parathyroid hormone abnormalities	–	–
Vitamin D administration	–	+
Inflammation	+	+

Abbreviations: +, association; –, no association.
Adapted from Goodman WG, London G, Amann K, et al. Vascular calcification in chronic kidney disease. Am J Kidney Dis 2004;43(3):575.

Table 2
Relative advantages for the use of electron-beam computed tomography or multidetector computed tomography in the assessment of coronary calcification

Advantages	EBCT	MDCT
High temporal resolution	+	–
High in-plane spatial resolution	–	+
Low occurrence of motion artifacts	+	–
Low image noise	–	+
Widespread availability	–	+
Used for other applications	–	+
Low radiation exposure	+	–
High interstudy reproducibility	+	+

Abbreviations: +, present; –, absent; EBCT, electron-beam computed tomography; MDCT, multidetector computed tomography.

digital subtraction angiography) have been applied to detect and measure VC. At present, electron-beam computed tomography (EBCT) and multidetector computed tomography (MDCT) are the most accurate techniques available for calcium quantification (Table 2). Calcium scoring with EBCT and MDCT does not require the use of contrast media, a potential serious contraindication in persons with renal failure.

EBCT has been used with good results for more than a decade to detect and quantify cardiovascular calcification and is currently considered the reference standard [47]. Most medical centers, however, do not have access to EBCT scanners because of their relatively high cost and limited applications other than the calcium scoring. MDCT scanners, which are more widely available and can be used for a number of cardiac and noncardiac applications, are therefore more practical for assessment of VC (Fig. 3) [48].

A variety of studies have compared EBCT and MDCT (4- and 16-slice) directly, demonstrating excellent correlation between these techniques for calcium quantification [49–51]. Three different methods of calcium quantification and scoring have been applied by various investigators: the Agatston method, the volumetric method, and the mass method [52–54]. The Agatston score has been the most commonly used index in clinical

investigations, and most epidemiologic data have been derived from it. Reproducibility, however, seems to be worst for the Agatston method, intermediate for the volumetric approach, and best for the mass method [55].

The coronary calcium score is a sensitive test for the presence of coronary artery disease, but it is not specific for prediction of significant coronary lesions [56,57]. The American Heart Association and American College of Cardiology recently published guidelines for the use of the coronary artery calcium score as a diagnostic tool for clinical decision making [47]. It is recommended that the coronary calcium score be used only to identify asymptomatic patients at low to intermediate risk who may benefit from more aggressive risk factor modification.

Coronary calcification closely correlates with the presence of calcium in the aorta (at thoracic and abdominal levels) and in the aortic valve, suggesting a common pathophysiologic mechanism for dystrophic calcification (Fig. 4) [58,59].

There is still controversy regarding the prognostic significance of coronary calcium. In recent years, several studies involving distinct target populations have investigated the prognostic value of calcium scoring [60]. As expected, coronary VC detected by EBCT was strongly associated with all-cause mortality [61,62]. On the other hand, evidence regarding the usefulness of coronary VC in

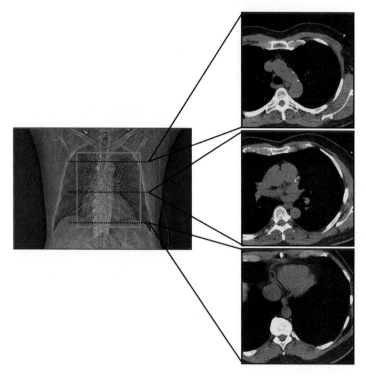

Fig. 3. MDCT (16-slice) for vascular calcium scoring. A continuous volume containing the heart and the thoracic aorta is scanned in one breathhold, ECG-gated acquisition. The postprocessing of the resulting axial images allows the quantification of calcium score at level of the coronaries, the thoracic aorta, and the cardiac valves.

predicting severe cardiovascular events (myocardial infarction and cardiac death) is conflicting [63–65]. Although a number of methodologic limitations (ie, large loss of patients to follow-up and lack of a standardized method for calcium scoring) may account for some of this discrepancy, part of the explanation may relate to coronary VC's representing an "innocent bystander," at least in advanced lesions, rather than a direct determinant of cardiovascular risk [66,67].

Vascular calcification in patients who have end-stage renal disease

For many years, VC has been recognized as a common complication in patients who have ESRD [68,69]. Table 3 lists the available studies evaluating the presence of coronary VC in patients who have renal failure.

Braun and colleagues [70] first reported the use of EBCT in 49 hemodialysis patients, showing coronary calcium scores 2.5 to fivefold higher than in nonhemodialysis patients. Subsequent studies have revealed pronounced VC even in young adults with ESRD, who are otherwise not at risk for VC

[44,45]. In another report, Raggi and colleagues [71] studied a population of 205 patients receiving maintenance hemodialysis therapy; they observed high calcium scores at level of the coronary arteries, thoracic aorta, and cardiac valves. Furthermore, the coronary calcium score was significantly related to a previous history of myocardial infarction ($P < .0001$) and angina ($P < .0001$).

Vascular calcification in predialysis patients who have chronic kidney disease

Patients with predialysis CKD constitute a large population with a documented high risk for cardiovascular events [7]. Recent data reveal that advanced atherosclerosis (as demonstrated by the thickening of arterial wall) is already present in patients who have CKD before they require hemodialysis [72].

VC has been studied much less intensively in patients who have predialysis CKD than in patients receiving hemodialysis. Mehrotra and colleagues [73] recently used EBCT to study a group of 60 patients who had diabetic nephropathy. They found a higher prevalence and severity

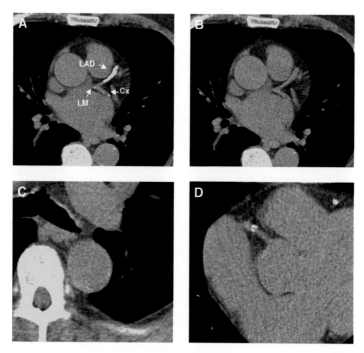

Fig. 4. Postprocessing analysis of MDCT images for quantification of calcium score at level of (*A*, *B*) coronary arteries, (*C*) thoracic aorta, and (*D*) aortic valve. Coronary calcifications are automatically detected by the software (*yellow areas in A*) and then are confirmed by the operator with the attribution to specific territories (*B*). Cx, left circumflex coronary artery; LAD, left anterior descending coronary artery; LM, left main coronary artery.

of coronary VC in these patients than in diabetic controls who had normal renal function. In the patients who had diabetic neuropathy, the high degree of VC was not related to measures of disordered mineral metabolism (see Table 3) [74].

No studies are available that used modern, fully quantifiable, CT-based technology to assess VC in unselected populations of patients who have CKD. As part of the Renal Research Institute (RRI)-CKD Study, the authors are evaluating the severity of VC at level of the coronary artery, thoracic aorta, and cardiac valves in a subgroup of approximately 100 patients studied by 16-slice MDCT [75]. This study is the first specifically designed to assess the prevalence and correlates of VC in an unselected population of patients who have CKD but do not require dialysis. The preliminary results seem to show a high prevalence of VC in this population, but no clear correlation with an index of abnormal mineral metabolism has been noted.

Progression in vascular calcification

VC progresses more rapidly in patients treated with dialysis than in the general population (Table 4) [44,76]. In asymptomatic persons who have normal renal function, the Agatston score progresses at an average rate of 33% per year [77]. Bursztyn and colleagues [78] reported a twofold greater progression in coronary calcium score (measured by MDCT) in hypertensive patients who have CKD than in hypertensive patients with normal renal function. It is possible (although still a hypothesis) that medial wall calcification plays a dominant role in the progression of VC in patients who have ESRD, whereas VC progression in patients who have normal renal function mainly reflects the evolution of atherosclerotic calcification [79].

Do alterations in calcium and phosphate metabolism affect progression in dialysis patients? In a group of patients receiving peritoneal dialysis studied by MDCT at baseline and after 1 year of follow-up, Stompor and colleagues [80] reported a significant correlation between the change in coronary calcium score and mean values of phosphate and calcium–phosphate product. Corroborating the association of VC progression with abnormal mineral metabolism, greater rates of VC progression have been demonstrated in patients who have ESRD treated with large oral

Table 3
Studies using electron-beam computed tomography or multi-detector computed tomography to assess coronary calcium score in patients who have renal failure

Study	Study population	Imaging modality	Correlates for coronary calcium score				
			Mineral metabolism				
			Ca	P	Ca–P product	PTH	Others
Braun et al, 1996 [70]	49 HD	EBCT	−	−	NA	−	Age, hypertension
Goodmann et al, 2000 [44]	39 HD	EBCT	−	−	+	−	Age, body mass index, cholesterolemia, dialysis vintage
Oh et al, 2002 [45]	39 ESRD (13 HD + 26 RT)	EBCT	−	−	+	+	C-reactive protein, homocysteine
Raggi et al, 2002 [71]	205 HD	EBCT	+	+	−	−	Age, diabetes mellitus
Moe et al, 2003 [46]	55 ESRD (33 HD + 38 RT)	MDCT	−	−	−	−	Age, longer dialysis
Haydar et al, 2004 [74]	46 HD	EBCT	NA	NA	NA	NA	Angiographic coronary artery disease
Mehrotra et al, 2004 [73]	60 CKD + DM	EBCT	−	−	−	−	Age, creatinine, GFR
Nitta et al, 2004 [13]	53 HD	MDCT	−	−	−	−	Age, C-reactive protein

Abbreviations: CKD, chronic renal disease; EBCT, electron-beam computed tomography; ESRD, end-stage renal disease; GFR, glomerular filtration rate; HD, hemodialysis; MDCT, multidetector computed tomography; NA, not applicable; PTH, parathyroid hormone; RT, renal transplantation.

doses of calcium-containing compounds, in comparison with patients treated with the calcium-free, phosphate-binding agent sevelamer [81].

There are limited data regarding the progression of VC in patients who have predialysis CKD [78]. A subgroup of approximately 50 patients enrolled in the RRI-CKD Study has been studied with 16-slice MDCT at baseline and after about 1 year of follow-up. Preliminary data reveal a high rate of VC progression in this unselected population (authors' unpublished observations).

Prognostic value of vascular calcification in patients who have renal failure

The usefulness of VC measurements by EBCT or MDCT as a predictor of adverse cardiovascular outcomes is yet to be demonstrated in patients who have renal failure. A number of issues relevant to the renal patients need to be studied carefully. These issues include the evolution of VC and its relationship to decline in renal function.

Although it is likely that medial and intimal VC may have different impacts on prognosis in CKD and for dialysis patients, the image resolution of EBCT and MDCT is currently insufficient to distinguish between these two processes [82].

Summary

The mortality from cardiovascular events in CKD and dialysis patients is substantially higher than in the general population. VC is ubiquitous and progresses rapidly in this patient population.

Although there has been progress in the understanding of the pathogenesis and correlates of VC, much work needs to be done in this area. The role of calcium and, probably, phosphate (obligatory participants) is unquestionable, but the understanding of the paracrine and molecular determinants of VC in renal failure is continuously evolving. VC is probably a dynamic process resulting from the imbalance between molecules that promote and those that inhibit VC. The understanding of latter area has recently evolved with identification of new signaling pathways with molecules such as osteoprotegerin, fetuin-A, and MPG.

From a clinical perspective, new modalities such as EBCT and MDCT allow noninvasive detection and quantification of VC. VC may represent a potential useful index for prognostic stratification and treatment planning in patients who have renal failure. At present, however, the data on the prognostic value of VC are available only in populations of patients who have normal renal function.

Table 4
Studies using electron-beam computed tomography or multidetector computed tomography to assess the progression in coronary calcium score in patients who have renal failure

Study	Study population	Duration of follow-up	Imaging modality	Findings
Tamashiro et al, 2001 [76]	24 HD	17 months	EBCT	Progression correlates with higher triglycerides and lower HDL cholesterol
Chertow et al, 2002 [81]	132 HD	11 months	EBCT	Progression reduced by sevelamer
Bursztyn et al, 2003 [78]	53 CKD + HTN	3 years	MDCT	Progression faster in CKD compared with non-CKD
Stompór et al, 2004 [80]	47 PD	1 year	MDCT	Progression correlates with higher C-reactive protein, serum phosphate, and calcium–phosphate product

Abbreviations: CKD, chronic renal disease; EBCT, electron-beam computed tomography; MDCT, multidetector computed tomography; HD, hemodialysis; HDL, high-density lipoprotein; HTN, hypertension; PD, peritoneal dialysis.

Large-scale, prospective, observational studies should be designed to identify the determinants of VC and to define the prognostic role of calcium scoring in cohorts of patients who have predialysis CKD and with ESRD.

References

[1] Meguid El, Nahas A, Bello AK. Chronic kidney disease: the global challenge. Lancet 2005;365(9456):331–40.

[2] Coresh J, Astor BC, Greene T, et al. Prevalence of chronic kidney disease and decreased kidney function in the adult US population: Third National Health and Nutrition Examination Survey. Am J Kidney Dis 2003;41(1):1–12.

[3] Shulman NB, Ford CE, Hall WD, et al. Prognostic value of serum creatinine and effect of treatment of hypertension on renal function. Results from the hypertension detection and follow-up program. The Hypertension Detection and Follow-up Program Cooperative Group. Hypertension 1989;13(5 Suppl):I80–93.

[4] Manjunath G, Tighiouart H, Ibrahim H, et al. Level of kidney function as a risk factor for atherosclerotic cardiovascular outcomes in the community. J Am Coll Cardiol 2003;41(1):47–55.

[5] Fried LF, Shlipak MG, Crump C, et al. Renal insufficiency as a predictor of cardiovascular outcomes and mortality in elderly individuals. J Am Coll Cardiol 2003;41(8):1364–72.

[6] Shlipak MG, Heidenreich PA, Noguchi H, et al. Association of renal insufficiency with treatment and outcomes after myocardial infarction in elderly patients. Ann Intern Med 2002;137(7):555–62.

[7] Go AS, Chertow GM, Fan D, et al. Chronic kidney disease and the risks of death, cardiovascular events, and hospitalization. N Engl J Med 2004;351(13):1296–305.

[8] Sarnak MJ, Levey AS, Schoolwerth AC, et al. Kidney disease as a risk factor for development of cardiovascular disease: a statement from the American Heart Association Councils on Kidney in Cardiovascular Disease, High Blood Pressure Research, Clinical Cardiology, and Epidemiology and Prevention. Circulation 2003;108(17):2154–69.

[9] Schwarz U, Buzello M, Ritz E, et al. Morphology of coronary atherosclerotic lesions in patients with end-stage renal failure. Nephrol Dial Transplant 2000;15(2):218–23.

[10] Jungers P, Massy ZA, Khoa TN, et al. Incidence and risk factors of atherosclerotic cardiovascular accidents in predialysis chronic renal failure patients: a prospective study. Nephrol Dial Transplant 1997;12(12):2597–602.

[11] Moe SM, Chen NX. Calciphylaxis and vascular calcification: a continuum of extra-skeletal osteogenesis. Pediatr Nephrol 2003;18(10):969–75.

[12] London GM, Marchais SJ, Guerin AP, et al. Arterial structure and function in end-stage renal disease. Nephrol Dial Transplant 2002;17(10):1713–24.

[13] Nitta K, Akiba T, Suzuki K, et al. Assessment of coronary artery calcification in hemodialysis patients using multi-detector spiral CT scan. Hypertens Res 2004;27(8):527–33.

[14] Stary HC, Chandler AB, Dinsmore RE, et al. A definition of advanced types of atherosclerotic lesions and a histological classification of atherosclerosis. A report from the Committee on Vascular Lesions of the Council on Arteriosclerosis, American Heart Association. Circulation 1995;92(5):1355–74.

[15] Beckman JA, Ganz J, Creager MA, et al. Relationship of clinical presentation and calcification of culprit coronary artery stenoses. Arterioscler Thromb Vasc Biol 2001;21(10):1618–22.

[16] Huang H, Virmani R, Younis H, et al. The impact of calcification on the biomechanical stability of atherosclerotic plaques. Circulation 2001;103(8):1051–6.

[17] Loree HM, Kamm RD, Stringfellow RG, et al. Effects of fibrous cap thickness on peak circumferential stress in model atherosclerotic vessels. Circ Res 1992;71(4):850–8.

[18] Abedin M, Tintut Y, Demer LL. Vascular calcification: mechanisms and clinical ramifications. Arterioscler Thromb Vasc Biol 2004;24(7):1161–70.

[19] Bostrom K, Watson KE, Horn S, et al. Bone morphogenetic protein expression in human atherosclerotic lesions. J Clin Invest 1993;91(4):1800–9.

[20] Fitzpatrick LA, Severson A, Edwards WD, et al. Diffuse calcification in human coronary arteries. Association of osteopontin with atherosclerosis. J Clin Invest 1994;94(4):1597–604.

[21] Moe SM, O'Neill KD, Duan D, et al. Medial artery calcification in ESRD patients is associated with deposition of bone matrix proteins. Kidney Int 2002;61(2):638–47.

[22] Shanahan CM, Cary NR, Metcalfe JC, et al. High expression of genes for calcification-regulating proteins in human atherosclerotic plaques. J Clin Invest 1994;93(6):2393–402.

[23] Hujairi NM, Afzali B, Goldsmith DJ. Cardiac calcification in renal patients: what we do and don't know. Am J Kidney Dis 2004;43(2):234–43.

[24] Shanahan CM, Cary NR, Salisbury JR, et al. Medial localization of mineralization-regulating proteins in association with Monckeberg's sclerosis: evidence for smooth muscle cell-mediated vascular calcification. Circulation 1999;100(21):2168–76.

[25] Jono S, Nishizawa Y, Shioi A, et al. Parathyroid hormone-related peptide as a local regulator of vascular calcification. Its inhibitory action on in vitro calcification by bovine vascular smooth muscle cells. Arterioscler Thromb Vasc Biol 1997;17(6):1135–42.

[26] Simonet WS, Lacey DL, Dunstan CR, et al. Osteoprotegerin: a novel secreted protein involved in the regulation of bone density. Cell 1997;89(2):309–19.

[27] Kaden JJ, Bickelhaupt S, Grobholz R, et al. Receptor activator of nuclear factor kappaB ligand and osteoprotegerin regulate aortic valve calcification. J Mol Cell Cardiol 2004;36(1):57–66.

[28] Avbersek-Luznik I, Malesic I, Rus I, et al. Increased levels of osteoprotegerin in hemodialysis patients. Clin Chem Lab Med 2002;40(10):1019–23.

[29] Jono S, McKee MD, Murry CE, et al. Phosphate regulation of vascular smooth muscle cell calcification. Circ Res 2000;87(7):E10–7.

[30] Ducy P, Zhang R, Geoffroy V, et al. Osf2/Cbfa1: a transcriptional activator of osteoblast differentiation. Cell 1997;89(5):747–54.

[31] Chen NX, O'Neill KD, Duan D, et al. Phosphorus and uremic serum up-regulate osteopontin expression in vascular smooth muscle cells. Kidney Int 2002;62(5):1724–31.

[32] Giachelli CM. Vascular calcification mechanisms. J Am Soc Nephrol 2004;15(12):2959–64.

[33] Ketteler M, Bongartz P, Westenfeld R, et al. Association of low fetuin-A (AHSG) concentrations in serum with cardiovascular mortality in patients on dialysis: a cross-sectional study. Lancet 2003;361(9360):827–33.

[34] Mehrotra R, Westenfeld R, Christenson P, et al. Serum fetuin-A in nondialyzed patients with diabetic nephropathy: relationship with coronary artery calcification. Kidney Int 2005;67(3):1070–7.

[35] Farzaneh-Far A, Proudfoot D, Weissberg PL, et al. Matrix Gla protein is regulated by a mechanism functionally related to the calcium-sensing receptor. Biochem Biophys Res Commun 2000;277(3):736–40.

[36] Luo G, Ducy P, McKee MD, et al. Spontaneous calcification of arteries and cartilage in mice lacking matrix GLA protein. Nature 1997;386(6620):78–81.

[37] Wada T, McKee MD, Steitz S, et al. Calcification of vascular smooth muscle cell cultures: inhibition by osteopontin. Circ Res 1999;84(2):166–78.

[38] Steitz SA, Speer MY, McKee MD, et al. Osteopontin inhibits mineral deposition and promotes regression of ectopic calcification. Am J Pathol 2002;161(6):2035–46.

[39] Giachelli CM, Bae N, Almeida M, et al. Osteopontin is elevated during neointima formation in rat arteries and is a novel component of human atherosclerotic plaques. J Clin Invest 1993;92(4):1686–96.

[40] Speer MY, McKee MD, Guldberg RE, et al. Inactivation of the osteopontin gene enhances vascular calcification of matrix Gla protein-deficient mice: evidence for osteopontin as an inducible inhibitor of vascular calcification in vivo. J Exp Med 2002;196(8):1047–55.

[41] Goodman WG, London G, Amann K, et al. Vascular calcification in chronic kidney disease. Am J Kidney Dis 2004;43(3):572–9.

[42] Zimmermann J, Herrlinger S, Pruy A, et al. Inflammation enhances cardiovascular risk and mortality in hemodialysis patients. Kidney Int 1999;55(2):648–58.

[43] Raggi P. Effects of excess calcium load on the cardiovascular system measured with electron beam tomography in end-stage renal disease. Nephrol Dial Transplant 2002;17(2):332–5.

[44] Goodman WG, Goldin J, Kuizon BD, et al. Coronary-artery calcification in young adults with end-stage renal disease who are undergoing dialysis. N Engl J Med 2000;342(20):1478–83.

[45] Oh J, Wunsch R, Turzer M, et al. Advanced coronary and carotid arteriopathy in young adults with childhood-onset chronic renal failure. Circulation 2002;106(1):100–5.

[46] Moe SM, O'Neill KD, Fineberg N, et al. Assessment of vascular calcification in ESRD patients using spiral CT. Nephrol Dial Transplant 2003;18(6):1152–8.

[47] O'Rourke RA, Brundage BH, Froelicher VF, et al. American College of Cardiology/American Heart Association Expert Consensus document on electron-beam computed tomography for the diagnosis and prognosis of coronary artery disease. Circulation 2000;102(1):126–40.

[48] Cury RC, Ferencik M, Hoffmann U, et al. Epidemiology and association of vascular and valvular calcium quantified by multidetector computed tomography in elderly asymptomatic subjects. Am J Cardiol 2004;94(3):348–51.

[49] Becker CR, Kleffel T, Crispin A, Knez A, et al. Coronary artery calcium measurement: agreement of multirow detector and electron beam CT. AJR Am J Roentgenol 2001;176(5):1295–8.

[50] Stanford W, Thompson BH, Burns TL, et al. Coronary artery calcium quantification at multi-detector row helical CT versus electron-beam CT. Radiology 2004;230(2):397–402.

[51] Horiguchi J, Yamamoto H, Akiyama Y, et al. Coronary artery calcium scoring using 16-MDCT and a retrospective ECG-gating reconstruction algorithm. AJR Am J Roentgenol 2004;183(1):103–8.

[52] Agatston AS, Janowitz WR, Hildner FJ, et al. Quantification of coronary artery calcium using ultrafast computed tomography. J Am Coll Cardiol 1990; 15(4):827–32.

[53] Callister TQ, Cooil B, Raya SP, et al. Coronary artery disease: improved reproducibility of calcium scoring with an electron-beam CT volumetric method. Radiology 1998;208(3):807–14.

[54] Ohnesorge B, Flohr T, Fischbach R, et al. Reproducibility of coronary calcium quantification in repeat examinations with retrospectively ECG-gated multisection spiral CT. Eur Radiol 2002;12(6): 1532–40.

[55] Rumberger JA, Kaufman L. A Rosetta stone for coronary calcium risk stratification: Agatston, volume, and mass scores in 11,490 individuals. AJR Am J Roentgenol 2003;181(3):743–8.

[56] Sangiorgi G, Rumberger JA, Severson A, et al. Arterial calcification and not lumen stenosis is highly correlated with atherosclerotic plaque burden in humans: a histologic study of 723 coronary artery segments using nondecalcifying methodology. J Am Coll Cardiol 1998;31(1):126–33.

[57] Nallamothu BK, Saint S, Bielak LF, et al. Electron-beam computed tomography in the diagnosis of coronary artery disease: a meta-analysis. Arch Intern Med 2001;161(6):833–8.

[58] Yamamoto H, Shavelle D, Takasu J, et al. Valvular and thoracic aortic calcium as a marker of the extent and severity of angiographic coronary artery disease. Am Heart J 2003;146(1):153–9.

[59] Cury RC, Ferencik M, Hoffmann U, et al. Epidemiology and association of vascular and valvular calcium quantified by multidetector computed tomography in elderly asymptomatic subjects. Am J Cardiol 2004;94(3):348–51.

[60] Raggi P, Callister TQ, Cooil B, et al. Identification of patients at increased risk of first unheralded acute myocardial infarction by electron-beam computed tomography. Circulation 2000;101(8):850–5.

[61] Shaw LJ, Raggi P, Schisterman E, et al. Prognostic value of cardiac risk factors and coronary artery calcium screening for all-cause mortality. Radiology 2003;228(3):826–33.

[62] Raggi P, Shaw LJ, Berman DS, et al. Prognostic value of coronary artery calcium screening in subjects with and without diabetes. J Am Coll Cardiol 2004;43(9):1663–9.

[63] Detrano RC, Wong ND, Doherty TM, et al. Coronary calcium does not accurately predict near-term future coronary events in high-risk adults. Circulation 1999;99(20):2633–8.

[64] Arad Y, Spadaro LA, Goodman K, et al. Prediction of coronary events with electron beam computed tomography. J Am Coll Cardiol 2000;36(4):1253–60.

[65] Greenland P, LaBree L, Azen SP, et al. Coronary artery calcium score combined with Framingham score for risk prediction in asymptomatic individuals. JAMA 2004;291(2):210–5.

[66] Pletcher MJ, Tice JA, Pignone M, et al. What does my patient's coronary artery calcium score mean? Combining information from the coronary artery calcium score with information from conventional risk factors to estimate coronary heart disease risk. BMC Med 2004;2(1):31.

[67] O'Malley PG, Taylor AJ, Jackson JL, et al. Prognostic value of coronary electron-beam computed tomography for coronary heart disease events in asymptomatic populations. Am J Cardiol 2000; 85(8):945–8.

[68] Salusky IB, Goodman WG. Cardiovascular calcification in end-stage renal disease. Nephrol Dial Transplant 2002;17(2):336–9.

[69] Davies MR, Hruska KA. Pathophysiological mechanisms of vascular calcification in end-stage renal disease. Kidney Int 2001;60(2):472–9.

[70] Braun J, Oldendorf M, Moshage W, et al. Electron beam computed tomography in the evaluation of cardiac calcification in chronic dialysis patients. Am J Kidney Dis 1996;27(3):394–401.

[71] Raggi P, Boulay A, Chasan-Taber S, et al. Cardiac calcification in adult hemodialysis patients. A link between end-stage renal disease and cardiovascular disease? J Am Coll Cardiol 2002;39(4):695–701.

[72] Shoji T, Emoto M, Tabata T, et al. Advanced atherosclerosis in predialysis patients with chronic renal failure. Kidney Int 2002;61(6):2187–92.

[73] Mehrotra R, Budoff M, Christenson P, et al. Determinants of coronary artery calcification in diabetics with and without nephropathy. Kidney Int 2004; 66(5):2022–31.

[74] Haydar AA, Hujairi NM, Covic AA, et al. Coronary artery calcification is related to coronary atherosclerosis in chronic renal disease patients: a study comparing EBCT-generated coronary artery calcium

scores and coronary angiography. Nephrol Dial Transplant 2004;19(9):2307–12.

[75] Perlman RL, Kiser M, Finkelstein F, et al. The longitudinal chronic kidney disease study: a prospective cohort study of predialysis renal failure. Semin Dial 2003;16(6):418–23.

[76] Tamashiro M, Iseki K, Sunagawa OT, et al. Significant association between the progression of coronary artery calcification and dyslipidemia in patients on chronic hemodialysis. Am J Kidney Dis 2001;38(1): 64–9.

[77] Budoff MJ, Lane KL, Bakhsheshi H, et al. Rates of progression of coronary calcium by electron beam tomography. Am J Cardiol 2000; 86(1):8–11.

[78] Bursztyn M, Motro M, Grossman E, et al. Accelerated coronary artery calcification in mildly reduced renal function of high-risk hypertensives: a 3-year

prospective observation. J Hypertens 2003;21(10): 1953–9.

[79] Callister TQ, Raggi P, Cooil B, et al. Effect of HMG-CoA reductase inhibitors on coronary artery disease as assessed by electron-beam computed tomography. N Engl J Med 1998;339(27):1972–8.

[80] Stompor TP, Pasowicz M, Sulowicz W, et al. Trends and dynamics of changes in calcification score over the 1-year observation period in patients on peritoneal dialysis. Am J Kidney Dis 2004;44(3):517–28.

[81] Chertow GM, Burke SK, Raggi P. Sevelamer attenuates the progression of coronary and aortic calcification in hemodialysis patients. Kidney Int 2002;62(1):245–52.

[82] London GM, Guerin AP, Marchais SJ, et al. Arterial media calcification in end-stage renal disease: impact on all-cause and cardiovascular mortality. Nephrol Dial Transplant 2003;18(9):1731–40.

ELSEVIER
SAUNDERS

Cardiol Clin 23 (2005) 385–391

CARDIOLOGY
CLINICS

Newer Paradigms in Renal Replacement Therapy: Will They Alter Cardiovascular Outcomes?

Kiran Kundhal, MD[a], Andreas Pierratos, MD, FRCPC[b], Christopher T. Chan, MD, FRCPC[a],*

[a]Division of Nephrology, Department of Medicine, Toronto General Hospital–University Health Network,
12 Eaton North, 200 Elizabeth Street, Toronto, Ontario M5G 2C4, Canada
[b]Division of Nephrology, Department of Medicine, Humber River Regional Hospital, 200 Church Street,
Weston, Ontario M9N 1N8, Canada

Cardiovascular disease remains the leading cause of death in patients with end-stage renal disease (ESRD) [1]. Etiologic factors include persistent myocardial injury exacerbated by volume and pressure overload as well as endothelial dysfunction [2,3]. Impaired endothelial-dependent dilation is becoming recognized as an early dysfunction in both non-ESRD and uremic populations [4,5] and has been associated with traditional cardiovascular risk factors such as insulin resistance [6], hypertension [7], and hyperlipidemia [8]. Patients receiving conventional hemodialysis (4 hours/session, three treatments/week) have impaired endothelial responsiveness, decreased vascular compliance, and activated vasoconstrictor systems [5,9]. Patients with severe endothelial dysfunction and vascular stiffness tend to also have left ventricular hypertrophy (LVH), impaired left ventricular systolic function, and accelerated atherosclerosis. These conditions are known to be independent risk factors for cardiac death in ESRD [10]. Indeed, in patients undergoing conventional hemodialysis, poor uremic control, hypertension, LVH, and impaired systolic function are markers for adverse cardiovascular events [3,11–13].

In addition, hyperphosphatemia and hyperparathyroidism have been shown to be independent cardiovascular risk factors in ESRD [14].

Elevated phosphate levels may contribute to the development of uremic calcific vasculopathy [15,16]. Furthermore, recent evidence suggests that hyperparathyroidism may cause interstitial cell activation, thereby leading to cardiac fibrosis [17]. It can be postulated that myocardial fibrosis reduces cardiac compliance, resulting in an increased tendency for arrhythmias.

To date, conventional hemodialysis has not significantly altered the aforementioned markers for adverse cardiovascular events. Patients with ESRD continue to suffer an astonishingly high annual mortality rate, approximately 20% [1].

Other alternatives to conventional hemodialysis include short daily hemodialysis (2 hours/session, six sessions/week) and nocturnal home hemodialysis (6 hours/session, five to six sessions/week). Short daily hemodialysis was first described in 1968 by DePalma et al [18]. The rationale for short daily hemodialysis is that it provides enhanced hemodynamic stability and increases solute removal by delivering dialysis when the plasma–dialysate gradient is highest. Nocturnal home hemodialysis was described in 1996 by Uldall et al [19]. It is delivered at home, 5 to 6 nights/week, at variable blood and dialysate flow rates. One of the rationales for the preference of nocturnal home hemodialysis is that it increases middle molecule clearance because of the increased frequency and length of dialysis treatments [20–22]. Increased middle molecule clearance has been associated with higher patient survival [23,24].

Both short daily hemodialysis and nocturnal home hemodialysis have been associated with significant clinical benefits. Specifically, nocturnal

---

* Corresponding author.

E-mail address: christopher.chan@uhn.on.ca (C.T. Chan).

0733-8651/05/$ - see front matter © 2005 Elsevier Inc. All rights reserved.
doi:10.1016/j.ccl.2005.03.001

home hemodialysis has been associated with improved solute removal [20–22], increased quality of life [23–26], and improved anemia control with decreasing erythropoietin requirements [27–29]. In addition, recent studies have demonstrated improvement in sleep disorders, as evidenced by an improvement in the number of apnea-hypopnea episodes [30], as well as reduced overall costs because of lowered fixed modality expenditures [31,32].

Furthermore, nocturnal hemodialysis has been associated with significant benefits in cardiovascular parameters. This article (1) reviews the documented effects of intensive hemodialysis on blood pressure control, cardiac geometry and left ventricular systolic function, lipid profiles, calcium–phosphate metabolism and parathyroid hormone (PTH) levels, homocysteine levels, and sleep apnea and autonomic modulation of heart rate, and (2) provides possible mechanistic explanations to account for these observed changes.

Blood pressure

Hypertension related to ESRD has been recently reviewed [33]. From a simplified hemodynamic standpoint, elevated arterial pressure may be caused by either extracellular volume expansion or increased total peripheral resistance. Volume and pressure overload have been classically associated with the development of hypertension [34]. Volume overload in usually attributed to sodium and water retention [35], whereas pressure overload is attributed to increased peripheral resistance and increased arterial stiffness [36]. Renal replacement therapy improves volume overload by removing excess extracellular fluid and thus lowering blood pressure.

Both short daily hemodialysis and nocturnal hemodialysis have been shown to result in improved blood pressure control in ESRD. In 1999, Woods et al [37] reported in a retrospective review that 75% of patients receiving short daily hemodialysis had normal blood pressure values without the concomitant use of antihypertensive agents [37]. Likewise, Fagugli et al [38] reported in their cross-over prospective design that short daily hemodialysis resulted in improvements in blood pressure control and decreased antihypertensive requirements. Systolic blood pressures fell from 148 ± 19 mm Hg to 128 ± 12 mm Hg ($P < 0.01$). Similarly, diastolic blood pressures fell from 73 ± 5 mm Hg to 67 ± 8 mm Hg ($P = 0.01$). Both investigators measured the change in extracellular fluid content and attributed the reductions in blood pressure to a decrease in extracellular fluid volume.

In a similar fashion, nocturnal home hemodialysis has been consistently associated with improved blood pressure control along with decreased antihypertensive requirements. Raj et al [39] described superior blood pressure control coincident with a decrease in the number of antihypertensive agents in patients switching from conventional hemodialysis to nocturnal home hemodialysis. In a controlled cohort design, investigators at the University of Toronto studied 28 patients undergoing nocturnal home hemodialysis for a minimum of 2 years and compared these patients with 13 self-care conventional hemodialysis patients [40]. Systolic blood pressures fell from 145 ± 20 mm Hg to 122 ± 13 mm Hg ($P < 0.001$), and diastolic pressures fell from 84 ± 15 mm Hg to 74 ± 12 mm Hg ($P = 0.02$). These decreases occurred even though the use of antihypertensive medications was reduced (from 1.8 per patient to 0.3 per patient; $P < 0.05$). Unlike the studies of short daily hemodialysis, the Toronto experience did not find significant changes in extracellular volume. Similar results were reported by Nesrallah et al [41] at the University of Western Ontario. They found that both short daily hemodialysis and nocturnal hemodialysis resulted in blood pressure normalization, but extracellular fluid control was significant only in short daily hemodialysis. This finding suggests that short daily hemodialysis improves blood pressure through improved control of extracellular volume, whereas other mechanisms, such as enhanced solute removal or decreased neurohormonal factors, may be involved in the nocturnal home hemodialysis cohort. Chan and colleagues [42] tested this hypothesis by studying 18 consecutive patients who switched from conventional to nocturnal home hemodialysis. They found that as the dialysis dose per session (Kt/V) increased after 2 months, mean arterial pressure decreased from 102 ± 3 to 90 ± 2 mm Hg. There was an associated decrease in total peripheral resistance (from 1967 ± 235 to 1499 ± 191 dyne.s.cm^{-5}; $P < 0.01$) and in plasma norepinephrine levels (from 2.66 ± 0.4 to 1.96 ± 0.2 nmol; $P = 0.04$). Although endothelium-dependent vasodilation could not be elicited during conventional hemodialysis, it was restored after a 2-month period of nocturnal hemodialysis. In addition, brachial artery responsiveness to nitroglycerin improved from $6.9 \pm 2.8\%$ to $15.7 \pm 1.6\%$ ($P < 0.05$). No significant change in weight and extracellular volume was demonstrated.

Cardiac geometry and systolic function

As with hypertension, volume and pressure overload has been associated with the development of LVH [34,43–45] and with increased cardiovascular mortality in patients with ESRD [46]. Volume and pressure overload is characterized by a generalized increase in left ventricular mass, enlargement in left ventricular end-diastolic diameters, or an increase in left ventricular wall thickness [43,44]. These factors culminate in a combination of eccentric and concentric LVH. Although ventricular hypertrophy is an initial beneficial adaptive response, continuous hemodynamic overload leads to a maladaptive hypertrophic phenotype that results in congestive heart failure [13,47,48]. At the cellular level, there is a demonstrable increase in myocardial size, mass, and interstitial collagen content. At the molecular level, fetal gene expression occurs along with abnormal protein production. Hence, congestive heart failure is the end result of LVH progression, as systolic and diastolic dysfunction develops. Patients with congestive heart failure benefit from volume removal through renal replacement therapy. Their ventricular preload is decreased, resulting in improved left ventricle filling, and stroke volume is decrease because of diastolic ventricular interaction [49].

Similar to the beneficial antihypertensive outcomes, the Toronto experience demonstrated a significant regression in left ventricular mass index (LVMI) from 147 g/m^2 to 122 g/m^2 when patients switched from conventional hemodialysis to nocturnal home hemodialysis [40]. A consistent finding was the positive correlative between systolic blood pressure and LVMI.

In addition to the beneficial changes in blood pressure control and LVMI regression, the Toronto experience has also demonstrated the positive impact of nocturnal home hemodialysis on impaired left ventricular ejection fraction [50]. In a cohort study, six ESRD patients with coexistent congestive heart failure switched from conventional hemodialysis to nocturnal home hemodialysis. Along with a significant decrease in systolic blood pressure (from 138 $\pm$ 10 mm Hg to 120 $\pm$ 9 mm Hg; P = 0.04), these patients had a significant increase in their left ventricular ejection fraction (from 28 $\pm$ 12% to 41 $\pm$ 18%; P = 0.01). These changes occurred even though the number of

vasoactive medications was decreased (from 2.2 to 0.7/patient; P = 0.02) and without a change in extracellular fluid volume. These findings show that, for improved cardiovascular indices, enhanced uremic clearance and hemodynamic effects are more important than decreased extracellular volume content.

Lipid profile

In the general population, a low high-density lipoprotein (HDL) level and a high triglyceride level are independent risk factors for the development of atherosclerosis and coronary artery disease [51–54]. More than 90% of hemodialysis patients have a characteristic dyslipidemia that includes increased concentrations of triglyceride-rich apolipoprotein B–containing lipoproteins, very-low-density lipoproteins, and intermediate-low-density lipoproteins and decreased HDL [55]. These changes promote atherosclerosis [56,57]. Bugeja and Chan [58] conducted a prospective study in a cohort of 11 patients with ESRD, studying their lipid profiles before and after conversion from conventional hemodialysis to nocturnal home hemodialysis [58]. They found a significant decrease in triglyceride concentrations (from 2.05 $\pm$ 0.30 to 1.01 $\pm$ 0.14 mmol/L; P < 0.001), a significant increase in HDL concentrations (from 1.17 $\pm$ 0.13 to 1.65 $\pm$ 0.14 mmol/L; P < 0.001), and a significant increase in the HDL/trigliceride ratio (from 0.26 $\pm$ 0.03 to 0.35 $\pm$ 0.02; P < 0.001). Although the exact mechanisms for these changes are unknown, the authors postulated that superior uremic clearance allowed the restoration of lipase function and modification of lipoprotein composition by removing uremic inhibitors such as pre-B-HDL.

Calcium–phosphate metabolism and hyperparathyroidism

An elevated calcium–phosphate product and hyperphosphatemia can contribute to cardiovascular disease in ESRD patients through vascular calcifications and hardening. Increasing evidence suggests that improving phosphate control reduces the incidence in vascular calcifications [59]. Conventional hemodialysis results in suboptimal removal of phosphate because phosphate is mobilized slowly from the deep tissues during dialysis. This slow mobilization results in an early decline in the serum phosphate levels during dialysis and subsequent loss of the serum–dialysate concentration gradient. During the last hour of dialysis and after its termination, serum phosphate levels rebound [60]. Although high-flux dialyzers and the convective process can increase phosphate removal, the main determinant of phosphate removal is the duration of dialysis. High-frequency dialysis likewise increases phosphate removal because it allows daily equilibration of serum phosphate levels, thereby restoring the blood–dialysate gradient [22]. Nocturnal home hemodialysis has been shown to double the weekly phosphate removal as compared with conventional hemodialysis. In fact, many patients are able to discontinue phosphate binders within 1 week after initiating nocturnal home hemodialysis and can take an unrestricted-phosphate diet [61]. Dissolution of tumoral extra-osseous calcifications has been reported in one patient receiving nocturnal hemodialysis every 24 hours [62].

Because patients receiving nocturnal home dialysis no longer require calcium-containing phosphate binders, they are typically in a negative calcium balance and often require a higher dialysate calcium level than patients receiving conventional hemodialysis [63,64]. Dialysate calcium levels can be adjusted by adding powdered calcium chloride into the acid concentrate to achieve the desired pre- and postdialysis calcium and PTH levels. The average dialysate calcium level was 1.6 ± 0.1 mmol/L at one center [63]. This relatively increased calcium bath led to a significantly lower PTH level after 6 months (from 580 ± 590 ng/mL to 228 ± 295 ng/mL).

Homocysteine levels

Hyperhomocysteinemia is a documented risk factor for atherosclerotic outcomes, and homocysteine level have been shown to be elevated in more than 85% of hemodialysis patients. High-flux or super-flux hemodialysis has consistently failed to normalize total homocysteine (tHcy) levels. There are limited data examining the effects of nocturnal home hemodialysis on tHcy levels. Friedman et al [65] compared predialysis plasma tHcy levels in 23 patients undergoing nocturnal home hemodialysis with those of 31 patients undergoing conventional hemodialysis [65]. The tHcy levels for the nocturnal home hemodialysis patients were significantly lower (12.7 versus 20.0 μM, $P < 0.0001$), as was the prevalence of mild-to-moderate hyperhomocysteinemia (>12 μM; nocturnal home hemodialysis, 57%; conventional hemodialysis, 94%; $P = 0.002$). The authors concluded that tHcy levels are significantly lower

among nocturnal home hemodialysis patients than in patients receiving conventional dialysis. Similarly, a study conducted by Nesrallah and colleagues [66] found that patients who underwent either short daily hemodialysis or nocturnal home hemodialysis had significantly lower homocysteine levels than patients receiving conventional dialysis [66].

Nocturnal hypoxemia

Nocturnal hypoxemia is a known trigger of the sympathetic nervous system, which is in turn associated with the development of concentric LVH [67]. Zoccali and colleagues [68] recently postulated that nocturnal hypoxemia may be an overlooked cardiovascular risk factor linked to mortality in ESRD. The correction of sleep apnea is yet another modality that may lower cardiovascular mortality risk in ESRD patients [69]. Sleep studies were performed on 14 subjects who were enrolled in the first nocturnal hemodialysis project in Toronto [30]. Seven of these patients had sleep apnea as defined by the apnea–hypopnea index of more than 15 episodes/h. The apnea–hypopnea index in these patients decreased from 46 ± 19 to 9 ± 9 per hour ($P = 0.006$). There was an associated increase in the minimal oxygen saturation from $89.2 \pm 1.8\%$ to $94.1 \pm 1.6\%$ ($P = 0.005$). There was no effect on daytime sleepiness when measured before and after conversion to nocturnal hemodialysis.

Decreased heart-rate variability has been correlated with cardiovascular mortality in healthy subjects and following myocardial infarction [70]. ESRD patients have been shown to have decreased heart variability and increased sympathetic activity, factors that are correlated with increased mortality [71]. Chan et al [72] analyzed heart-rate variability during stage II sleep in nine ESRD patients when receiving conventional hemodialysis and 6 to 15 months after conversion to nocturnal hemodialysis. Patients receiving nocturnal hemodialysis had a significantly reduced duration of nocturnal hypoxemia and increased heart-rate variability during sleep. At present, it is unclear how these observations may affect clinical outcomes.

Cardiovascular events and survival outcomes

Because nocturnal home hemodialysis is a relatively new modality, few outcome studies examining cardiovascular events and survival outcomes are available; in fact, no hard data are available to date. Patient survival in 83 patients at the Humber

River Regional Hospital has been reported to be 81% over a 5-year period [73]. One retrospective study reported lower hospitalization rates in patients receiving daily hemodialysis than in patients receiving conventional hemodialysis [74]. Similar findings were found in a prospective study comparing two cohorts of patients receiving conventional and nocturnal hemodialysis [75]. One should be careful in interpreting these results, because the higher-than-expected survival rates and the lower-than-expected hospitalization rates may be related to a case-mix bias.

Physiologic link between nocturnal home hemodialysis and cardiovascular improvements

Both short daily hemodialysis and nocturnal home hemodialysis improve blood pressure readings. The mechanism for short daily hemodialysis seems to be related primarily to improved removal of extracellular volume achieved through more frequent renal replacement therapy.

Nocturnal home hemodialysis, however, has not been shown to decrease extracellular volume significantly. Its superior effects may be attributed to improved clearance of uremic solute through the greater frequency and duration of renal replacement therapy. The physiologic impact of nocturnal home hemodialysis on cardiovascular outcomes is being actively investigated at the University of Toronto. Conventional hemodialysis creates tremendous fluctuations in extracellular volume and biochemical status [76]. Nocturnal home hemodialysis more closely approximates the natural physiology of the kidneys than do other modalities of renal replacement therapy, and this closer approximation of natural function may be an important factor [77]. Indeed, beneficial effects have been described in improved endothelial-dependent and -independent vasodilation, decreased total peripheral resistance, decreased plasma norepinephrine levels, correction of sleep apnea, improved autonomic modulation of heart rate during sleep, and normalization of calcium–phosphate–PTH balance.

Future directions

A randomized, controlled trial is currently underway through the National Institute of Health–sponsored Frequent Hemodialysis Network trial. Patients enrolled in this trial will be randomly assigned to receive nocturnal home hemodialysis, short daily dialysis, or conventional hemodialysis

in accordance with the current Kidney/Dialysis Outcome Quality Initiative adequacy guidelines. The cardiovascular effects of intensive hemodialysis modalities will be compared with standard therapy. This study, and others, are required to understand more clearly the impact of frequent intensive hemodialysis on cardiovascular event rates in ESRD patients.

References

[1] Foley RN, Parfrey PS, Arnak MJ. Clinial epidemiology of cardiovascular disease in chronic renal disease. Am J Kidney Dis 1998;32:S112–9.

[2] London GM, Guerin AP, Marchais SJ, et al. Cardiac and arterial interactions in end-stage renal disease. Kidney Int 1996;50:600–8.

[3] Zoccali C, Mallamaci F, Tripepi G. Traditional and emerging cardiovascular risk factors in end-stage renal disease. Kidney Int Suppl 2003;85:105–10.

[4] Verma S, Anderson TJ. Fundamentals of endothelial function for the clinical cardiologist. Circulation 2002;105:546–9.

[5] Pannier B, Guerin AP, Marchais S, et al. Postischemic vasodilation, endothelial activation, and cardiovascular remodeling in end-stage renal disease. Kidney Int 2000;57:1091–9.

[6] McVeigh GE, Brennan GM, Johnston GD, et al. Impaired endothelium-dependent and independent vasodilation in patients with type 2 (non-insulin-dependent) diabetes mellitus. Diabetologia 1992; 35:771–6.

[7] Panza JA, Casino PR, Kilcoyne CM, et al. Role of endothelium-derived nitric oxide in the abnormal endothelium-dependent vascular relaxation of patients with essential hypertension. Circulation 1993;87:1468–74.

[8] Seiler C, Hess OM, Buechi M, et al. Influence of serum cholesterol and other coronary risk factors on vasomotion of angiographically normal coronary arteries. Circulation 1993;88:2139–48.

[9] Fathi R, Haluska B, Isbel N, et al. The relative importance of vascular structure and function in predicting cardiovascular events. J Am Coll Cardiol 2004;43:616–23.

[10] Lopez-Gomez JM, Verde E, Perez-Garcia R. Blood pressure, left ventricular hypertrophy and long-term prognosis in hemodialysis patients. Kidney Int Suppl 1998;68:S92–8.

[11] Owen WF Jr, Chertow GM, Lazarus JM, et al. Dose of hemodialysis and survival: differences by race and sex. JAMA 1998;280:1764–8.

[12] Foley RN, Parfrey PS, Harnett JD, et al. The prognostic importance of left ventricular geometry in uremic cardiomyopathy. J Am Soc Nephrol 1995;5: 2024–31.

[13] Foley RN, Parfrey PS, Kent GM, et al. Serial change in echocardiographic parameters and cardiac failure

in end-stage renal disease. J Am Soc Nephrol 2000;
11:912–6.

[14] Block GA, Hulbert-Shearon TE, Levin NW, et al. Association of serum phosphorus and calcium x phosphate product with mortality risk in chronic hemodialysis patients: a national study. Am J Kidney Dis 1998;31:607–17.

[15] London GM. Vascular disease and atherosclerosis in uremia. Blood Purif 2001;19:139–42.

[16] Indridason OS, Quarles LD. Hyperphosphatemia in end-stage renal disease. Adv Ren Replace Ther 2002; 9:184–92.

[17] Amann K, Ritz E, Wiest G, et al. A role of parathyroid hormone for the activation of cardiac fibroblasts in uremia. J Am Soc Nephrol 1994;4: 1814–9.

[18] DePalma JR, Pecker EA, Gordon A, et al. A new compact automatic home hemodialysis system. Trans Am Soc Artif Intern Organs 1968;14:152–9.

[19] Uldall R, Ouwendyk M, Francoeur R, et al. Slow nocturnal home hemodialysis at the Wellesley Hospital. Adv Ren Replace Ther 1996;3:133–6.

[20] Clark WR, Leypoldt JK, Henderson LW, et al. Quantifying the effect of changes in the hemodialysis prescription of effective solute removal with a mathematical model. J Am Soc Nephrol 1999;10(3): 601–9.

[21] Goldfarb-Rumyantzev AS, Cheung AK, Leypoldt JK. Computer simulation of small-solute and middle-molecule removal during short daily and long thrice-weekly hemodialysis. Am J Kidney Dis 2002;40(6):1211–8.

[22] Pierratos A. Effect of therapy time and frequency on effective solute removal. Semin Dial 2001;14(4): 284–8.

[23] Leypoldt JK, Cheung AK, Carroll CE, et al. Effect of dialysis membranes and middle molecule removal on chronic hemodialysis patient survival. Am J Kidney Dis 1999;33(2):349–55.

[24] Cheung AK, Levin NW, Greene T, et al. Effects of high-flux hemodialysis and clinical outcomes: results of the HEMO study. J Am Soc Nephrol 2003;14(12): 3251–63.

[25] Brissenden JE, Pierratos A, Ouwendyk M, et al. Improvements in quality of life with nocturnal hemodialysis. J Am Soc Nephrol 1998;9:168A.

[26] Kooistra MP, Vos J, Koomans HA, et al. Daily home hemodialysis in the Netherlands: effects of metabolic control, haemodynamics, and quality of life. Nephrol Dial Transplant 1998;13(11):2853–60.

[27] Woods JD, Port FK, Orzol S, et al. Clinical and biochemical correlates of starting "daily" hemodialysis. Kidney Int 1999;55(6):2467–76.

[28] Ting GO, Kjellstrand C, Freitas T, et al. Long-term study of high-comorbidity ESRD patients converted from conventional to short daily hemodialysis. Am J Kidney Dis 2003;42(5):1020–35.

[29] Schwartz D, Pierratos A, Richardson RMA, et al. Impact of nocturnal home hemodialysis on anemia

management in patients with end-stage renal disease. Clin Nephrol 2005;63:202–8.

[30] Hanly PJ, Pierratos A. Improvement of sleep apnea in patients with chronic renal failure who undergo nocturnal hemodialysis. N Engl J Med 2001; 344(2):102–7.

[31] McFarlane PA, Pierratos A, Redelemeier DA. Cost savings of home nocturnal versus conventional in-center hemodialysis. Kidney Int 2002; 62(6):2216–22.

[32] Kroeker A, Clark WF, Heidenheim AP, et al. An operating cost comparison between conventional and home quotidian hemodialysis. Am J Kidney Dis 2003;41(1 Suppl):49–55.

[33] Horl MP, Horl WH. Hemodialysis-associated hypertension: pathophysiology and therapy. Am J Kidney Dis 2002;39:227–44.

[34] London GM. Cardiovascular disease in chronic renal failure: pathophysiologic aspects. Semin Dial 2003;16:85–94.

[35] Lins RL, Elseviers M, Rogiers P, et al. Importance of volume factors in dialysis related hypertension. Clin Nephrol 1997;48:29–33.

[36] Onesti G, Kim KE, Greco JA, et al. Blood pressure regulation in end-stage renal disease and anephric man. Circ Res 1975;36:145–52.

[37] Woods JD, Port FK, Orzol S, et al. Clinical and biochemical correlates of starting "daily" hemodialysis. Kidney Int 1999;55:2467–76.

[38] Fagugli RM, Reboldi G, Quintaliani G, et al. Short daily hemodialysis: blood pressure control and left ventricular mass reduction in hypertensive hemodialysis patients. Am J Kidney Dis 2001;38: 371–6.

[39] Raj DS, Charra B, Pierratos A, et al. In search of ideal hemodialysis: is prolonged frequent dialysis the answer. Am J Kidney Dis 1999;34:597–610.

[40] Chan CT, Floras JS, Miller JA, et al. Regression of left ventricular hypertrophy after conversion to nocturnal hemodialysis. Kidney Int 2002;61: 2235–9.

[41] Nesrallah G, Suri R, Moist L, et al. Volume control and blood pressure management in patients undergoing quotidian hemodialysis. Am J Kidney Dis 2003;41(1 Suppl):13–7.

[42] Chan CT, Harvey PJ, Picton P, et al. Short-term blood pressure, noradrenergic, and vascular effects of nocturnal home hemodialysis. Hypertension 2003;42:925–31.

[43] Chaigon M, Chen WT, Tarazi RC, et al. Effect of hemodialysis on blood volume distribution and cardiac output. Hypertension 1981;3:327–32.

[44] Zoccali C, Mallamaci F, Benedetto FA, et al. Cardiac natriuretic peptides are related to left ventricular mass and function and predict mortality in dialysis patients. J Am Soc Nephrol 2001;12:1508–15.

[45] London G, Guerin A, Pannier B, et al. Increased systolic pressure in chronic uremia. Role of arterial wave reflections. Hypertension 1992;20:10–9.

[46] Klassen PS, Lowrie EG, Reddan DN, et al. Association between pulse pressure and mortality in patients undergoing maintenance hemodialysis. JAMA 2002;287:1548–55.

[47] London GM, Guerin AP, Marchais SJ, et al. Cardiac and arterial interactions in end-stage renal disease. Kidney Int 1996;50:600–8.

[48] Katz AM. Cardiomyopathy of overload. A major determinant of prognosis in congestive heart failure. N Engl J Med 1990;322:100–10.

[49] Atherton JJ, Moore TD, Lele SS, et al. Diastolic ventricular interaction in chronic heart failure. Lancet 1997;349:1720–4.

[50] Chan CT, Floras JS, Miller JA, et al. Improvement in ejection fraction by nocturnal hemodialysis in end-stage renal failure patients with coexisting heart failure. Nephrol Dial Transplant 2002;17:1518–21.

[51] Gordon T, Castelli W, Hjortland M, et al. High density lipoprotein as a protective factor against coronary heart disease. The Framingham Study. Am J Med 1977;62:707–14.

[52] Castelli W. Cardiovascular disease and multifactorial risk: challenge of the 1980s. Am Heart J 1983; 106(5 Pt 2):1191–200.

[53] Hokanson J, Austin M. Plasma triglyceride level is a risk factor for cardiovascular disease independent of high-density lipoprotein cholesterol level: a meta-analysis of population-based prospective studies. J Cardiovasc Risk 1996;3:213–9.

[54] Jeppesen J, Hein H, Suadicani P, et al. Triglyceride concentration and ischemic heart disease: an eight-year follow-up in the Copenhagen Male Study. Circulation 1998;97:1029–36.

[55] Wanner C. Importance of hyperlipidemia and therapy in renal patients. Nephrol Dial Transplant 2000;15(Suppl 5):92–6.

[56] Shoji T, Nishizawa Y, Kawagishi T, et al. Atherogenic lipoprotein changes in the absence of hyperlipidemia in patients with chronic renal failure treated by hemodialysis. Atherosclerosis 1997;131:229–36.

[57] Attman P, Samuelsson O, Alaupovic P. Lipoprotein metabolism and renal failure. Am J Kidney Dis 1993;21:573–92.

[58] Bugeja AL, Chan CT. Improvement in lipid profile by nocturnal hemodialysis in patients with end-stage renal disease. ASAIO J 2004;40:1–4.

[59] Block GA, Hulbert-Shearon TE, Levin NW, et al. Association of serum phosphors and calcium x phosphate product with mortality risk in chronic hemodialysis patients: a national study. Am J Kidney Dis 1998;31(4):607–17.

[60] DeSoi CA, Umans JG. Phosphate kinetics during high-flux hemodialysis. J Am Soc Nephrol 1993; 4(5):1214–8.

[61] Mucsi I, Hercz G, Uldall R, et al. Control of serum phosphate without any phosphate binders in patients treated with nocturnal hemodialysis. Kidney Int 53(5):1399–1404.

[62] Kim SJ, Goldstein M, Szabo T, et al. Resolution of massive uremic tumoral calcinosis with daily nocturnal home hemodialysis. Am J Kidney Dis 2003; 41(3):E12.

[63] Pierratos A, Hercz G, Sherrard DJ, et al. Calcium, phosphorus metabolism and bone pathology on long term nocturnal hemodialysis. J Am Soc Nephrol 2001;12:274A.

[64] Al Hejaili F, Kortas C, Leitch R, et al. Nocturnal but not short hours quotidian hemodialysis requires an elevated dialysate calcium concentration. J Am Soc Nephrol 2003;14(9):2322–8.

[65] Friedman AN, Bostom AG, Levey AS, et al. Plasma total homocysteine levels among patients undergoing nocturnal versus standard hemodialysis. J Am Soc Nephrol 2002;13(1):265–8.

[66] Nesrallah G, Suri R, Moist L, et al. Volume control and blood pressure management in patients undergoing quotidian hemodialysis. Am J Kidney Dis 2003;42(1 Suppl):13–7.

[67] Zoccali C, Benedetto FA, Mallamaci F, et al. Left ventricular hypertrophy and nocturnal hypoxemia in hemodialysis patients. J Hypertens 2001;19: 287–93.

[68] Zoccali C, Mallamaci F, Tripepi G. Nocturnal hypoxemia predicts incident cardiovascular complications in dialysis patients. J Am Soc Nephrol 2002; 13:729–33.

[69] Zoccali C, Mallamaci F, Tripepi G. Nocturnal hypoxemia: a neglected cardiovascular risk factor in end-stage renal disease? Blood Purif 2002;20:120–3.

[70] Tsuji H, Larson MG, Venditti FL Jr, et al. Impact of reduced heart rate variability on risk for cardiac events. The Framingham Heart Study. Circulation 1996;94(11):2850–5.

[71] Fukuta H, Hayano J, Ishihara S, et al. Prognostic value of heart rate variability in patients with end-stage renal disease on chronic hemodialysis. Nephrol Dial Transplant 2003;18(2):318–25.

[72] Chan CT, Hanly P, Gabor J, et al. Impact of nocturnal hemodialysis on the variability of heart rate and duration of hypoxemia during sleep. Kidney Int, in press.

[73] Pierratos A. Daily nocturnal home hemodialysis. Kidney Int 2004;65(5):1975–86.

[74] Mohr PE, Neumann PJ, Franco SJ, et al. The case for daily dialysis: its impact on costs and quality of life. Am J Kidney Dis 2001;37(4):777–89.

[75] McFarlane PA, Pierratos A, Redelmeier DA. Cost savings of home nocturnal versus conventional in-center hemodialysis. Kidney Int 2002;62(6):2216–22.

[76] Kjellstrand CM, Evans RL, Petersen RJ, et al. The "unphysiology" of dialysis: a major cause of dialysis side effects? Kidney Int Suppl 1975;2: 30–4.

[77] Chan CT. Nocturnal hemodialysis: an attempt to correct the "unphysiology" of conventional intermittent renal replacement therapy. Clin Invest Med 2002;25:233–5.

ELSEVIER
SAUNDERS

Cardiol Clin 23 (2005) 393–399

CARDIOLOGY
CLINICS

Index

Note: Page numbers of article titles are in **boldface** type.

Changing Your Address?

Make sure your subscription changes too! When you notify us of your new address, you can help make our job easier by including an exact copy of your Clinics label number with your old address (see illustration below.) This number identifies you to our computer system and will speed the processing of your address change. Please be sure this label number accompanies your old address and your corrected address—you can send an old Clinics label with your number on it or just copy it exactly and send it to the address listed below.

We appreciate your help in our attempt to give you continuous coverage. Thank you.

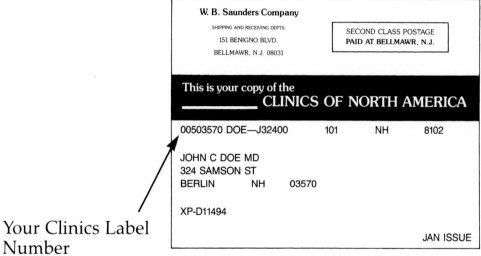

Your Clinics Label Number
Copy it exactly or send your label along with your address to:
W.B. Saunders Company, Customer Service
Orlando, FL 32887-4800
Call Toll Free 1-800-654-2452

Please allow four to six weeks for delivery of new subscriptions and for processing address changes.